International He

and Aid Policies

The Need for Alternatives

International Health and Aid Policies

The Need for Alternatives

Jean-Pierre Unger

Pierre De Paepe

Kasturi Sen

Werner Soors

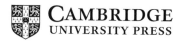

CAMBRIDGE UNIVERSITY PRESS
Cambridge, New York, Melbourne, Madrid, Cape Town, Singapore, São
Paulo, Delhi, Dubai, Tokyo

Cambridge University Press
The Edinburgh Building, Cambridge CB2 8RU, UK

Published in the United States of America by
Cambridge University Press, New York

www.cambridge.org
Information on this title: www.cambridge.org/9780521174268

© Institute of Tropical Medicine 2010

First published 2010

Printed in the United Kingdom at the University Press, Cambridge

*A catalog record for this publication is available from the
British Library*

Library of Congress Cataloging in Publication Data

International health and aid policies : the need for alternatives /
[edited by] Jean-Pierre Unger ... [et al.].
   p. cm.
Includes bibliographical references and index.
ISBN 978-0-521-17426-8 (pbk.)
1. Public health–International cooperation. 2. World health. 3. Poor–Medical
care. 4. Medically underserved areas. 5. Medical care–Developing countries.
I. Unger, Jean-Pierre, 1954–II. Title.

RA441.I565 2010
362.1–dc22   2010021038

ISBN 978-0-521-17426-8 Paperback

Contents

Preface

This book explores health policies through examining patterns of commercialization that have underpinned the vast majority of these policies in different regions of the world, at the same time providing the reader with both concepts in public health and techniques to develop health services with a social mission. The chapters in the book include case studies and an extensive review of the literature.

We began this task with one main purpose: to explore the extent to which donors and international agencies have, over the past two decades, shared the same underlying motivation: that is to primarily commercialize the health sector of low-income countries (LIC) and middle-income countries (MIC), despite the stated aim of improving access to health care and addressing issues of poverty and exclusion. In this book, we provide evidence showing the contradictions between access to care and strengthening health systems on the one hand and increased commercialization on the other.

The ideas and evidence presented in this book thus call for an exploration of the contradictions of commercialized health care delivery under the guise of maintaining public provision. The book challenges the discourse and status quo among national bodies, in global policy circles, among donors and northern governments. It argues for

- the creation of health care services that have a social rather than a commercial motivation, and
- delivery of publicly oriented health care based on (professionally defined) 'needs' and on the (population) 'demand' to access quality, polyvalent health care, rather than on health interventions efficiency only.

Biographies

Authors

Jean-Pierre Unger (MD 1979 and PhD 1991, Free University of Brussels; DTM&H 1980, ITM Antwerp; MPH 1983, Harvard School of Public Health) is senior lecturer at the Institute of Tropical Medicine, Antwerp. He started his career in 1981, as a doctor, in the ITM Kasongo project, Congo, then gained experience in health systems and academic development mainly in Africa (in the 1980s and early 1990s) and in Latin America thereafter. He researched strategies to develop publicly oriented health care services (in Africa, Latin America, Asia, Middle East, and Europe), and, since 2000, studies international health policies.

Pierre De Paepe (MD 1977, Antwerp; MPH 1985, Buenos Aires; certificate in health economics 2005, York) spent 25 years in Latin America (Haiti, Peru, Argentina and Ecuador) and has worked at the ITM since 2003 at the Public Policy and Management Unit. His professional experience focused on the implementation of primary health care programmes, health systems analysis, the documentation of country case studies of Latin America, health systems funding, and financing. He is currently studying Colombian and Brazilian health policies.

Kasturi Sen (Dip Soc. Pol, PhD) is a social scientist who has worked on issues of public health and development for the past 25 years. She helped set up a network of seven countries to monitor the public health implications of health reforms in the late 1990s in India and also worked with statisticians, economists and epidemiologists to collect one of the largest data sets on household level impact of changes in the organization of health services in three states of India, on safety nets, on quality and on access to care. Kasturi has taught in public health departments at London (1991–1995), Cambridge (1996–2004) and at Oxford (2005–2008) where she helped establish a course on public health and development. She is working on a collaborative project on global health policies at ITM.

Werner Soors was born in 1955 in Antwerp (MD 1986, University of Antwerp, DTM&H) and worked in Nicaragua up until 2003, with a strong focus on public health care and community participation. Back in Antwerp, he attained his MPH and has been with ITM since 2004. He works in ITM's Department of Public Health on health systems and reform analysis (Public Policy and Management Unit) and on social protection in health (Health Policy and Financing Unit).

Contributors

Luis Abad MD (State University of Cuenca, Ecuador), MPH (National North East University, Argentina), has been district medical officer for the Azogues Health Area, Cañar Province in southern Ecuador, since 1992. He has been a public health advisor of the 'Primary Health Care – APS project' by the Belgian Technical Cooperation Organisation in Ecuador (1994–2003). He also lectures on occasion in public health and health systems organization in the Masters in Public Health Course of the Pontificia Universidad Católica del Ecuador, PUCE, Ecuador.

Oscar Arteaga MD, MSc, DrPH. Health Policy and Management Unit, School of Public Health, Faculty of Medicine, University of Chile. Academic Director of University of Chile's Master in Public Health Programme.

Lennart Bogg MSc, PhD economist, BA (Sinology), MScBA (Uppsala University). Served with UNICEF in Burma and in China (1982–1988); from 1988 with Swedish International Development Cooperation Agency (SIDA), Stockholm, first as Financial Controller in the Finance Department and later as Economist (Health Policy) with the Department of Eastern Europe and Central Asia, with UNRWA as Finance Director (Gaza), and with the World Bank Baltic Regional Office as social sector economist. Since 2004 Senior Researcher, Division of Global Health (HCAR), Karolinska Institute (research addressing rural health insurance in Asia, barriers to maternal health in China), and Senior Lecturer (Financial Management), School of Sustainable Development of Society and Technology (HST), Mälardalen University, Sweden.

Rene Buitrón MD, MPH, MSc, physician and epidemiologist by training, has directed the Institute of Public Health, Pontificia Universidad Católica del Ecuador, Quito, where he is now Professor of pre- and postgraduate courses and Vice Dean of the medical faculty.

Daniel Burdet MD (Free University of Brussels 1977), general practitioner working in a multidisciplinary primary care team (Maison Médicale Forest), is training supervisor in general practice, quality coordinator, health care manager and a member of the Health Promotion and Quality workgroup (EPSQ) in the Fédération des Maisons Médicales.

Bart Criel MD, DTM&H, MSc, PhD, senior lecturer at the Department of Public Health of the Institute of Tropical Medicine (ITM) in Antwerp, Belgium. He worked as medical officer in rural Democratic Republic of Congo (1983–1990) and joined the ITM in 1990. He has extensive experience in health systems research with a special focus on district health systems and on arrangements for social protection in health in sub-Saharan countries and in the Indian sub-continent.

Umberto d'Alessandro MD (Pisa 1982), MSc (London 1990) and PhD (London 1996) is Professor of parasitology and head of the epidemiological parasitology unit (Institute of Tropical Medicine, Antwerp). He has extensively studied malaria control and clinical trials in malariology.

Tony De Groote MD, DTM&H, MPH, worked mainly in sub-Saharan Africa and Latin America. He is Assistant Professor at St. George's University in Grenada.

Paul De Munck MD, MPH, DTM&H, general practitioner, has 14 years' experience in family and community medicine in a Brussels multidisciplinary, self-managed primary health care centre. Since 1997 he has worked as a public health doctor to support health systems in sub-Saharan Africa.

Moussa Diao is a retired nurse (Ecole Nationale des Infirmiers d'Etat, Dakar). He has had extensive experience in the field of primary health care and has been supervisor of the primary health care Kolda district in Senegal during the 1990s.

Dong Hengjin BA in Public Health (1978–1983, Shanghai Medical University), MSc (in Health Statistics and Social Medicine 1983–1986), MA in Health Management, Planning and Policy (1990–1991, Nuffield Institute for Health, Leeds University), PhD (Karolinska

Institute, area of Health Services Research). Professor and director of the Department of Hospital Management, vice-director of Health Technology Assessment (HTA) and Research Centre, Dean Assistant of School of Public Health at Shanghai Medical University (SMU) (1997–2000). Senior research fellow in Health Economics Research Group, Brunel University, UK (2004–2006) and senior lecturer at Heidelberg University (2000–2004). Currently leader of the Junior Group of International Health Economics and Technology Assessment at Heidelberg University, Germany.

Sylvie Dugas MD, MPH, has experience in health services organization in Zimbabwe and Guinea and was Research Assistant at the Department of Public Health (Institute of Tropical Medicine, Antwerp). She currently works for the Ministère de la santé, de la famille et des personnes handicapées in France.

Patricia Ghilbert RN, MCommH, MPH is a nurse specialized in public health. She has been a research assistant at the Institute of Tropical Medicine, Antwerp, and is currently working for the Federal Service of Health, Food Chain Safety and Environment, Directorate-General for the Organization of Health Care Establishments, Belgium.

Andrew Green BA, MA, PhD, is Professor of International Health Planning at Leeds University, UK, and until recently, was head of its Nuffield Centre for International Health and Development. He teaches health policy, planning, and economics on undergraduate and postgraduate courses both at Leeds and as a guest lecturer in other institutions. His interest, research and publications focus on health planning, health policy processes, and the role of NGOs in health. He has held positions in Western and Southern Africa and the UK NHS as well as having conducted research and short-term consultancy in other parts of Africa, Asia, South America and the Caribbean.

Pierre Leemans has been working as a general practitioner for more than 25 years. He has been practical trainer at the Free University of Brussels since 1991 and has responsibilities in the local GPs' organization (Brussels Region).

Bruno Marchal MD, DTM&H, MPH, PhD, worked as district hospital director in Kenya between 1993 and 1999 and is currently a research fellow at the Department of Public Health, Institute of Tropical Medicine, Antwerp. His current research focuses on the role of (health workforce) management on hospital performance and evaluation of complex interventions in health care.

Amadou Mbaye MD (Dakar University), MPH (ITM, Antwerp) is currently attached as a health specialist to the Union Economique et Monétaire Ouest Africaine (UEMOA).

Imrana Qadeer is a J. P. Naik senior fellow at the Centre for Women's Development Studies at present and was Professor at the Centre of Social Medicine and Community Health (Jawaharlal Nehru University, New Delhi) that she joined after working at the AIIMS, Department of Paediatrics until 1971. She served as a member of the Review Committee for the National Rural Health Mission, Population Commission and several health and nutritional planning sub-groups in the Planning Commission of India. Current areas of research include the organization of health services in India, political economy of health, women's health, epidemiology, and interdisciplinary research methodology. She also continues to work with people's organizations working for health of the marginalized.

Edgar W. Rojas González MD (1988), MPH (1996), born in Azogues, Ecuador, was with the Ministry of Health from 1988 to 1997 as a clinician, and director of several services. Since 1999 he has been Professor on the MPH program and at the Nursing Faculty of the Pontificia Universidad Católica del Ecuador. He has also worked as a national and international advisor and consultant in public health. He is currently Director of Nutrition in Ecuador's National Program 'Alimentate Ecuador' for the Ministry of Economic and Social Inclusion.

Abla Mehio Sibai is Professor at the Department of Epidemiology and Population Health at the American University of Beirut, Lebanon. She has been involved in a number of major international research projects on population health and was scientific coordinator of the multi-centre EC-funded research on the impact of conflict on population health in Lebanon (1996–2000), the National Burden of Disease Study (2003), and more recently the NCD Risk Factors study in Lebanon. She is currently on several advisory committees, national, regional and international, to support the establishment of a database for reporting of morbidity and for policy formulation for the elderly population of Lebanon. She is a founder member and director of the Centre for Studies on Ageing in Lebanon.

Giorgio Solimano, physician by training, is director of the School of Public Health, University of Chile, Santiago, and professor of public health. He has been professor associate and then professor from 1988 to 2006 at the School of Public Health, Health Sciences Faculty, Columbia University, New York. He has written numerous books and articles on public health and nutrition.

Jacques Unger MD 1973, PhD 1983. Head of the Thyroid Unit Academic Hospital 1987–1994, Head of the Internal Medicine Department César de Paepe 1994–1997, Molière Hospital Brussels 1997–2001, Professor of Endocrinology 1990–1994 and of Internal Medicine 1998–2001.

Jean Van der Vennet, is a medical sociologist (Free University of Brussels), who has been working for many years on the Belgian health system. He joined ITM as a medical sociologist in 1991. From 1993 to 1997 he was a Technical Adviser to the Regional Health Services of the Department of Cochabamba, Bolivia, based at the University Mayor de San Simon. At ITM he is currently working on the development of Local Health Systems in Belgium and also teaching Public Health and is responsible for the ITM's Alumni network. He also provides support to Masters students at the School of Public Health in Lubumbashi, in the Democratic Republic of the Congo.

Patrick Van Dessel was born in 1964 in Antwerp, MD 1991, Ghent, Belgium, DTM&H 1992, and MPH 1997, ITM Antwerp, worked for more than a decade in Africa (Malawi, Rwanda) and Latin America (Bolivia) with a main interest in integrated health system organization and primary health care. He has experience with epidemiology and health care accessibility in neglected urban areas in Belgium (2004–2008) and has been working with ITM's Public Policy and Management Unit since 2008. His current focus in Antwerp is on health system research, public institutional capacity building and teaching public health in a globalized context.

Monique Van Dormael PhD in Sociology, started her career studying primary care group practices in Belgium and Europe. Since 1987 she has been involved in teaching and research in public health at the Institute of Tropical Medicine in Antwerp, with a special emphasis on human resources for health in developing countries.

Ingrid Vargas Lorenzo BA Econ, MSc, PhD, is a health economist, researcher at the Health Policy Unit of the Consorci Hospitalari de Catalunya, Barcelona, Spain, with experience in health policy analysis, health financing, equity and IHN. Published PhD Thesis: 'Barriers and facilitators for continuity of IHN in Colombia.'

Maria Luisa Vázquez MD, PhD, MSc, Public Health specialist, is currently Head of Research of the Health Policy Research Unit of the Consorci Hospitalari de Catalunya, Barcelona, Spain. She started her career as a researcher at the Institute of Tropical Hygiene and Public Health, University of Heidelberg, and then continued as a lecturer at the Liverpool School of Tropical Medicine (UK), before moving to Spain in 1998. During the past 25 years she has gained wide experience in health systems and policy research in Latin America and Spain. She has published many national and international articles. Her particular areas of interest include access to health care, integrated health care, health policy analysis, and care to migrant populations.

Marie-Jeanne Wuidar sociologist (Free University of Brussels, 1972), MD 1980. From 1980 onwards she has worked as a general practitioner at the Marconi Medical Centre, Brussels. She also has experience in the organization of the primary health services, Yanbu, Saudi Arabia.

Walter Zocchi, MD (Milan University, 1974), DTM&H (ITM, 1996), MPH (ITM Antwerp, 2002), has worked as a surgeon and a general practitioner in Italy, Mozambique, Algiers, Burkina Faso and Sierra Leone. Since 1996 Walter Zocchi has worked with several NGOs in Haiti, Somalia, Montenegro, Serbia, Bosnia, Zimbabwe, Eritrea, Ecuador, Afghanistan, and India.

Notices

The majority of the papers in this collection have been published already. However, the interest they created inspired us to combine them into one volume aimed at students and public health professionals.

Acknowledgements

This book would not have been possible without the efforts of several people within our unit and outside. First, Patrick Van Dessel, in addition to being co-author of several of the chapters, has been instrumental in the completion of this project, contributing to the edition and the bibliographic research. Indranil Mukhopadhyay, from the Centre of Social Medicine and Community Health (CSMCH) of the Jawaharlal Nehru University, New Delhi, India, undertook the edit of a first draft, working closely with Jean-Pierre Unger and Kasturi Sen. We have also had invaluable help from medical student, Casper Van der Veer, who managed with great skill all the technical aspects of the manuscript from the illustrations to formatting and referencing. His efforts especially during the final stages have been integral to the completion of this project. His work has been supported and complemented by our highly skilled secretary Linde De Kinder. The contractual negotiations were also managed, with care and attention, by the legal advisor to the Institute, Jef Van Lint. The task of seeing this through various committees and Cambridge in-house rules was carefully and consistently undertaken by series editor Richard Marley aided by Editorial Assistant, Rachael Lazenby, and Jane Seakins, Publishing Assistant, Medicine. All of the editors of this text have worked hard to complete this marathon project in a short time. The views expressed in the articles and chapters are the authors' own and do not reflect those of the Institute of Tropical Medicine (ITM) or that of the publisher, Cambridge University Press.

Professor Em. Pierre Mercenier and Professor Harrie Van Baelen, physicians and professors of public health at the Institute of Tropical Medicine, Antwerp (ITM), pioneered numerous concepts formulated in this book (e.g., holistic, continuous and integrated care; integrated health services and systems). Our intellectual debt to them is immense.

Finally, we are indebted to the Belgian Directorate-General of Development Cooperation for the funding of several research endeavours presented in this book.

List of Abbreviations

ACT	Artemesinine Combination Therapy
ADB	Asian Development Bank
AHDR	Arab Human Development Report
ARI	Acute Respiratory Infection
ART	Antiretroviral Therapy
ASeMeCo	Asociación de Servicios Médicos Costarricense (Costa Rican Association of Medical Services)
BI	Bamako Initiative
CAFTA	Central American Free Market Agreement
CCSS	Caja Costarricense de Seguro Social (Costa Rica, Social Security Administration; see SSAC)
CHC	Comprehensive Health Care
CHW	Community Health Worker
CMH	Commission on Macroeconomics and Health (WHO)
CMP	Common Minimum Programme (India)
(N)CMS	(New) Cooperative Medical System (China)
COMAC-HSR	(European) 'Concerted action' on Health Services Research
CPHC	Comprehensive Primary Health Care
CSC	Civil Service Cooperative (Lebanon)
CSDH	Commission on Social Determinants of Health (WHO)
CSMCH	Centre of Social Medicine and Community Health of the Jawaharlal Nehru University, New Delhi, India
CT (Scan)	Computed Tomography (Scan)
CUP	Cambridge University Press
DAC	Development Assistance Committee (OECD)
DALY	Disability-Adjusted life year
DANIDA	Danish International Development Agency
DCP(s)	Disease-Control Programme(s)
DFID	Department for International Development
DGDC	(Belgian) Directorate-General for Development Cooperation
DOTS	Directly Observed Treatment Short Course
DPH	Department of Public Health at the Prince Leopold Institute of Tropical Medicine Antwerp
DSP(s)	Disease-specific Programme(s)
EBAIS	Equipos Básicos de Atención Integral en Salud (Costa Rica; primary health care clinics)
ECP	Essential Clinical Package
EPI	Extended Programme on Immunisation (WHO)
ESAFs	Enhanced Structural Adjustment Facilities (International Monetary Fund)
ESE	Empresas Sociales del Estado (Colombia; Public Hospital and Health Centres)

EU	European Union
FDI	Foreign Direct Investment
FMP/A	Fund for Military Personnel / Army (Lebanon)
FONASA	Fondo Nacional de Salud (Chile; National Health Fund)
FWP	Family Welfare Programme (India)
GATS	General Agreement on Trade in Services
GCI	Global Competitiveness Index (World Economic Forum, 2006)
GDP	Gross Domestic Product
G.E.R.M.	Groupe d'Etude pour une Réforme de la Médecine
GFATM	Global Fund to Fight AIDS, Tuberculosis and Malaria
GHI	Global Health Initiative (or Global Health Partnership)
GHP	Global Health Programme
GMR	Global Monitoring Report (World Bank)
GNP	Gross National Product
GOBI	Growth monitoring of young children, Oral rehydration therapy, promotion of Breast-feeding, and Immunisation programme (UNICEF)
GP	General practitioner
GPPP(s)	Global Public–Private Partnership(s)
GSF	General Security Forces (Lebanon)
HCDI	Health care Delivery Institutions (Colombia; Instituciones Prestadores de Servicios de Salud, IPS)
HDR	Human Development Report (WHO, 2003)
HFLC	High Frequency Low Cost
HIC	High-Income Country
HIV/AIDS	Human Immunodeficiency Virus / Acquired Immune Deficiency Syndrome
HMO	Health Maintenance Organization
HPE	Health Promoting Enterprises (Colombia; Empresas Promotores de Salud, EPS)
HSR	Health Services Research / Health Service Region / Health Sector Reform
IDP(s)	Internally displaced person(s)
IDWSSD	International Drinking Water Supply and Sanitation Decade
IFI(s)	International Financing Institution(s)
IFPA	Interface Flow Process Audit
IHP	International Health Partnership
IMF	International Monetary Fund
IMR	Infant Mortality Rate
IPPI	Intensified Pulse Polio Immunization
ISAPRES	Private insurers (Chile)
ISF	International Security Forces (Lebanon)
ITM	(Prince Leopold) Institute of Tropical Medicine Antwerp
LA	Latin America(n)
LDC	Less-Developed Country
LFHC	Low Frequency High Cost
LIC	Low-Income Country

LMIC	Low- and Middle-Income Country
lpcd	liters per capita per day
MAP	Minimum Activities Package
MDG(s)	Millennium Development Goal(s)
MHO(s)	Mutual Health Organization(s)
MIC	Middle-Income Country
MMR	Maternal Mortality Rate
MNC(s)	Multinational Corporation(s)
MNP	Minimum Needs Programme (India)
MoH	Ministry of Health
MOPH	Ministry of Public Health (Lebanon)
MRI	Magnetic Resonance Imaging
NCAER	National Council of Applied Economic Research
NCD(s)	Non-Communicable Disease(s)
NCMS	New Cooperative Medical System
NFHS	National Family Health Surveys
NGO(s)	Non-governmental organization(s)
NHA	National Health Accounts (Lebanon)
NHES	National Household Expenditure Survey (Lebanon, 2000)
NHHEUS	National Household Health Expenditures and Utilisation Survey (Lebanon, 2000)
NHP	National Health Policy (India)
NHS	National Health System / National Health Service (Great Britain) / National Household Survey (Colombia, 1992; Encuesta Nacional de Hogares, ENH)
NQLS	National Quality of Life Survey (Colombia, 1997)
NRHM	National Rural Health Mission
NSS	National Sample Survey (Kerala, India)
NSSF	National Social Security Fund (Lebanon)
NTP(s)	National Tuberculosis Programme(s)
ODA	Official Development Assistance / Official Donor Assistance
OECD	Organization for Economic Co-operation and Development
OHP	Obligatory Health Plan (Colombia)
OR	Odds Ratio
PAHO / OPS	Pan American Health Organization / Organización Panamericana de la Salud
PDS	Public Distribution System
PFI	Private Finance Initiative
PHC	Primary Health Care
PHS	Population and Housing Survey (Lebanon)
PP(s)	Private provider(s)/practitioner(s)
PPM-DOTS	Public-Private Mix for Directly Observed Treatment, Short Course
PPMU	Public Policy and Management Unit (ITM Antwerp)
PPP(s)	Public–Private Partnership(s)
PPS	Pre-payment System

PRSP	Poverty Reduction Strategy Paper/Program Requirements Support Plan
QALY	Quality-Adjusted Life Year
RMB	Chinese Renminbi (People's Republic of China currency)
SAPs	Structural Adjustment Programmes (World Bank)
SARS	Severe Acute Respiratory Syndrome
SDC	Swiss agency for Development and Cooperation
SIDA	Swedish International Development Cooperation Agency
SPHC	Selective Primary Health Care
SSA	Subsidised System Administrators (Colombia; Administradores de Regimen Subsidiado, ARS)
SSAC	Social Security Administration of Costa Rica (see CCSS)
SSF	State Security Forces (Lebanon)
TBHBC	Tuberculosis High Burden Countries
TNC(s)	Transnational Corporation(s)
TPDS	Targeted Public Distribution System
TRIPS	Trade Related Intellectual Property Rights
UN	United Nations
UNAIDS	(Joint) United Nations Programme on HIV/AIDS
UNICEF	United Nations Children's Fund
UNRISD	United Nations Research Institute for Social Development
WB	World Bank
WDR	World Development Report
WHA	World Health Assembly
WHO/OMS	World Health Organization / Organización Mundial de la Salud
WONCA	World Organization of Family Doctors
WTO	World Trade Organization

Reviews

International Health and Aid Policies: The Need for Alternatives, represents an important and comprehensive effort in gathering the evidence of the grave consequences on developing countries' health systems of some international health and aid policies that promote excessive reliance on disease-specific programmes and commercialized care. The book proposes alternative policy scenarios to begin reverting the for-profit on self-sustained and fragmented health care systems, and highlights the key role of health system researchers in influencing the development of pro-equity international health policies and the evaluation of their impact. The thorough review of historic data and trend analysis will serve scholars and decision makers alike.

Dr. Mirta Roses
Director
Pan American Health Organization
Regional Office of the World Health Organization

Timing is everything in comedy and in scholarship. One cannot imagine a better timing for this book's publication.

The title of the book promises to make a call for health services with a clear social mission; and this it fully delivers. Here is a book that paves the way in a direction using the right political analyses. It tells us that it has been donors who have pushed the patterns of commercialization of health in poor countries; and that aid policies share a large responsibility for the breakdown of the health systems of many of the poor countries we currently see. It highlights the contradictions of public provision under the guise of commercialized health care looking at two decades of neoliberal policy that has systematically undermined access to quality health care services for a majority of the world population. This, it rightly claims, receives far too little attention in the literature.

The book is clear about the need for a policy shift that re-establishes the right to access to quality health care. It proposes a health policy based on a political philosophy in an attempt to reconcile professional, cultural and political ethics. It clearly states that health policy is political in the sense that it refers to actions (deeds) meant to challenge the structures of power and social organization from an ethical perspective.

For all these reasons, the People's Health Movement feels the principles of its People's Charter for Health are here represented; our worldwide membership would want to read it.

Bridget Lloyd
People's Health Movement Co-ordinating Commission

This important book challenges the dominant discourse on global health and the growing commoditization of health care to the detriment of poor people all over the world. The serious and evidence-based questions and facts raised by the authors on the relentless promotion of private sector growth in health must now be answered.

Ann Marriott
Development Finance and Public Services Team
Oxfam GB

This book comes at a time of a highly needed reform in the Global Health Governance and the International Health Aid Architecture. The attention to health has been enhanced in global fora and health aid has tripled in the last decade. We all share responsibility and the challenge to address the highly fragmented health landscape. The EU is developing a new policy framework aimed at greater equity and coherence in the EU role in global health. The agreed global commitment to universal coverage rescuing the Alma Ata principles and applying the principles of partnership and ownership to health in development aid are clear opportunities. The reflections of this book will be a valuable reference for our debate and the enhanced EU role in the global health challenges.

Juan Garay
Public Health Physician
Health Team coordinator
DG Development
European Commission

Introduction – Overview and purpose

> Confident in the infinity of time, a certain conception of history discerns only the rhythm, faster or slower, at which men and times move along the path of progress.
> Walter Benjamin, 1915. La vie des étudiants. In: W. Benjamin, Œuvres I, Folio Essais, Editions Gallimard, 2000, p. 125.

> Plato was the first to discern between those who know without acting and those who act without knowing while in the past, action was divided in enterprise and achievement: the result was that the knowledge of action to accomplish and its implementation became two radically different concepts.
> H. Arendt. Condition de l'homme moderne. Calmann Levy Ed., Paris, 1983, p. 286.

After 15 years of neoliberal international health policy, data from 26 sub-Saharan countries reveals that more than 50% of the poorest children receive no health care when sick (Marek et al., 2005). Data from 44 low- to middle-income countries (LMICs) suggest that the greater the participation of the private sector in primary health care (PHC), the higher the exclusion from treatment and care (Macintosh & Koivusalo, 2005) across sectors.

This is a textbook about public health with a difference. Firstly, it addresses policies relating to the delivery of health care – while the study of public health has historically evolved around issues of disease control. This book makes a case for alternative policies that could shape the structure and provision of universally accessible, polyvalent, discretionary health care, rather than making it work through its commodification[1] and the priorities of cost-effective interventions in public services. Secondly, the articles we have included are critical of the debates over the political and technical paradigms of such discussion, often predicated, in our view, on international political ties and commercial relationships. Thirdly, a strong current of thinking in the book is the view, often neglected, that policies have a direct impact on the motivation and practice of professionals in the health sector and that such professionals can, and should, contribute towards developing health services with a social mission whatever the national health policy might dictate. In other words, the book approaches many of the contradictions of current policies from the perspective of practice. It thus offers a combination of theory, evidence from four continents and practice interwoven with guidance directed at policy makers, researchers, doctors, and nurses on ways and means to achieve comprehensive health care (CHC) provision in order to strengthen health systems.

Consequently, this is a textbook also on health services organization, designed to open avenues for reflection and action for the reader. Its targeted audience includes students, researchers, and practitioners of public health as well as health professionals with a practice in LMICs.

Whilst hierarchy conveys a top-down flow of authority, information, and ideology, this book aims at providing health professionals with action perspectives to amend (inter)national health policies in an experience-based perspective, in order to encourage the development of publicly oriented health services under any circumstance, wherever the health practitioners may be posted and whatever might be the national health policy. The book thus offers the reader arguments

---

[1] To turn into, or treat as, a commodity; make commercial.

reversing the well-established hierarchical flows of information that sustain a normative order. It provides in its place a fresh policy perspective, a methodology, and strategies to develop publicly oriented health services, to implement a more equitable care delivery and tentatively influence national policies.

Origins

Some 10 years ago, the Public Policy and Management Unit (PPMU) at the Department of Public Health (DPH) of the ITM began in-depth research into international health policies in order to understand some of the factors behind the incompatibility of existing health care management techniques with policies that were being advocated worldwide, despite the variations in context. This resulted in a series of papers and articles, highlighting the linkages and contradictions between integrated, co-managed health services delivering comprehensive care and existing policies that were rooted in systems of segmentation and fragmentation. We learned from our experience that the latter results in poor quality and high cost health care that leads to the exclusion of large elements of the population from health services.

Six concerns governed the preparation of this book:

1. There is a need to explore whether there is an underlying commonality to the policies advocated by multilateral organizations as diverse as the World Health Organization (WHO), the United Nations Children's Fund (UNICEF), the European Union (EU), Organisation of Economic Co-operation and Development (OECD), the World Bank, the International Monetary Fund (IMF) and others, despite their declared diversity of perspective on health services.

2. The nature and type of links between these policies and the prevailing fragmentation of the health sector in LMICs is examined. In particular the policy of limiting the problem-solving capacity of LMIC public services to disease control (under the guise of prioritization and efficient use of limited resources) is clearly linked to attempts to expand health markets. As put by a Rockefeller Foundation report, 'If public health agencies are encouraged to expand their focus on specific populations and interventions, at the expense of general primary and chronic care, the private sector may fill the void' (Lagomarsino et al., 2009).

3. The analysis of the nature and impact in terms of the cost, accessibility and the quality of health care provision of international health policies may be best undertaken through interdisciplinary tools and not by economic analysis alone.

4. Given the current impasse and seemingly irreversible changes to the health sector, we question the extent to which it is possible to posit alternative options with an emphasis on comprehensive care and on the health system as a whole. This perspective is based on the understanding that the credibility of an option may depend not just on the existence of successful case studies, but also on the 'know-how' and the evidence gained from actual experience in the delivery and management of health care.

5. It is increasingly acknowledged that there are shades of grey between health services in public and in private ownership. In most cases it is never exclusively one or the other. Despite shared characteristics in different regions and contexts such as in the need for profit, there are different types of private provision of care (Baru, 1998; Bhat, 1999; Maarse, 2006; Marriott, 2009; Newbrander & Rosenthal, 1997). In addition the traditional

typology of health services may also be blurred by the confusion often generated between their statutes and mission or practice (Giusti et al., 1997). Commercial provision in the health sector is premised on the primary need for profit (the quest for maximization of financial return) even if it is engaged in partnership with many not-for-profit providers or if it consists of individual physicians providing family medicine.

6. Services are often not subject to an effective regulatory system which would encourage them to operate in line with the criteria of a publicly oriented, social mission.

Following two decades of privatization policies and repeated calls for regulation, most developing countries still appear not to have the regulatory structures to appropriately monitor medical care and enforce quality standards (Asiimwe & Lule, 1992; Hozumi et al., 2008; Yesudian, 1994). The Rockefeller Foundation recently observed that 'While comprehensive regulatory regimes are absent in most low income countries, a few narrow regulatory programmes have been somewhat successful … in the domain of pharmaceuticals distribution' (!). The report listed a number of obstacles to decent regulation in LMICs (Lagomarsino et al., 2009). It states that 'Without a mechanism to intervene and control health markets, this distribution of wealth and disease perpetuates the inequitable delivery and financing of care' because 'Health markets favor wealthier segments of the population.' However, and paradoxically, the report recognizes that 'Progress toward stewardship of mixed health systems – especially the non-state sector – is a long-term aspiration rather than a short-term goal.' In other words, it suggests that regulation in LMICs could prove to merely be a lure for continued privatization.

Having examined the evidence this book thus contends that health policies and systems should be categorized into those with a social motive (their standards are described in Section 5, Chapter 14) and those with a commercial incentive (for-profit, aiming at maximizing return). With others, it argues that publicly oriented providers, strengthened, coordinated, and democratized in each country context, are needed to improve population health and access to health services (Blam & Kovalev, 2005; Drache & Sullivan, 1999; Evans, 1997; Macintosh & Koivusalo, 2005; Sen, 2003; Whitfield, 2001; World Health Organization, 2009). Their social motivation can be enhanced with appropriate financing and contracts.

Content

What, then, is the underlying theme of the book?

Section 1: Identifying international policies and paradigms

Based on a review of both published and grey literature, produced by the key institutional players in international health policy making over the past two decades, the two chapters in the first section summarize their doctrine and our concerns about their implications worldwide. This then serves as an introduction to the whole book.

WHO, the World Bank and the European Union do have a doctrine on aid and international health policy. They divide up health institutions into government and private and classify health interventions into health care and disease control. Whenever possible, they allocate disease control to the public and curative health care to the private sector. Such policies are neoliberal in their promotion of commoditization and privatization as they tend to restrict public services to the delivery of disease-control programmes.

Section 2: Demonstrating the epidemiological consequences of international policies

This section addresses the failure to control epidemiological challenges ('disease control'), although this has been the paradigm of international policies for LMICs for the past three decades. Together with other factors, disease-specific programmes are responsible for the lack of effectiveness of disease control and for many avoidable deaths in LMICs, as suggested by the monitoring of Millennium Development Goals (MDG) attainment. The failure mechanism is as follows. On a data set of Mali, a mathematical model allows us to see that to be effective, the malaria control programme – and others relying on clinical interventions – need to be integrated in health facilities where there are patients, representing a pool for early detection and continuity of care (Section 2, Chapter 3). Unfortunately, disease-control programmes undermine access to care in these facilities where they are implemented, via several mechanisms, e.g., multiplication of disease-specific divisions in national health administrations; failure to clarify the lines of command and opportunity costs (Section 2, Chapter 4). This chapter also illustrates that the organization of the services delivering disease-control interventions has been affected by the commercial constraints of the General Agreement on Trade in Services (GATS) and of regional commercial agreements such as ALCA/TLC, which undermine access to polyvalent multi-function health care. In theory this contradiction could have been solved by privatizing disease control. However, the first attempts to contract out tuberculosis control fell short of their goal even where private services represented the bulk of health care services as in India (Section 2, Chapter 5) because the professional, private sector was not very interested in such a prospect, owing to the lack of profitability, the opportunity costs involved and because it was scarce in LMIC rural and poor urban areas. Notice that these observations also hold for maternal care (Unger et al., 2009).

We therefore continue to question why access to comprehensive health care (CHC) was not included as part of the MDGs and why CHC continues to remain largely excluded from aid programmes.

Section 3: International health policies and their impact on access to health in middle-income countries: some experiences from Latin America

International policies are neoliberal in that they promote the commodification of health insurance and health care. This section suggests that this policy is not evidence-based. The analysis of Costa Rican, Colombian and Chilean policies does not confirm what a rapid WHO classification of country performances suggested in 2000 (World Health Organization, 2000): that health care privatization would yield significant efficiency gains. Instead these reform experiences confirm that health policies based on well-financed publicly oriented services are both effective and efficient, a conclusion also reached about European health care systems, as early as 2004 (European Commission, 2004). Costa Ricans spend nine times less on health than US citizens and enjoy a better health status. Hence the question: Why does the Costa Rican model not serve as a model for international policies? (Section 3, Chapter 6). Colombia has carefully applied the recommendations of Bretton Woods agencies since 1993 and has failed dramatically to secure access to decent quality versatile care and to control costs (Section 3, Chapter 7). Finally, we show that the good output of the Chilean health system is to be attributed to the public services, which managed to survive Pinochet's dictatorship, and by no means to the private sector (Section 3, Chapter 8). While Colombia and Chile are still cited as 'model' experiments (Lagomarsino et al., 2009) by those foundations promoting neoliberal policies (Lagomarsino et al., 2009), these Latin American case studies show that, being neoliberal in essence, the international health and aid policies to date have a share of responsibility in the failure to secure universal access to care. The demonstrated failure of the Colombia and Chile private sectors to deliver undermines the credibility of a key argument to privatize health care: if mixed health system stewardship mechanisms – regulation, commercial risk-pooling, and purchasing – failed in these two MICs presented as models, they are unlikely to operate in LICs.

One of the main questions raised in this book is whether current international health policies being implemented in other countries have actually taken into account the evidence gained from these experiments of health reform, in order to formulate their objectives and strategies. Our initial findings based on the case studies and reviews suggest that this may not be the case, despite the fact that so-called evidence-based policy has evolved almost into a discipline by itself, serving as a guiding rhetoric for most donors and funding institutions.

Section 4: An analysis of the political, commercial and historical determinants of international policies

The three case studies in Section 4 provide an opportunity to scrutinize the effects of bringing in different disciplines to explore the determinants and implications of neoliberal health policies: sociology and political sciences in India; economic analysis in China and history in Lebanon, where many commercial interests have found it all too easy to penetrate into the health sector with a weak political organization of the poor, powerful mechanisms of corporate lobbying and support from experts and local elites (Section 4, Chapters 9, 10 and 11). These case studies also allow one to challenge the one-sided nature of the evidence base that is utilized for policy making and illustrate with a powerful lens their long-term consequences for population health and equity in access to care. This section reinforces the evidences for the blanket nature of reforms (current and past) and the inability or unwillingness of donors and national policy makers to learn from lessons.

We have not included case studies from the African region (except for some elements of the second section). This region, despite its diversity, presents many LICs and some typically fragile states. Most have extremely limited access to care; a focus on essential packages rather than comprehensive care; substantial rural–urban and rich–poor divides in the availability of services and low levels of public expenditure on health per capita. Their health system, though not applicable to every country in the region, may be described as an over-riding pattern of donor assistance, accompanied by high levels of bureaucratization of public structures and an almost exclusive focus on disease control in the public health sector. The demise of the public sector in most countries of the region over the past 20 years is partly linked to Structural Adjustment Programmes (SAPs) that encouraged debt repayment as a priority, over support for public services. This strategy, among other impacts, actively encouraged an exodus of medical staff (internal and international migration) from this sector in most countries. Now widely documented, it is causing a crisis of professional human resources throughout LMICs, and particularly in Africa (Buckley & Baker, 2008).

Therefore, the four first chapters identify some of the dismal consequences of policies premised on neoliberal thinking that have been imposed on LMIC health sectors. Firstly, there are conditions associated with (inter)national trade which oblige LMICs to privatize health care delivery while they are structurally unable to regulate it. Secondly, disease-control programmes have yielded a worldwide institution of bureaucracy of unprecedented size. Thirdly, there is a cost to LMIC states which have frequently had to subsidize the international policies by providing human resources and infrastructure. The expansion of private provision and donor-supported public–private global health initiatives caused an internal brain-drain of medical personnel from the public to the private sector and to the aid-funded disease-specific programmes. Fourthly, in turn, this has been detrimental to their health services and to their ability to deliver health care. Access to care was eroded to a large degree because the private sector did not replace the collapsing public health systems. In addition, to the vast majority of users throughout low- and many middle-income countries, the private sector did not mean more than unregulated drug outlets, unlicensed nurses, and village health workers. The reduced access to care has led to suffering and deaths that could have been avoided and to catastrophic health expenditure. In many LMICs the cost of health care became a primary cause of falling into poverty.

Although reached with radically different methodologies, these observations are in line with those of a recently released and debated (Moszynski, 2009) Oxfam report (Marriott, 2009), which argues that health policies based on privatization and commercialization packages are not only costly, but have also failed to deliver on their own aims as well as causing much suffering, particularly for those most dependent upon public providers. It contends that the private sector is not a single entity but that the cost and quality of provision is very uneven. The report also shows that the private sector often survives through public subsidy, conveniently named public–private partnerships (PPPs) that have been advocated as the dominant mode of provision by lenders such as the World Bank since the publication of its 2004 report 'Making Services Work for the Poor' (World Bank, 2004). It claims that, although attracting much international attention and investment, the registered private sector is not a significant provider of care in many LICs: 'Oxfam's analysis of the data used by the International Finance Corporation (IFC) finds that nearly 40% of the private provision it identifies is just small shops selling drugs of unknown quality.' Moreover, those accessing trained health workers represent a small fraction of this sector clientele. In India, where 82% of outpatient care is privately delivered, only half the mothers get any medical assistance during childbirth. The private sector does not provide (as is often argued) additional investments to cash-starved public health systems but rather manages to attract significant public subsidy. In South Africa the majority of private medical scheme members receive a higher subsidy from the government through tax exemption than is spent per person dependent on publicly provided health services. Private participation in health care is associated with higher expenditure, as shown in the report through a comparison of Lebanon and Sri Lanka (e.g., due to the difficulty of regulating private providers in developing countries). There is a lack of evidence to support claims for the superior quality of the private health care sector, and in particular that it is any more responsive or any less corruptible than the public sector. Rather than helping to reach the poor, private provision can increase inequity of access because it naturally favours those who can afford treatment.

SAPs and international financing institutions used loans as a leverage to reorient LMIC health policies towards health care privatization. Today both regional economic treaties (such as TLC between Latin American countries and USA) and World Trade Organization (WTO) GATS negotiations force developing countries to implement such policies and open their market to international health care trade – with potentially catastrophic consequences. The similarity between international trade treaties and the rationale of international aid suggests that capital return and profits for industrialized countries were the real motives for contemporary design of international aid – which is elaborated further in Section 1.

However, international health policies have not been alone in promoting these policies. The expansion of commercial health care has often favoured the LMIC minority urban middle class. This elite supported the status quo, as it thought it was protected against the rising cost of care by private insurances. Often the ability to afford private provision was viewed as a mark of distinction from the rest of the population. The experience of the United States (Himmelstein et al., 2001), Chile and Colombia suggest that such policies lead to escalating costs, well beyond the limits of insurance. All this has led some to contend that many of the policies advocated in recent decades are rooted in ideology and commercial interest, rather than upon evidence of effectiveness, quality and equitability in the provision of health care (Buckley & Baker, 2008, Kessler, 2003, Pollock & Price, 2000).

Section 5: Principles for alternative policies for planning, management and delivery

As an alternative aid and international health policy, we propose an integrated, social and democratic strategy based on the financing of – and technical support to – publicly oriented (not-for-profit, socially motivated) health services. The kind of medical care these would deliver, and the sort of management needed to run them, is specific. This implies that there is not one medicine but two, and not one managerial science for health but two, according to whether the motive is profit or not. In parallel we plead for a specific disease-control organization, likely to protect access to polyvalent health care.

Section 5 provides principles for the development of such a sector. These principles encompass a paradigm shift in functions of public services and methodologies to identify them (Section 5, Chapter 12); the design of integrated health policies (Section 5, Chapter 13); health care delivery and management with a social objective (Section 5, Chapter 14); the planning of health services and systems (Section 5, Chapter 15); and the management of disease-control programmes in order to avoid undermining access to health care in public services (Section 5, Chapter 16).

Community participation and co-management among users of publicly oriented services is an important cross-cutting theme throughout the proposed policy. It is applicable only to health facilities with a social, rather than a commercial mission. The rationale of participation is partly technical since the effectiveness of health interventions ideally requires an individual and sometimes a collective *dialogue* between professionals and users of those services. It also has a political function since co-management contributes to making public health services more democratic, accountable, and responsive. Furthermore, health services development relying on community participation needs to recognize and build on popular cultures[2] rather than, as has often been the case, upon the power of local elites and non-governmental organizations (NGOs) making up the 'civil society.' We would argue that a contribution to the cultural dynamics as well as to social progress of a particular locality or region needs to be a criterion

---

[2] The term 'culture' has many meanings: 1. The symbolic organization of a group, the transmission of its knowledge and values enabling self-representation and encompassing its relationships with the universe. 2. It also describes the group traditions, beliefs, language, ideas, as well as its environmental organization – its material culture. 3. Another definition also conveys a political dimension: the potential for collective action, inherited from traditions and revealed by exceptional individuals, such as artists, poets and philosophers, who often cross the boundaries of privilege to reflect the universal value of humanity.

when assessing policies for health services, alongside the quest for equity, solidarity and the struggle against social injustice.

Section 6: A public health, strategic toolkit to implement these alternatives

This section focuses on a learning process for strategic action derived from professional practice. On this basis, it challenges policy makers to make use of the best experiments from the field to design national health policies.

In Colombia, where neoliberal reforms have been completed, professionals now complain of poor salaries, lack of professional stability, reduced professional responsibilities, over-standardization of clinical decision making related to managed care, and deteriorating ethics. Just as professionals were instrumental in promoting neoliberal policies, in our view, they could help reverse the trend if equipped with appropriate knowledge – management strategies to develop and run publicly oriented health systems and public health academic units. Although covering a limited area of their decision making, these strategies were conceived to reduce uncertainty in decision making and encourage creative thinking, while at the same time being specific in terms of targeted action and processes of change. These strategies encompass the development of family and community health in publicly oriented services (Section 6, Chapter 17); the promotion of publicly oriented hospitals with systemic responsibilities; the organization of districts and local health systems (Section 5, Chapter 15); the use of reflexive methods to bridge the gap between medical and public health identities of health professionals and improve practice (Section 6, Chapter 19); the improvement of access to health care (Section 6, Chapter 18, Part 1) and drugs (Section 6, Chapter 18, Part 2); social control at the peripheral level to increase accountability and responsiveness in publicly oriented facilities; the reorientation of international research, university teaching (Section 6, Chapter 20) and in-service training efforts.

National (tax-based or social insurance) and additional international sources are required to provide viable financing for this alternative strategy. Supply-side subsidies and contracting of not-for-profit health facilities responsible for care delivery (and disease control) are concrete ways to implement the widely advocated strengthening of health systems. Finally, our proposed policy also calls for networking and lobbying in the international arena. Whilst we are certainly not the first to undertake this task, with our proposals we hope we introduce a particular set of philosophical values in the practice of health services.

Relevance – why now?

International health policies appear to be in a period of transition, and this book aims at providing conceptual and knowledge ammunitions to those who wish to promote change. A decade following the launch of the MDGs, multilateral agencies have begun to examine their achievements and some even recognize the conceptual mistake of not considering 'access to health care' as a core MDG and the negative implications of the commercialized discourse predominant in health policies of recent years (Action for Global Health, 2009; Chan, 2008; Economic Governance for Health, 2009). In 2003 the Pan American Health Organization

(PAHO) was among the first multilateral organizations advocating a change in international policy orientations (Pan American Health Organization, 2003). In 2008 WHO followed suit (World Health Organization, 2008).

During the second half of 2008, while holding the EU presidency, France considered CHC in LMICs as one of its main priorities – a sign of possible change in the strategy put forward by the influential 1993 World Bank report 'Investing in Health.' However, the way such thinking and strategy will unfold and whether it will be devoid of commercial undertones is uncertain. Moreover, once-confident financial institutions, such as banks, have been visibly shaken by the financial worldwide crisis in 2008, which has had a devastating impact on all other sectors, notably those of employment, housing, health, social security, and pensions. The cascade effects of the international crisis on the social sectors indicate an escalation in costs of premiums, medical equipment and pharmaceuticals. The full impact of the financial and economic crisis on fragile health systems (e.g., 1.02 billion people are undernourished today, with 100 million more between 2006 and 2008) (Food and Agriculture Organization of the United Nations, 2009) and upon access to health care are yet to unfold.

The book questions the extent to which large sections of the scientific community who have been working closely with donors (Behague & Storeng, 2008), preparing aid policies and seeing through their implementation, are also prepared for change; that is from promoting the idea of markets in health care, to supporting comprehensive and accessible health care. Though this does not encompass the whole scientific community, it is clear that over the past two decades substantial sections of it have argued the case of dismantling public and CHC in favour of provider choice and supposed quality in private provision, despite strong evidence to the contrary. Whether we are right to raise the issue in this manner is a question that is best judged by the readership, premised on the evidence that is provided and on an understanding of the underlying motives of international health policies. Whilst many international NGOs continue to rather uncritically apply international health policies as they exist in their domains, there are also signs of change in this sector. Christian Aid among a handful of others have documented the negative effects of health policies that promote commercialized care upon access for the majority of people in countries where they have become the mainstay of the health sector. This applies especially to conflict zones such as Afghanistan and Iraq where the need for public provision is at its greatest (Christian Aid, 2004). More recently, the above quoted Oxfam report (Marriott, 2009) delivered a damning critique of the policies of disinvestment in public provision and the policy of privatizing health care particularly in LICs.

Nowadays, the health sector represents some 17% of the US gross domestic product (GDP) – most of it in the hands of private interests – and has probably the potential to grow to a similar proportion of the world GDP if the US model continues to be exported worldwide. There is much to be gained by the insurance business and the medical industry and lobbying by private interests will remain active. Public investment would thus go on 'maturing' markets through creating further restrictions on public services, and expensive health care for the middle classes will offer outlets for the booming corporate care, in partnership with biomedical and pharmaceutical industries.

It would be easy for aid to continue to remain project-based – with a wealth of evaluations, consultant firms and reports. Its epistemological paradigm could remain focused on high-tech medicine for the rich and alleged 'trickle-down' economic development, and disease control for the poor rather than on the reconstruction of systems providing access to family and community medicine, hospital care and on democratization of public services that require a sense of social solidarity and political commitment.

Declarations from the WHO in favour of strengthening health systems through the strategy of PHC may, as a result, be unable to reverse the trend. Access to quality health care could remain a commodity, instead of a human right with a strong potential for the redistribution of wealth. Thus these are ever more reasons why health professionals require support to develop knowledge awareness and avenues for action, to counteract a powerful economical determinism, and to take advantage of the signs of change among policy makers who have begun to realize that the lack of access to quality health care could in reality generate a great deal of political instability across many LMICs.

Definitions in health care and disease control

Some definitions are crucial to understanding the ideas contained in the forthcoming chapters. The following are definitions of disease-specific programmes (DSPs) and CHC.

Disease-specific programmes

Coherent sets of activities, know-how, and resources designed to control a single or a limited number of related disease(s) are known as disease-control programmes (Cairncross et al., 1997) or disease-specific programmes. They include:

- clinical (curative and preventive) interventions delivered in professional health facilities;
- health promotion activities carried out outside the health services;
- mass distribution of drugs (also called community distribution);
- water and sanitation interventions including vector control activities (e.g., of Simulium and Tsetse flies).

The portfolios of disease-specific programmes are huge and problematic. Funding levels for HIV/AIDS, for example, have been known often to exceed the entire national health budget (Shiffman, 2008) in several sub-Saharan African countries. In theory DSPs are designed to address major health problems and epidemiological challenges. In practice they also tackle conditions as well as diseases that cause a lesser burden on the population. Cost-effectiveness analysis was intended to determine priority control interventions but in practice, proved to be an illusion (see Section 5, Chapter 12).

Global health initiatives (GHIs)

Over the past decade, in LICs and fragile states, GHIs (or Global Health Partnerships) emerged as key donors in the health sector alongside bilateral and multilateral agencies. Funded by public and private partners, they have contributed to a significant amplification of health sector aid. Development assistance for health has increased from just over USD 6 billion in 1999 to USD 13.4 billion in 2005 (OECD, 2008).

Comprehensive health care (CHC)

CHC includes care delivered at the patient's initiative as well as care initiated by health professionals and DSPs. This care is delivered by polyvalent (versatile, multi-functional) services and includes hospital medicine able to handle at least medical, obstetrical and surgical emergencies. In LMICs first-line health services would include family and community medicine, which encompass individually tailored prevention and promotion activities in health institutions as well as mass prevention and clinical interventions that are part of the DSPs. Such care may be delivered by an array of professionals from physicians and assistant medical officers, to clinical officers or nurses, but not by community health workers. CHC has been demoted in LICs through political moves, but also with the collaboration of scientists (e.g., use of the cost–benefit model).

Community health workers (CHW) are community members, trained often for a few weeks depending on location and context (whether LIC or not). Historically they have played a useful role in remote villages, e.g., in participating in professional mobile preventive clinic activities, and in contributing to the continuity of health care and the distribution of drugs.[3] To operate properly, they need to be regularly supervised. There is a risk that in the future the concept of PHC remains limited to the deployment of an army of CHW and excludes professional services from its scope – to secure the status quo of commercial interests.

CHC does not usually include water and sanitation, or interventions such as vector control, but may exceptionally include some of these (bed net distribution, for instance).

Patient-centred care is discretionary by definition. It responds to the patient's demand for the alleviation of pain and suffering, anxiety, and perceived risk of death. It is often triggered by signs or symptoms (say a cough). The related care is often curative and polyvalent (versatile), and includes first-line services (family/community medicine) and specialized hospitals. Another type of care may be described as provider-led and is active in the early detection of patients in communities (e.g., patients suspected of trypanosomiasis/sleeping sickness). Government support for patient-initiated care may be limited in terms of a system's tiers (for instance limited to health centres and district or regional hospitals) and/or scope (e.g., excluding aesthetic surgery).H. Arendt. Condition de l'homme moderne. Calmann Levy Ed., Paris, 1983, p. 286.

References

Action for Global Health. (2009). Back to Basics: Primary Health Care Renewal at the 62nd World Health Assembly. http://www.actionfo rglobalhealth.eu/news/back_to_basics_ primary_health_care_renewal_at_the_62nd_ world_health_assembly.

Asiimwe D. & Lule J. C. (1992). *The Public Private Mix in Financing and Provision of Health Services in Uganda. 1992.* Kampala, Uganda: Makarere Institute of Social Research. Research paper Makerere Institute of Social Research.

Baru R. V. (1998). *Private Health Care in India: Social Characteristics and Trends.* New Delhi: Sage Publications.

Behague D. P. & Storeng K. T. (2008). Collapsing the vertical-horizontal divide: An ethnographic study of evidence-based policymaking in maternal health. *American Journal of Public Health*, **98**(4), pp. 644–9.

Bhat R. (1999). Characteristics of private medical practice in India: A provider perspective. *Health Policy and Planning*, **14**(1), pp. 26–37.

Blam I. & Kovalev S. (2005).On Shadow Commercialization of Health Care in Russia. *In Commercialization of Health Care: Global and Local Dynamics and Policy Responses.* Hampshire, UK: Macmillan Publishers Limited, pp. 117–35.

---

[3] Mass drug distribution consists of prophylactic drug distribution to entire communities. It generally targets tropical diseases (e.g., with ivermectin, albendazole). We call it multifunction when several drugs are delivered together by one organization, in order to cut down on operating costs. Mass drug distribution can also be viewed as the object of a vertical organization led independently from health care services.

Buckley R. P. & Baker J. (2008). IMF policies and health in sub-Saharan Africa. http://austlii.law.uts.edu.au/au/journals/UNSWLRS/2008/14.html.

Cairncross S., Periés H., & Cutts F. (1997). Vertical health programmes. *Lancet,* **349**(Supplement III), pp. 20–2.

Chan M. (2008). Return to Alma-Ata. *Lancet,* **372**(9642), pp. 865–6.

Christian Aid. (2004). *The Politics of Poverty – Aid in the New Cold War.* London, UK: Christian Aid.

Drache D. & Sullivan T. (1999). *Health Reform. Public Success, Private Failure.* London, UK: Routledge / Taylor & Francis Group.

Economic Governance for Health. (2009). Economic Governance for Health Newsletter 5, 10th May 09. http://www.eg4health.org/2009/05/11/1052/#more-1052.

European Commission. (2004). *European Competitiveness Report.* Brussels: European Commission.

Evans R. G. (1997). Going for the gold: The redistributive agenda behind market-based health care reform. *Journal of Health Politics, Policy and Law,* **22**(2), pp. 427–65.

Food and Agriculture Organization of the United Nations. (2009). *The State of Food Insecurity in the World: Economic Crisis – Impacts and Lessons Learned.* Rome: Food and Agriculture Organization of the United Nations.

Giusti D., Criel B., & de Béthune X. (1997). Viewpoint: Public versus private health care delivery: Beyond the slogans. *Health Policy and Planning,* **12**(3), pp. 192–8.

Himmelstein D. U., Woolhandler S., & Hellander I. (2001). *Bleeding The Patient: The Consequences of Corporate Health Care.* Monroe, ME: Common Courage Press.

Hozumi, D., Frost, L., Suraratdecha, C., Pratt, B.A., Sezgin, Y., Reichenback, L., & Reich, M. (2008). *The role of the private sector in health: A landscape analysis of global players' attitudes toward the private sector in health systems and levers that influence these attitudes.* Washington, DC: Results for Development Institute.

Kessler T. (2003). *Review of 2004 World Development Report. Critical Analysis of the WDR 2004. Silver Spring, MD: Results for Development Institute.*

Lagomarsino G., Nachuk S., & Singh Kundra S. (2009). *Public Stewardship of Private Providers in Mixed Health Systems. Synthesis from the Rockefeller Foundation.* Washington, DC: Results for Development Institute.

Maarse H. (2006). The privatization of health care in Europe: An eight-country analysis. *Journal of Health Politics, Policy and Law,* **31**(5), pp. 981–1014.

Macintosh M. & Koivusalo M. (2005). *Commercialization of Health Care: Global and Local Dynamics and Policy Responses.* Hampshire, UK: Macmillan Publishers Limited.

Marek T., O'Farrell C., Yamamoto C., & Zable I. (2005). *Trends and Opportunities in Public–Private Partnerships to Improve Health Service Delivery in Africa.* World Bank. Africa Region Human Development Working Paper Series.

Marriott A. (2009). *Blind Optimism: Challenging the Myths About Private Health Care in Poor Countries.* Oxford, UK: Oxfam International.

Moszynski P. (2009). Health care in poor countries must be defended against privatisation, Oxfam says. *British Medical Journal,* **339**, b2737.

Muntaner C. & Chung H. J. (2008). Macrosocial determinants, epidemiology, and health policy: Should politics and economics be banned from social determinants of health research? *Journal of Public Health Policy,* **29**(3), pp. 299–306.

Newbrander W. & Rosenthal G. (1997). Quality of care issues in health sector reform. In *Private Health Sector Growth in Asia, Issues and Implications.* New York: John Wiley & Sons, pp. 177–217.

OECD. (2008). *Development Co-operation Report 2007. Chapter Three: Aid Effectiveness Implementing the Paris Principles. Development Co-operation Report.* Paris: OECD, p. 53.

Pan American Health Organization. (2003). *Primary Health Care in the Americas: Lessons Learned over 25 Years and Future*

Challenges. Washington, DC: World Health Organization.

Pollock A. M. & Price D. (2000). Rewriting the regulations: How the World Trade Organisation could accelerate privatisation in health care systems. *Lancet*, **356**(9246), pp. 1995–2000.

Sen K. (2003). *Restructuring Health Services: Changing Contexts and Comparative Perspectives*. London, UK: Zed Books.

Shiffman J. (2008). Has donor prioritization of HIV/AIDS displaced aid for other health issues. *Health Policy and Planning*, **23**(2), pp. 95–100.

Unger J. P., Van Dessel P., Sen K., & De Paepe P. (2009). International health policy and stagnating maternal mortality: Is there a causal link? *Reproductive Health Matters*, **17**(33), pp. 91–104.

Whitfield D. (2001). *Public Services or Corporate Welfare. Rethinking the Nation State in the Global Economy*. London, UK: Pluto Press.

World Bank. (2004). *World Development Report 2004: Making Services Work for Poor People*. Washington, DC: Oxford University Press.

World Health Organization. (2000). *World Health Report 2000: Health Systems. Improving Performance*. Geneva: World Health Organization.

World Health Organization. (2008). *The World Health Report 2008 Primary Health Care – Now More Than Ever*. Geneva: World Health Organization.

World Health Organization. (2009). WHO Statistical Information System (WHOSIS). 2009.

Yesudian C. A. K. (1994). Behaviour of the private sector in the health market of Bombay. *Health Policy and Planning*, **9**(1), pp. 72–80.

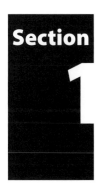

Section 1

Paradigms of international policies

Introduction to Section 1

This section outlines the doctrine of international health policies that have prevailed over the past 25 years, acknowledging that implementation has varied a great deal from place to place and over time. Chapter 1 delineates the paradigm of contemporary international health policies. Chapter 2 provides a summary of our concerns about them. This section thus serves as the basis for, and as an introduction to, the main elements of the book.

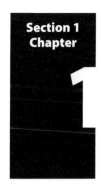

Donor led policies: analysis of an underlying doctrine

Chapter 1 contains material previously published in:
De Paepe P., Soors W., Unger J. -P. International Aid Policy: Public Disease Control and Private Curative Care? Cadernos de Saude Publica 2007; 23(Suppl. 2): S273–281.

Introduction

Many authors advocate integrating vertical programmes into local health facilities in order to achieve reasonable prospects for successful disease control (Bossyns, 1997; Loretti, 1989; Oxfam, 2003; Tulloch, 1999). An editorial in the influential *New England Journal of Medicine* (Mulholland & Adegbola, 2005) on bacterial infections (as a major cause of death among children in Africa), for example, stressed the need for comprehensive, integrated and accessible health services to address health needs and questioned the narrow, disease-based approach that has prevailed to date.

Whilst there is a need for some non-integrated vertical programmes in most countries (Criel et al., 1997), any health policy allocating public health activities and disease-control programmes to Ministry of Health (MoH) structures and general health care to private facilities remains highly problematic since it precludes the integration of disease control with general health care.

Through a review of multilateral aid policies, this chapter examines whether current international aid policies have supported the allocation of health care and disease control to different health facilities rather than integrating them into one. In other words this section will focus on outlining the doctrines informing policy rather than describing their implementation, which will be addressed in later sections. The actual implementation may differ due to specific political, social, geo-strategic, and economic factors. The analysis of the doctrine however is relevant per se, since it will clarify health policies promoted by international organizations, which have influenced national policy design in developing countries for decades (Koivusalo & Ollila, 1998; Ollila et al., 2000). First we examine some historical factors, followed by a more detailed focus upon cases in order to explore the nature and function of the doctrine that has been an underlying feature of international health policies.

To what extent have international aid agencies allocated health care and disease control to different health facilities?

The background

The history of international aid is one of action and reaction: the restoration of an order established in the 1950s – disease control at that time being the core of health policies conceived by industrialized countries mainly for the then colonies – and reconfirmed in the 1990s, as opposed to the Primary Health Care (PHC) strategy that was advocated in the 1970s. We contend that the allocation of disease control and health care to separate sectors is the result of both this history and an explicit doctrine.

Citizens of most colonies had little political weight and limited access to health care, which had never been viewed as a priority by the colonial powers. These diseases were managed in isolation, as a quick and cheap way of dealing with health problems without having to provide a comprehensive service. During the 1950s and even in the 1960s, policies for disease control in many African countries focused on vertical programmes with a disease-oriented approach. The most important achievement of this approach was the eradication of smallpox in 1979. This success eventually was used as a major argument for continuing with this strategy: Foege et al., for example, suggested organizing health services along the lines of fire brigades, based on epidemiological surveillance and modelled after smallpox control (Foege et al., 1976). This proposal failed to recognize the specificity of health service organizations and underestimated the epidemiological features of smallpox, characterized by very slow transmission. So far, successful disease eradication has not been repeated (the failure of the malaria eradication campaign is a good example), although the burden of poliomyelitis, dracunculiasis, onchocerciasis, and measles was greatly reduced owing to disease-control programmes.

In 1978 a challenging new approach was approved in Alma Ata (World Health Organization, 1978), under the leadership of the World Health Organization (WHO) and its Director-General Halfdan Mahler: PHC promoted comprehensive care and community participation in public services, which echoed the mood of the 1970s and the politics of participatory democracy. This new vision of health promoted community participation to democratize publicly oriented services, with users being called to co-manage health services together with professionals and civil servants. This 'health for all' concept brought WHO several head-on confrontations with multinational companies (for example, on breast milk, essential drugs and substitutes), with the United States even withholding its contribution to the WHO's regular budget in 1985 (Walt, 1993).

This caused a return to the strategies of the 1950s – vertical programmes – at least for developing countries. One year after the Alma Ata conference (1978) Walsh & Warren, from the Rockefeller Foundation, wrote a paper in the *New England Journal of Medicine* to reduce the scope of PHC to the control of four or five diseases, a strategy labelled 'Selective Primary Health Care' (SPHC) (Walsh & Warren, 1979). This was officially promoted by the Rockefeller Foundation and United Nations Children's Fund (UNICEF), which contended that the public sector should be selective in the services it offers and that most health care is better delivered and financed privately. This policy, however, was criticized on the grounds that Comprehensive Primary Health Care (CPHC), including the same disease-control objectives but securing access to health care, incurred the same costs as SPHC (Unger & Killingsworth, 1986). The numerous scientists who had mobilized around the world against this initiative failed to sway US policy. Instead, soon after, the World Bank (WB) followed the United States. Its 1987 report, Financing Health Services in Developing Countries: An Agenda for Reform (World Bank, 1987) (p. 38), began to distinguish between health care and disease control: 'For some types of health care, especially simple curative care, private providers may well be more efficient than the government and offer comparable or better services at lower unit cost,' and 'many health-related services such as information and control of contagious disease are public goods.' The paper argued in favour of greater reliance on private-sector health care provision and the reduction of public involvement in health services delivery. As a United Nations Research Institute for Social Development (UNRISD) report states: 'What is not in doubt is the scale of the policy pressures over the last two decades from, particularly, multilateral donors to commercialize health care. The WB has been particularly influential in promoting the concept of health care as largely private good, hence deliverable through the market, all the while downplaying the well-understood perverse incentives structures in health care markets' (Mackintosh, 2003) (p. 6).

In 1993, echoing the SPHC policy, the WB report Investing in Health (World Bank, 1993) proposed a basic service package to be provided by public health services, and other curative care by private for-profit providers. The report, WB's most comprehensive document regarding health, viewed health care not as a need, much less as a right, but as a demand, defined by the consumers' ability and willingness to pay (Nair et al., 2006). As observers in developing countries noticed, the Bank's 1993 report opened avenues for private investment in formerly public programmes (Turshen, 1999; World Bank, 1999).

A 1996 WB discussion paper recommended governments not to tie public finance to public provision, 'though that does not necessarily mean eliminating public provision, which will sometimes be the best solution' (Musgrove, 1996) (p. 56). The objective of the paper was to 'minimise deadweight losses from public intervention and leave as much room as possible for private choices.'

The 1997 Strategy Paper for the World Bank Health, Nutrition, and Population Program was even more explicit (Human Development Network, 1993). It stated that 'in low-income countries, where private sector activities often dominate, governments will be encouraged to focus their attention on the provision of: services with large externalities (preventive health services); essential clinical services for the poor; and more effective regulation for the private sector, and to promote greater diversity in service delivery systems by providing funding for civil society and non-governmental providers on a competitive basis, instead of limiting public funds to public facilities' (p. 26). The minimal package for the poor to be provided or mandated by governments would include 'basic immunization, management of sick children, maternal care, family planning, targeted nutrition, school health, communicable disease control' (p. 26). Excluded from the package were family medicine, or patient-centred care with an assessment of social, family, psychological, and somatic factors that may influence the problem and its solution, and 'expensive' hospital care.

In its 1997 report 'The State in a Changing World,' the WB recognized that markets undersupply a range of collective goods, among which public health goods (World Bank & Chibber, 1997). Instead the report favoured the private sector as the provider of choice for individual health care. It focused on programmes that would take a vertical approach to disease control while ignoring the effect of non-specific mortality in deprived groups. The results were expert-decided standardized disease control over context-dependent priority setting by the local community and national MoH, and a failure to support an integrated approach to health services.

The history of competition between the WB and WHO for leadership in international health can be written as the record of neoliberal ideology capturing international policy. Neoliberalism refers to political–economical policies that de-emphasize or reject government intervention in domestic economies, but favour the use of political power to open up foreign nations to entry by multinational corporations. In a broader sense it is used to describe the movement towards using the market to achieve a wide range of social ends that were previously filled by government. Arguments for the effectiveness of this movement follow the neoliberal paradigm that markets perform best in allocating and using resources, even in the field of public health (Armada et al., 2001). It is the story of market values replacing the vision of medical ethos and humanitarian aid, of industry controlling the scientific community, of free-market philosophy overtaking social and democratic ideals. WHO's third function, advocacy for changes in health policy, which came to the fore with the launch of Health for All in 1977, had been taken over by the Bank while WHO had retreated into its technical and biomedical shell (Godlee, 1994).

The WHO, in its well-known report Health Systems: Improving Performance in 2000, emphasized the increasing demands on health systems and the limits as to what governments can finance (World Health Organization, 2000). It then recommended a 'public process of priority setting to identify the contents of a benefit package available to all, which should reflect local disease priorities and cost-effectiveness' (p. 15). In this way, it implicitly separated disease control and individual curative care. It also reaffirmed the key role of government as stewardship, to 'row less and steer more,' and promoted quality-based competition among providers, together with a combination of public subsidy and regulation for private providers in middle-income countries.

A good example of the powerful influence of the WB on WHO was the 2001 report on Macroeconomics and Health: Investing in Health for Economic Development (Commission on Macroeconomics and Health, 2001). Investing in Health, the subtitle of this Commission's report, echoed the Bank's controversial World Development Report 1993: Investing in Health (World Bank, 1993). The Report on Macroeconomics and Health updated the earlier Rockefeller Foundation campaigns (Commission on Macroeconomics and Health, 2001) against endemic infections, which were deemed necessary to improve labour productivity. It recommended, against criticisms from several sources (Banerji, 2002), a vertical approach to the eradication of specific diseases, rather than encouraging the development of integrated health care systems.

The authors of the report, all of them commissioned by WHO but most having had extensive experience with the WB, International Monetary Fund (IMF) or other multilateral economic organizations (Katz, 2004), argued that investment to improve health was a key strategy towards economic development. This development meant reform: 'streamlining the public sector, privatization, public funding of private services, introduction of market principles based on competition' (Waitzkin, 2003) (p. 523). The proposed system would involve a mix of state and non-state health service providers, with financing guaranteed by the state. 'In this model, the government may own and operate service units, or it may contract for services with for-profit and not-for-profit providers' (Waitzkin, 2003) (p. 524). One of the working papers of the Commission on Macroeconomics and Health (CMH) bluntly stated that in order to make progress in liberalizing health services in the current round of General Agreement on Trade in Services (GATS), more member countries would need to schedule this sector (Chanda, 2001). 'Given privatization trends and greater public–private cooperation in the delivery of health services around the world, often necessitated by declining public sector resources, more countries may be willing to table health services in this round of GATS discussions' (Chanda, 2001) (p. 88).

This formula was accepted without much critical analysis and was seen as a desirable goal in the WHO-funded paper, despite reports of poor results of health sector reform in countries such as Chile and Colombia, which had applied them comprehensively (Holst et al., 2004; Navarro, 2004; Chapters 6 and 8 of Section 3). Trade agreements, in particular the GATS/World Trade Organization (WTO) and the plethora of regional and bilateral treaties (Free Trade Agreement of the Americas, Association of Southeast Asian Nations etc.) since the Doha round, also limited the ability of governments to control markets through regulatory measures (Feedman, 2005). Whilst discussion on Trade Related Intellactual Property Rights (TRIPS) have taken precedence over those related to trade in services (GATS) and are more visible in the public domain, the underlying threat to public services from GATS could prove to be more pernicious.

The European Union (EU) did not lag behind. A 2002 communication from The Commission to the European Council (p. 14) stated: 'The European Community will work closely with development partners including government, civil society, and the private sector,' 'exploring opportunities to work with the private, not-for-profit and for-profit sectors.' A more active approach would be adopted for 'community work with the private for-profit health sector,' and mechanisms would be sought to 'enhance co-operation with private investors to improve their responsibility for health in developing countries.'

The World Development Report 2004 (p. 215), entitled 'Basic Services for the Poor,' separated 'highly transaction-intensive and individual-oriented clinical services,' requiring individually tailored diagnostics and treatment, from 'population-oriented outreach services; services that can be standardized and include vector control, immunisation or vitamin A supplementation' (World Bank, 2004) (p. 133). These were new ways of denominating and, at the same time, administratively and operationally segregating curative individual medicine and disease-control programmes. The report stated that even governments with limited capacity could provide the latter (or write contracts with public or private entities to provide them, which now opens the door for private sector involvement in disease-control programmes), while the former were best left to private initiative.

The report stressed the public sectors' difficulties in providing clinical services for the poor, though both the long route, which requires the policymaker to monitor the provider, and the short route of direct control of the patient over his provider fail. The first fails because of the complexity of clinical services and the heterogeneity of health needs, which make it difficult to standardize service provision and to monitor performance. The second fails because of the lack of accountability of public providers. It did not mention that the long route is the one that worked in Northern European countries, nor that the short route in private practice may not be so short because of information asymmetry, supplier-induced demand, and the opportunity cost for communities of monitoring health care providers.

The World Development Report (WDR) 2004 recommended private provision of clinical services, except for the few countries with a strong public ethos, pro-poor policies, and enforcements of rules (World Bank, 2004). The Bank maintained its bias against government-provided services, presenting obstacles to improving traditional public services as ample justification for shifting to new institutional arrangements, yet, obstacles to market-based approaches, even if severe, were characterized as challenges that could be met. For instance, according to the WDR, in a situation in which a public sector regulator is not independent from a policy-maker, it justifies the contracting-out of care. However, when the issue is privatization, the absence of regulatory experience (monitoring quality and compliance of private providers) only leads to recommendations for regulatory capacity building.

The last decade: the persistence of 'market deficiencies'

Attempts to remediate market deficiencies and to control diseases have featured in international policies tailored for LMICs during the first decade of the millennium. They ended up in an unprecedented bureaucratic growth while failing to achieve epidemiological objectives. Therefore, some donors reconsidered the value of applying markets without restraint while many others didn't but amended their strategical recommendations.

Global health initiatives and disease-control programmes

Global Health Initiatives are Public–Private Partnerships (PPPs) geared towards the control of diseases in LMICs. They have contributed to a significant increase of aid to the health sector. Development assistance for health was stable at around 5% of total ODA or around USD 3 billion during the beginning of the 1980s and remained virtually unchanged until the end of the 1990s. Since then it has started to grow and has increased from just over USD 6 billion in 1999 to USD 13.4 billion in 2005 and to USD 16.7 billion in 2006 (OECD, 2008). This expansion has to a large extent fed a rapidly increasing number of DSPs, and in particular HIV/AIDS. In 2006 HIV/AIDS (and other sexually transmitted diseases) were already representing about 50% of total health ODA commitments (Piva & Dodd, 2009).

PPPs are at the core of DSPs. They emerged from ventures organized in the mid-1990s through pharmaceutical industry initiatives and have also resulted from increased awareness of the heavy burden caused by some major diseases. In 2007 about 80 PPPs existed world wide, some with relatively small portfolios while others were managing sizeable ones. They have reportedly now increased to over 100. In the Congo alone, for example, in 2008 there were as many as 52 DSPs.

Although the typology is not clear-cut, GHIs may be classified into four main categories: those focusing on research and development, including discovery and development of new therapies; technical assistance/service support, including drug donations; advocacy at national and international levels; and those focusing on financing, including the provision of funds for specific programmes (Carlson, 2004). GHIs are central to the contemporary aid architecture. Their interests span from jobs to capital return, from academic to NGO activities and from trade to consultancy. They vary owing to their choice of disease target and product focus (drugs, vaccines, diagnostics, microbicides, and other health products) (Widdus & White, 2004). The portfolios of the DSPs are thus huge. The funding levels for HIV/AIDS alone approximate or exceed the entirety of the national health budget in several sub-Saharan African countries (Shiffman, 2008).

The rationale of the choice of intervention area has often been based on economic factors and/or a reflection of the fear of industrialized countries' of LDC borne pandemics. Therefore, GHI do not only address large health problems, but also conditions and diseases that cause lesser disease burden. For instance, top killers such as acute respiratory infections and shigellosis, cancers, cardio- and cerebro-vascular diseases have been largely overlooked (Shiffman et al., 2002).

GHI mobilized funds and, admittedly, in some cases took the lead in innovation. A Department for International Development (DFID) report (2004) identified several positive features of GHIs as follows (Caines et al., 2004): 'The R&D Global Health Programme (GHP) components generally appear as a particularly fruitful way to foster research and development for new diagnostics, drugs and vaccines. Some GHPs – such as the Global Alliance for Vaccines and Immunisation, the TB Global Drug Facility and the Green Light Committee for multidrug-resistant TB – have successfully secured commodity price reductions, and fostered both competition and research, though antiretroviral price reductions may stem more from increased competition from generic manufacturers and global pressure than the Accelerating Access Initiative.' However, the same authors continue: 'The more taxing concerns relate to GHP operations at country level.' Concerns that GHPs may weaken LMIC health systems arose as it could be assumed that the clinical activities of DSPs compete with those of general health care for limited system resources, particularly staff time (crowding-out effects) (Aylward et al., 2000; Travis et al., 2004) (see Section 2, Chapter 4). The numerous and often highly paid employees of DSPs have been responsible for a major internal brain-drain, especially in low-income countries (LICs). These concerns

	Maternal mortality	AIDS prevalence	TB mortality	Malaria risk
Latin America	moderate	moderate	low	moderate
Sub-Saharan Africa	very high	high	high	high
South Asia	high	low	moderate	moderate
South-East Asia	high	low	moderate	moderate

☐ Progress sufficient to reach the target if prevailing trends persist

☐ Progress insufficient to reach the target if prevailing trends persist

■ No progress or deterioration

Figure 1.1. Millennium Development Goals: Progress or deterioration? *Note*: The data for malaria was not available in the 2008 MDG progress chart, the data shown are data from the 2007 MDG progress chart. *Source*: Adapted by authors from MDG progress charts 2007 and 2008 (United Nations). TB, tuberculosis.

are crucial since the large increase in total ODA in health has not delivered the expected outcome – to significantly progress on MDGs (Figure 1.1).

Regulating health care markets in LMICs?

During the past decade, international policies stressed the need for improved regulation. While they assume that existing regulatory arrangements can be significantly improved, there are reasons to believe that this plea could be a straw man argument to justify continued privatization.

As early as 1994, most developing countries already had the basic legislation for regulation but there were difficulties in enforcing such controls (Bennett et al., 1994). Although calls to LMIC States to develop regulation in LMICs were heard since 1993, when the World Development Report addressed a crucial need for strengthening capacity of government to regulate the private sector, progress was either extremely slow or inexistent. This happened even in some middle-income countries (MICs) (see Section 3, Chapters 6 and 8) cited as 'success stories' where the private sector benefited from public subsidies. Enforcement of law and regulations against non-compliant health care providers remained thus usually weak (Matsebula et al., 2005) – because it was perverted by powerful vested interests (Bennet et al., 2005).

Anyway, legal interventions alone would have little influence on the behaviour of for-profit providers (Cassels, 1995) since bureaucratic control, sanctions, and penalties would tend to be ineffective unless there are underlying financial incentives (Ferrinho et al., 2004; La Forgia & Couttolenc, 2008). Unfortunately, financing the private sector and purchasing care for the poor are of limited practicability since LMIC public finances to support private providers has long been constrained by the weight of public services wages. Furthermore, the few countries which managed to release funds for the private sector such as Chile and Colombia did not manage to make it work for public goals (see Section 3).

In fact, and paradoxically, countries with a 'bad' regulatory governance record (e.g., because of insecure property rights and contracts (Qian, 2002) and because their health sector is less open to private initiative than the majority of the others) are those which get the best achievements (Grindle, 2007).

In conclusion, there are many reasons why the Rockefeller Foundation could depict 'non-model countries' (that is the large majority of them) with an 'absence of near-term government capacity for broad stewardship of health markets' and could state that 'Progress toward steward-ship of mixed health systems – especially the non-state sector – is a long-term aspiration rather than a short-term goal' (Lagomarsino et al., 2009). However, the Foundation report did not recommend treating as a long-term aspiration the commoditization of health care in LMICs.

Maturing markets and policies

During the past decade, several strategies attempted to remedy some of the deficiencies of health care markets in LMICs. These 'corrective' strategies spanned from market maturation to argumentation meant to explain past setbacks and offer avenues for further privatization. We will examine the concepts of social security under neoliberal health policies, community mutual aid associations, 'diagonal' organization, and strategic purchasing.

Bismarckian health policies were a response to political threats at the end of the nine-teenth century posed to the economical establishment by the working class organizations and to the State by the socialist movement (Rimlinger, 1971). At the end of World War II it was again the combined threat of a strong, armed resistence movement led by communist parties and the existence of a powerful Soviet block which led European governments to decently finance health care for the under-priviledged (Pauwels, 2002).

The concepts of social insurance and social protection for LMICs were verbally promot-ed by international aid agencies and industrialized governments (e.g., Arjona et al., 2001; Bennett et al., 1998). Like in European countries where mutual aid associations (the British 'friendly societies') had flourished without significant State financial support, and where mere solidarity amongst the poor never permitted real improvements in access to care nor reduc-tion in catastrophic health expenditure (de Swaan, 1988), successes in LMICs were expectedly rare. Thus, in French speaking Africa, compulsory insurance systems never contributed for more than 20% of overall health sector financing (Sery & Letourmy, 2006), and with a few exceptions, their coverage rate remained between 3 and 6% of the population (ibid, p 204). Although mutual aid associations were relatively old (Ndiaye, 2006), their members in 11 African French speaking countries represented only 0.58% of the total population of these countries in 2003 (ibid. p 326). Finally, while international organizations had hoped that com-munity associations would compensate for the lack of State regulation and funds, in practice, these associations did not even manage to influence quality of care where they existed (Criel et al., 2006).

As in the nineteenth century, social insurance remains conceived to purchase private health care (de Roodenbeke, 2005). The link appears clearly in the concept of 'diagonal organ-ization' (Sepúlveda, 2006) as labelled to describe the Mexican way of social insurance, the Plan Oportunidades. This organizational pattern was presented as a way to reconcile 'artificial dichotomies ... between the vertical approach focusing on specific disease priorities, and the horizontal approach aimed at strengthening the overall structure and functions of the health system' (Frenk, 2006). In practice this benefit package designed for 'the poor' encompassed a series of disease-specific programmes representing by their number a compromise between 'vertical' and Comprehensive Health Care (CHC) supposed to strengthen health systems. Just as vertical is not synonymous of 'disease specific' but rather refers to the type of admin-istration (Section 2, Chapter 4), the administrative costs of organizations managing health funds proved to be as high as those of disease-specific programmes (see transaction costs of the Colombian system, Section 3, Chapter 7).

These facts, together with the frequently observed paradox of increased health insurance coverage and reduced access to health care, lead us to two conclusions. Firstly, the feasibility of developing the social insurance model seems to have found little root in most LMICs. Secondly, the concept of social protection applied to health and often used for the expansion of social insurance appears to be little more then a lure to justify privatization. This is because, in reality, its practice will require a purchaser–provider split as has happened in Colombia and Chile (Section 3, Chapters 7 and 8).

Finally, 'strategic purchasing' is becoming a concept replacing 'contracting out' in neoliberal policies – which was acknowledged to have failed in the vast majority of LMICs (Lagomarsino et al., 2009) – by amplifying the range of purchased care and expanding the array of providers to complex organizations, in spite of manifest regulatory breakdown and government failure to control simple health care delivery in LMICs.

Is an international health policy reorientation in the pipeline?

In 2007, a new type of initiative, the International Health Partnership (IHP), aiming at the coordination of activities among donors and putting the principles of the Paris Declaration 2005 (harmonization of aid programmes) into practical action, appeared as a key element in the global aid architecture. This was intended to tackle the challenges of health systems, and its disintegration through disease-specific programmes – but without explicitly aiming at improving access to comprehensive care. It included some of the most resourceful actors such as the WHO, the WB, the Joint United Nations Programme on HIV and AIDS (UNAIDS), UNICEF, the Global Fund to Fight AIDS, Tuberculosis and Malaria (GFATM), the European Union (EU) as well as bilateral donors including the United Kingdom (UK), France, Germany, Italy, The Netherlands, and Norway. One aim was to speed up efforts to reach the MDGs by pooling resources, also from DSPs, into one national plan, with one single policy and results framework, one budget, and one monitoring system (the 'four ones'). A pilot study of the aid effectiveness was conducted in several countries between 2003 and 2007, with a budget of more than USD 1 billion. Its preliminary evaluation was completed in 2008. The results were uneven (OECD/DAC 2008). Although the move to coordinate aid initiatives is certainly a welcome one, international health policies continue to remain donor driven to a large extent and are unlikely, in the immediate future, to alter the damage caused by the effects of disease-specific programmes on health systems worldwide. Today multilateral agencies have begun to recognize the contradictions of not considering 'access to health care' as a core MDG and of the negative implications of this upon disease-control achievements (Action for Global Health, 2009; Economic Governance for Health, 2009). In 2003 the Pan American Health Organization (PAHO) began advocating a return to PHC (Macinko et al., 2007; Pan American Health Organization, 2003; Pan American Health Organization; 2005). In 2008 WHO also followed suit, indicating a shift in international policy directions (World Health Organization, 2008; World Health Organization, 2009). However, the way this strategy will unfold and whether it will be devoid of commercial tones is uncertain. As said earlier, there still is a risk, especially in Africa, of viewing the PHC strategy as limited to the introduction of village health workers without any attempt to change the health care system or improve access to health care.

Conclusion

To what extent does international aid have an underlying 'doctrine'? The answer appears to be an undeniable one: the general trend has been the allocation of public health and disease-control activities to MoH, and health care to the private sector as part of a neoliberal doctrine. That has become embedded in the health sector of many LMICs.

Multilateral agencies have tended to promote disease-control programmes without considering the possibility of integrating them into first-line health services. International financing and trade organizations also favoured the privatization of discretionary health care delivery, and supported a limited role for public sector activities, focusing mainly on unprofitable but necessary public health functions – mainly disease control (Waitzkin, 2003).

However, despite recognizing an underlying doctrine, these conclusions need to be interpreted carefully, in the light of this study's methodology. Firstly, our literature review is limited to multilateral aid, while bilateral aid was not reviewed. Secondly, the international agencies that formulated this doctrine did not implement it bluntly or homogeneously everywhere. International investments in public facilities have also occurred in many cases. In fact international agencies have complex decision making mechanisms, with different countervailing forces operating on different subjects at different points in time, as shown by the following examples. The WB policy note of the WDR 1993 was not fully reflected in actual WB health disbursements. Neither was this doctrine applied when private expenditures were so low that no investors were interested in a particular market (for instance in some West and Central African countries).

In addition, it is unclear whether the recent acknowledgement of policy failure in the health sector by WHO director, M Chan (2009), implies a policy reorientation. The role of international organizations has been that of a catalyst. Commoditization of health care has been the product of social and economical factors, as will be seen in the India and Lebanon case studies. However, a deconstruction of the paradigm of international health policies is central to understanding their limitations and failures in different contexts, as will be illustrated later.

References

Action for Global Health. (2009). Back to Basics: Primary Health Care Renewal at the 62nd World Health Assembly. http://www.actionforglobalhealth.eu/news/back_to_basics_primary_health_care_renewal_at_the_62nd_world_health_assembly.

Arjona R., Ladaique M., & Pearson M. (2001). *Growth, Inequality and Social Protection.* Paris: OECD, Directorate for Employment, Labour and Social Affairs.

Armada F., Muntaner C., & Navarro V. (2001). Health and social security reforms in Latin America: The convergence of the World Health Organization, the World Bank, and Transnational Corporations. *International Journal of Health Services, 31*(4), pp. 729–68.

Aylward R. B., Hull H. F., Cochi S. L., Sutter R. W., Olive J. M., & Melgaard B. (2000). Disease eradication as a public health strategy: A case study of poliomyelitis eradication. *Bulletin of the World Health Organization, 78*(3), pp. 285–97.

Banerji D. (2002). Report of the WHO Commission on Macroeconomics and Health: A critique. *International Journal of Health Services, 32*(4), pp. 733–54.

Bennett S., Dakpallah G., Garner P., et al. (1994). Carrot and stick: State mechanisms to influence private provider behavior. *Health Policy and Planning, 9*(1), pp. 1–13.

Bennett S., Creese A., & Monasch R. (1998). *Health Insurance Schemes for People Outside Formal Sector Employment.* ARA paper number 16, WHO/ARA/CC/98.1. Geneva: World Health Organization, Division of Analysis, Research and Assessment.

Bennet S., Hanson K., Kadama P., & Montagu D. (2005). *Working with the Non-state Sector to Achieve Public Health Goals.* Making Health Systems Work. Working paper no. 2. Geneva: World Health Organization.

Bossyns P. (1997). Big programmes, big errors? *Lancet, 350*(9093), pp. 1783–4.

Caines K., Buse K., Carlson C., et al. (2004). Assessing the impact of global health partnerships. *Synthesis of Findings From the 2004 DFID Studies: Global Health Partnerships: Assessing the Impact*. London: DFID Health Resource Centre.

Carlson C. (2004). *GHP Study Paper 1: Mapping Global Health Partnerships: What They Are, What They Do and Where They Operate*. Global health partnership study paper series. London: DFID Health Resource Centre.

Cassels A. (1995). Health sector reform: Key issues in less developed countries. *Journal of International Development*, 7(3), pp. 329–47.

Chanda R. (2001). *Trade in Health Services*. Working paper series n WG4: 5. New Delhi: Commission on Macroeconomics and Health.

Commission on Macroeconomics and Health. (2001). *Macroeconomics and Health: Investing in Health for Economic Development*. Geneva: World Health Organization.

Criel B., De Brouwere V., & Dugas S. (1997). *Integration of Vertical Programmes in Multi-Function Health Services*. Antwerp: ITG Press.

Criel B., Blaise P., & Ferette D. (2006). Mutuelles de santé en Afrique et qualité des soins dans les services: une interaction dynamique. In *L'Assurance Maladie En Afrique Francophone. Améliorer L'Accès Aux Soins Et Lutter Contre La Pauvreté. Série: Santé, Nutrition Et Population*, ed. G. Dussault et al., eds. Washington, DC: Banque Mondiale, pp. 353–72.

de Roodenbeke E. (2005). Purchasing hospital services: Key questions for policymakers. In: Langenbrunner J. & Langenbrunner J. C., eds. *Spending Wisely: Buying Health Services for the Poor*, ed. Geneva: World Bank, pp. 213–34.

de Swaan A. (1988). Workers' mutualism: An interlude on self-management. In: *In Care of the State: Health Care, Education and Welfare in Europe and the USA in the Modern Era*. Oxford, UK: Oxford University Press,

Economic Governance for Health. (2009). Economic Governance for Health. *Newsletter* 5, 10th May 09. http://wwweg4health.org/2009/05/11/1052/#more-1052.

Feedman L. P. (2005). Achieving the MDGs: Health systems as core social institutions. *Development*, 48(1), pp. 19–24.

Ferrinho P., Van Lerberghe W., Fronteira I., Hipolito F., & Biscaia A. (2004). Dual practice in the health sector: review of the evidence. *Human Resources for Health*, 2(1), p. 14.

Foege W. H., Hogan R. C., & Newton L. H. (1976). Surveillance projects for selected diseases. *International Journal of Epidemiology*, 5(1), pp. 29–37.

Frenk J. (2006). Bridging the divide: Global lessons from evidence-based health policy in Mexico. *Lancet*, 368(9539), pp. 954–61.

Godlee F. (1994). WHO in retreat: Is it losing its influence? *British Medical Journal*, 309(6967), pp. 1491–5.

Grindle M. S. (2007). Good enough governance revisited. *Development Policy Review*, 25(5), pp. 553–74.

Holst J., Laaser U., & Hohmann J. (2004). Chilean health insurance system: A source of inequity and selective social insecurity. *Journal of Public Health*, 12, pp. 271–82.

Human Development Network. (1993). *Health, Nutrition and Population*. Washington, DC: World Bank.

Katz A. (2004). The Sachs report: Investing in Health for Economic Development – or increasing the size of the crumbs from the rich man's table? Part I. *International Journal of Health Services*, 34(4), pp. 751–73.

Koivusalo M. & Ollila E. (1998). *Making a Healthy World: Agencies, Actors and Policies in International Health*. London, UK: Zed Books.

La Forgia G. M. & Couttolenc B. (2008). *Hospital Performance in Brazil: The Search for Excellence*. Washington, DC: World Bank.

Lagomarsino G., Nachuk S., & Singh Kundra S. (2009). *Public Stewardship of Private Providers in Mixed Health Systems. Synthesis from the Rockefeller Foundation*. Washington, DC: Results for Development Institute.

Loretti A. (1989). Leprosy control: The rationale of integration. *Leprosy Review*, 60(4), pp. 306–16.

Macinko J., Montenegro H., & Nebot C. (2007). *Renewing Primary Health Care in the*

Americas: A Position Paper of the Pan American Health Organization/World Health Organization (PAHO/WHO). Washington, DC: Pan American Health Organization/ World Health Organization (PAHO/WHO).

Mackintosh M. (2003). *Health Care Commercialisation and the Embedding of Inequality. RUIG/UNRISD Health Project Synthesis Paper*. Geneva: United Nations Research Institute for Social Development.

Matsebula T., Goudge J., & Gilson L. (2005). Regulating the Pharmaceutical Sector: Coping With Low Capacity While Maintaining Regulatory Independence. Health Economics & Financing Programme working paper.

Mulholland E. K. & Adegbola R. A. (2005). Bacterial infections. A major cause of death among children in Africa. *New England Journal of Medicine*, **352**(1), pp. 75–7.

Musgrove P. (1996). *Public and Private Roles In Health – Theory and Financing Patterns*. Washington: The International Bank for Reconstruction and Development / The World Bank, pp. 339.

Nair S., Sexton S., & Kirbat P. (2006). A decade after Cairo: Women's health in a free market economy. *Indian Journal of Gender Studies*, **13**(2), pp. 171–93.

Navarro V. (2004). The world situation and WHO. *Lancet*, **363**(9417), pp. 1321–3.

Ndiaye P. (2006). Le d'veloppement des mutelles de santé en Afrique. In: Dussault G., et al., eds. *L'Assurance Maladie En Afrique Francophone: Ameliorer L'Acces Aux Soins Et Lutter Contre La Pauvrete*. Geneva: World Bank, p. 314.

OECD. (2008). *Development Co-operation Report 2007. Chapter Three: Aid Effectiveness Implementing the Paris Principles*. Development Co-operation Report. Paris: OECD, p. 53.

Ollila E., Koivusalo M., & Hemminki E. (2000). International actors and population policies in India, with special reference to contraceptive policies. *International Journal of Health Services*, **30**(1), pp. 87–110.

Oxfam International. (2003). *False Hope or New Start? The Global Fund to Fight HIV/AIDS, TB and Malaria*. Rome: Oxfam International.

Pan American Health Organization. (2003). *Primary Health Care in the Americas: Lessons Learned over 25 Years and Future Challenges*. Washington, DC: World Health Organization.

Pan American Health Organization. (2005). *Declaración regional sobre las nuevas orientaciones de la atención primaria de salud (declaración de Montevideo)*. Washington DC: World Health Organization.

Pauwels J. (2002). *The Myth of the Good War: The USA in World War II*. Toronto: Lorimer.

Piva P. & Dodd R. (2009). Where did all the aid go? An in-depth analysis of increased health aid flows over the past 10 years. *Bulletin of the World Health Organization*, **87**(12), pp. 930–9.

Qian Y. (2002). How Reform Worked in China. 2002. *William Davidson Institute Working Paper series*.

Rimlinger G. V. (1971). Germany: Out of the Patriarchal Tradition. In: Rimlinger G. V., ed. *Welfare Policy and Industrialization in Europe, America and Russia*. New York: John Wiley & Sons, pp. 89–136.

Sepúlveda J. (2006). Foreword. In: Jamison D. T., et al, eds. *Disease Control Priorities in Developing Countries*. Washington, DC: Oxford University Press for the World Bank, pp. 13–5.

Sery J.-P. & Letourmy A. (2006). Couverture du risqué maladie en Afrique francophone: Etats des lieux, defis et perspectives. In: Dussalt G., et al., eds. *L'Assurance Maladie En Afrique Francophone: Ameliorer L'Acces Aux Soins Et Lutter Contre La Pauvrete*. Geneva: World Bank.

Shiffman J., Beer T., & Wu Y. (2002). The emergence of global disease control priorities. *Health Policy and Planning*, **17**(3), pp. 225–34.

Shiffman J. (2008). Has donor prioritization of HIV/AIDS displaced aid for other health issues. *Health Policy and Planning*, **23**(2), pp. 95–100.

Travis P., Bennett S., Haines P. A., et al. (2004). Overcoming health-systems constraints to achieve the Millennium Development Goals. *Lancet*, **364**(9437), pp. 900–6.

Tulloch J. (1999). Integrated approach to child health in developing countries. *Lancet*, **354**(Supplement 2), pp. SII16–SII20.

Turshen M. (1999). *Privatizing Health Services in Africa*. New Brunswick: Rutgers University Press.

Unger J. P. & Killingsworth J. R. (1986). Selective primary health care: A critical review of methods and results. *Social Science & Medicine*, **22**(10), pp. 1001–13.

Waitzkin H. (2003). Report of the WHO Commission on Macroeconomics and Health: A summary and critique. *Lancet*, **361**(9356), pp. 523–6.

Walsh J. A. & Warren K. S. (1979). Selective primary health care: an interim strategy for disease control in developing countries. *New England Journal of Medicine*, **301**(18), pp. 967–74.

Walt G. (1993). WHO under stress: Implications for health policy. *Health Policy*, **24**(2), pp. 125–44.

Widdus R. & White K. (2004). *Combating Diseases Associated With Poverty. Financing Product Development and the Potential Role of Public–Private Partnerships*. The Initiative on Public–Private Partnerships for Health (IPPPH).

World Bank. (1987). *Financing Health Services in Developing Countries: An Agenda for Reform*. A World Bank Policy Study. Washington, DC: World Bank. PUB-6563.

World Bank. (1993). *World Development Report 1993: Investing in Health*. Oxford: Oxford University Press.

World Bank. (1999). *Disinvesting in Health: The World Bank's Prescriptions for Health*. New Delhi: Sage Publications.

World Bank. (2004). *World Development Report 2004: Making Services Work for People*. Washington, DC: World Bank.

World Bank & Chibber A. (1997). *World Development Report 1997: The State in a Changing World*. Oxford, UK: Oxford University Press.

World Health Organization. (1978). Declaration of Alma-Ata. In *Report of the International Conference on Primary Health Care, Alma Ata, USSR, 6–12 September 1978*. Geneva: World Health Organization, pp. 2–6.

World Health Organization. (2000). *World Health Report 2000: Health systems. Improving performance*. Geneva: World Health Organization.

World Health Organization. (2008). *The World Health Report 2008 Primary Health Care – Now More Than Ever*. Geneva: World Health Organization.

World Health Organization. (2009). *62nd World Health Assembly. Agenda it 12.4: Primary Health Care, Including Health System Strengthening*. Geneva: World Health Organization.

Paradigms of international policies

The Achilles heel of international health policies in low- and middle-income countries

Chapter 2 contains material previously published in:
    Unger J.-P., De Paepe P., Ghilbert P., Soors W., Green A. 1. Disintegrated care: the Achilles heel of international health policies in low and middle-income countries. International Journal of Integrated Care 2006; 6. ISSN 1568–4156.

Introduction

It is clear to many health practitioners throughout the world, and, more recently, to WHO, that disease control, the favoured model of international aid, has failed to produce many of the desired results in LMICs despite intensive financing and political support. Following an insight of the related evidence, we will examine why international aid policies in our view share a large responsibility for this failure, with their promotion of the commodification of care, privatization of services, and a focus on disease control.

The poor performance of disease-control programmes (an update)

International health and aid policies have been highly restrictive because they ruled out as a priority access to family medicine and general hospital care. Furthermore, the definition of their priorities is questionable. The promotion of disease-specific programmes has been based on the concept of the 'burden of disease,' which functioned as the intellectual rationale for policies being implemented in its name. Its intrinsic logic was flawed (see Section 5, Chapter 12), and it was never used as a practical tool. Consequently, the international coalition[1] (established on the basis of working on the 'disease burden') has largely managed to evade the need for scientifically based definitions of priorities (Bossyns, 1997; Shiffman et al., 2002; Shiffman, 2006; Sridhar & Batniji, 2008).

- Acute respiratory infection (ARI) represented 25% of the world's 'burden of disease' but receives funds corresponding to 3% of total health-related overseas development aid;
- HIV/AIDS, which represents 5% of the 'burden,' received in 2002–2006 a share accounting for almost one-third (32%) of health aid (and this proportion is sharply on the rise, see Figure 2.1) (England et al., 2007; MacKellar, 2005; Norad, 2008);
- Shigellosis alone yielded up to 165 million cases annually and kills up to 1,100,000 (Kotloff et al., 1999) people a year – probably more than malaria (900,000 in Africa) (Stratton et al., 2008) – but receives no earmarked funds at all;

---

[1] Major donors including the WB, the IMF, and the WHO.

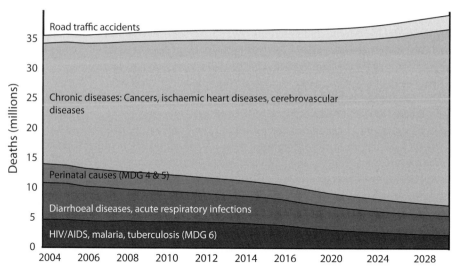

Figure 2.1. The shift towards non-communicable diseases and accidents as causes of death. *Source:* Adapted by authors from figure 1.8 World Health Report 2008.

- Cardiovascular diseases killed much more than tuberculosis (World Health Organization, 2008) (Figure 2.1) and receive little or no funds in LMICs (notice that close to 70% of the world's elderly live in these countries).

The MDGs issued in 2000 dramatically scaled down the ambitions of Alma Ata. While infant and maternal mortality (MDGs 4 and 5) mirror only a fraction of total avoidable mortality, the diseases addressed by MDG 3 represent only a limited proportion of the treatable diseases (Figure 2.1). And in spite of this reduction, the achievements to date have been very limited (see Section 5, Chapter 12).

Indeed, by 2008, the MDG situation as described by the WHO had not improved much (World Health Organization, 2006):

- In 2005, for example, 536,000 women were still dying of maternal causes, 99% in the self-same countries (World Health Organization, 2007b). The worst numbers were in sub-Saharan Africa, where coverage for maternal health had begun stagnating in the 1990s (Abouzahr & Wardlaw, 2001).
- Pneumonia and diarrhoea still kill 3.8 million children under 5 each year.
- 2.7 million people die each year of AIDS (UNAIDS, 2008).
- 1.6 million people died of tuberculosis in 2005 (World Health Organization, 2007a). The tuberculosis specific mortality rate among HIV negative people (per 100,000 population) was 45 in Africa in 2007 and slightly more, 48, among HIV positive people.
- In Africa, between 700,000 and 900,000 children are dying of malaria yearly (90% of total malaria-specific mortality).

We argue that these figures represent the failure of a policy rather than the 'developing' or the poor potential of conditions of LMICs to undertake such tasks, as is often argued. To demonstrate this failure we discuss a three-part hypothesis.

The vast majority of disease-control interventions are clinical in essence. To be effective they generally need to be integrated into health care delivery services. Such integration requires health facilities with patients: providing a sufficient pool of users needed by disease-control programmes for early detection.

In theory both public and private sectors can provide integrated disease-control activities. Yet international agencies have so far been reluctant to allocate disease control to the private for-profit sector – for good reasons.[2]

Instead, international agencies have promoted the continuing involvement of governments, NGOs and communities in disease control, while applying neoliberal principles of health care privatization, thereby precluding integration and leading to unacceptable disease control and health problems specific to performance.

Integration: a key to success for disease control

Disease-control activities implemented by specialized organizational structures and characterized by autonomous administration, sometimes bringing together several disease-control programmes (such as maternal and child health), are dubbed vertical programmes.

Many of the authors (Ageel & Amin, 1997; Bossyns, 1997; Loretti, 1989; Moerman et al., 2003; Tulloch, 1999; Wilkinson, 1999) of reports we cite in this book stress the need to integrate programmes into local health facilities in order to achieve a reasonable prospect for successful disease control. They also point to the merit of integrating curative and preventive care. Examples include the potential for detecting a patient with tuberculosis among those with coughs, or suggesting vaccination to a patient or to a population with whom the practitioner has established trust.

In specific cases, however, vertical programmes can be justified on technical grounds (Criel et al., 1997) such as in the need for:

- Vector control;
- The control of diseases too rare for generalists to maintain the necessary specialist skills, such as HIV/AIDS;
- Outreach to specific risk groups, such as commercial sex workers or drug addicts;
- The control of epidemics and emergencies;
- The provision of health activities for which there is no demand, such as epidemiological surveillance.

Nevertheless, the number of diseases requiring clinical interventions makes it impossible to consider vertical programmes as the gold standard template for disease-control organization, even where these programmes are closely coordinated amongst themselves (Molyneux & Nantulya, 2004). There are, for example:

- Diseases or health issues already addressed by programmes (such as AIDS, tuberculosis, malaria, onchocerciasis, immunizations, family planning, acute respiratory diseases, acute diarrhoeal diseases, poliomyelitis, leprosy, Chagas, Guinea worm);

---

[2] However more recently, the PPM-DOTS programme and the ongoing privatization of maternal care in Asia are both an exception to this and may be serving as pilots to a new policy in the near future.

- Virtually all neglected diseases (as they rely partly or completely on clinical components[3]);
- Chronic degenerative pathologies (cardiovascular and cerebrovascular diseases and diabetes).

Public rather than private disease control: the need for caution

In theory, both the public and the private sector can carry out disease-control activities, but historically the public sector has taken on this responsibility. Despite the widespread promotion of PPPs, international aid agencies have been cautious about contracting out disease control to the private sector. Instead such agencies have promoted the continued involvement of government facilities in disease control under the general label of 'prioritization' of their interventions. Their caution is understandable. The results of contracting out disease control to the private for-profit sector are not promising (Hanson, 2004; Lönnroth et al., 2003), except for tuberculosis control under specific conditions (Lönnroth et al., 2004) (see Section 2, Chapter 5). Furthermore, prospects for privatization of care for conditions attached to pregnancy look gloomy (Unger et al., 2009).

Public disease control and private health care: a circular trap

While disease control remains public, aid agencies have been encouraging a market approach to health care delivery in LICs for over a decade (see Section 1, Chapter 1). The transfer of 'public' care to the private for-profit sector is a core message of their policy on the grounds of the supposed higher efficiency of the for-profit sector and the poor responsiveness of the public one. Once predominantly providers, governments now have new roles as 'stewards', steering care by regulation and supervision. In theory such privatized care could be funded publicly (Figure 2.2).

This doctrine was introduced in LMICs where the market was seen as attractive, such as in parts of Asia and Latin America (George & Gould, 2000; Stocker et al., 1999). It was seen as less relevant in contexts where the market could not be developed easily, as in many parts of Africa. It was also not promoted in countries where geo-strategic considerations dictated an aid policy with clear social goals, as is the case in Jordan, the Southern Philippines, and some central Asian republics close to Afghanistan.

One outcome of this policy was a disease-control focus within Ministries of Health (MoH), with less support available for health care delivery. The continued concentration on disease control by the international aid community is reflected in the efforts to set up and channel significant aid through the GFATM, and which have been criticized strongly for ignoring the needs of, or even weakening, the wider health system (see Section 5, Chapter 12). Indeed

---

[3] This is shown by the following examples: soil transmitted helminths and schistosomiasis (prasiquantel, mebendazole, albendazole); lymphatic filariasis (diagnosis of acute adenolymphangitis attack, lymphoedema and scrotal swelling); leprosy (early diagnosis and multidrug therapy); visceral leishmaniasis (early diagnosis and treatment at hospital); onchocerciasis (blindness rehabilitation and ivermectin, not only in mass distribution); Guinea worm (early detection and treatment); trypanosomiasis (early diagnosis and treatment in specialized centres); trachoma (antibiotics if prevalence under 20%); cholera (rehydration, vaccination, antibiotics); rabies (curative vaccination); and Buruli ulcer (tuberculostatics).

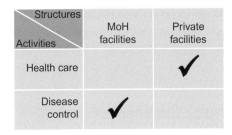

Activities \ Structures	MoH facilities	Private facilities
Health care		✔
Disease control	✔	

Figure 2.2. The roles of public and private sectors as promoted by neoliberal health policies.

disease-control programmes also strained first-line public health care delivery (see Section 2, Chapter 4). This occurred through pressure exerted by disease-control managers, through a multiplication of disease-specific divisions in (inter)national administrations; by vague priority-setting and increasing opportunity costs, unrealistic costing, inadequate budgets and financial overruns (Tulloch, 1999); failure to make clear the lines of command; tension between health care professionals over income disparity, treatment discrepancies, and opportunity costs; and problems with sustainability (Tulloch, 1999). Management by objective, the philosophical cornerstone of such programmes, transformed health organizations into what Mintzberg classifies as 'mechanistic bureaucracies' (Mintzberg, 1989).

This aid and health policy precluded effective integration in the field, which led to a catch-22: the bulk of general patients being cut off from public services, where most disease programmes are delivered, the pool of specific patients was cut off from disease-control interventions. In other words they ended up obtaining substandard detection and follow-up rates. This point has been demonstrated in a study published in 2006 (see Section 2, Chapter 3), where it was shown that, with a low utilization rate, adequate control that combined home treatment together with professional treatment was impossible, even when applying the best parameters from other countries. Thus, if malaria patients were to be treated and followed up early, basic health services needed also to deliver integrated care and have the attendance of a sufficient pool of users. Similarly, according to the WB, the essential clinical package (ECP) comprises tuberculosis (and others), but ignores a much larger morbidity caused by acute lower respiratory infections (ARI), chronic obstructive pulmonary disease (COPD) and asthma.

The narrow disease-control approach fails to deal with widely prevalent respiratory diseases as a group of symptoms and, thus, leaves at risk many patients. As stated earlier in order to detect a patient with tuberculosis, the programme clinician will need to access patients with a cough because patients generally ignore the aetiology of their condition (see Section 2, Chapter 3). This helps to explain why tuberculosis case findings decreased together with access to discretionary care, in the aftermath of neoliberal reform in Colombia (Lönnroth et al., 2003): disease-control programmes will lack effectiveness if they are carried out in (government) services that have been abandoned by patients due to a lack of resources and facilities.

Poor access to health care delivery

Access to health care in LMICs is also disappointing. Despite, or in some cases, because of, more than a decade of reforms, almost 50% of health systems did not provide adequate access to care for their citizens (Department of Economic and Social Affairs, 2000). Access to care is particularly difficult in China and in the republics of the former Soviet Union. It has also deteriorated in Latin America. A third of the world's population has no reliable access to essential drugs; this rate rises to above 50% in the poorest countries of Africa and Asia (World Health Organization, 2000).

In most LICs, the use and quality of government health facilities has fallen to an all-time low.[4] Uganda's University Hospital of Mbarara has been described by Kavalier as 'decades away from the end of the twentieth century' (Kavalier, 1998). Even in MICs the problem exists. Ellen Roskam asks: 'Where can you be treated by a doctor who, last year, worked 1,000 hours more than his official timetable, who has earned less than USD 15 per month, who has not been paid for 5 months, who has worked without drugs or bandages in an operating theatre with a leaking roof and where there has been no investment for many years? Maybe somewhere in Africa? No, in Eastern Europe.' (Walgate, 2002).

Meanwhile, care in private health facilities remained expensive, inefficient and unregulated (see Section 4, Chapters 10 and 11). Care suffered from accessibility and quality problems. Cream skimming, semi-monopolistic settings and corruption were widespread. The increase in unnecessary prescriptions, admissions, the length of stay, laboratory tests, and medical imaging exemplifies how profitability dominated evidence-based practice. In Brazil, for example, until recently the caesarean section rate reached 31% in the public sector, and 72% in the private sector (Potter et al., 2001).

Admittedly, poor access to decent health care in LICs is associated with multiple and interlinked determinants:

- An economic crisis, resulting in decreasing purchasing power, downsizing of public services and falling salaries, in most highly indebted poor countries. In Latin America deteriorating access to publicly delivered health care was associated with the public services' narrowing problem-solving capacity. Furthermore, professional associations sought part-time employment in public services, enabling private doctors to spot profitable patients and send them to their own clinics.
- Static or increasing social inequalities, as observed in the majority of countries in Latin America and the Caribbean, the region with the highest inequality in the world.
- A combination of external and internal adverse conditions. The simultaneous effect of Structural Adjustment Programmes (SAPs) and insufficient social control on administration, a lack of democracy, patronage, and nepotism, resulting in low priority given to the social sector.

However, the health policy promoted by international aid agencies may also have played a specific role through the promotion of the private sector.

The aid agencies' recommendations invariably appear to end in a dual system; with good clinical care for the wealthy and low quality 'essential' care for the poor. They have acted as though expansion of the private sector was fully compatible with public provision of the essential clinical package for the poor. Nevertheless, the two vessels are connected. Instead of adding extra capacity, the commercial presence of the private sector undermines public

---

[4] Here follow data found in (ITM) MPH theses and related to districts of at least 150,000 inhabitants: Guidiguis (Cameroon, 2006): 0.2 new cases per year per inhabitant; Ukerewe (Tanzania, 2007): 0.48 new cases per year per inhabitant; Nguelemendouka district (Cameroon, 2006): 0.14 new cases per year per inhabitant; Bogande district (Burkina Faso, 2006): 0.25 new cases per year per inhabitant; one district in Cambodia: 0.4 new cases per year per inhabitant; Dhenkanaldi district (Orissa State, India, 2006–2007): from 0.18 to 0.54 new cases per year per inhabitant according to health centres. Other highly preoccupying similar data were provided for China and the Philippines.

services by drawing away key medical personnel and picking the 'low-hanging fruit,' the healthiest and wealthiest consumers, destroying the possibility of cross-subsidization and risk pooling on which universal access is based.

We distinguish five different, sometimes complementary, ways in which the transfer of health care delivery to the private sector has been fulfilled:

- Governments underfinanced public services, allowing the private sector to offer care without having to deal with subsidized competition. Typically, this was the scenario adopted by sub-Saharan Africa and Andean countries where a paper assessed the relationship between public spending on health care and the health status of the poor, from demographic health surveys in 44 countries. It showed that public spending on health care has a consistent and significant impact on child mortality among the poor, as well as on infant mortality and birth attendance by skilled staff. In absolute terms (number of deaths per 1,000 live births), since child mortality is much higher among the poor, public spending had a larger impact on the poor. A 1% increase in public spending on health, according to these views, reduces child mortality nearly three times more among the poor as compared with the non-poor. This effect is strongest in LICs. Knowing that, in developing countries, public spending for the poor is mainly channelled through public services, these findings constitute a strong argument for continuing public investment in comprehensive public health services (Gupta et al., 2003).
- Governments, accepting the efficiency arguments of the international agencies, gradually reduced the operational role of the public sector to a greater focus on disease-control programmes. International agencies financed such programmes.
- Governments subcontracted health care to the private sector (in a very limited number of countries, such as Lebanon, Colombia, Zambia). In Latin America, International Financing Institutions (IFIs) also promoted and financed the privatization of health care.
- Governments leased or sold public hospitals to the private sector. The best-known experiences, promoted by WB authors as options of PPPs, are Stockholm's St. Goran's and a few converted Australian hospitals (Taylor & Blair, 2002). In LMICs this pathway was the exception rather than the rule. Examples included the former Soviet Union and Albania.
- Governments granted managerial autonomy to public hospitals, blurring the boundaries between public and for-profit objectives.

The main actors in setting and implementing policy have cited all but the first of these five pathways as beneficial. In practice, however, it was the underfunding of the public sector that most frequently led to privatization. This underfunding happened in many countries in the 1990s, as evidenced by the gap shown by the WHO Macroeconomic and Health Commission Report (Unger et al., 2003). The WB's SAPs and the IMF Enhanced Structural Adjustment Facilities (ESAFs) effectively reinforced the liberalization of services by starving them of public resources.

Thus in reality, the Bretton Woods institutions never effectively enforced the loan conditions to increase public–social spending, a responsibility also neglected by LMIC governments. International aid never compensated for the reduction in government health expenditures, but rather it reinforced the second scenario, driving a weakened public sector to focus largely on externally financed disease-control activities, thus straining the public delivery of care and creating a market opportunity for the private sector.

One consequence of this underfunding is now becoming apparent, with the haemorrhaging of professional staff to the private sector and increasingly to industrialized health systems, understandably attracted by the higher salary pull-factors (McCoy et al., 2008).

We thus raise the question, as we did for the poor performance of disease-control programmes, as to the extent to which international aid policy shares responsibility for this poor access to health care. Our analysis consists of three steps. Firstly, pilot local contracting-out experiments are analyzed. Following this, the national health care records of Colombia and Chile, two countries that have adopted contracting out as a basis for health care delivery, are contrasted with that of Costa Rica. Lastly, specific mechanisms of a failure of the policy in LMICs are explored (see demonstration in Section 3).

We turn now to discussion of contracting experiences drawing on pilot experiments and national data.

Evidence from pilot experiments: contracting out discretionary health care and managerial autonomy of hospitals

The PPP approaches were developed in the context of New Public Management. Thus PPP encompasses both Public Finance Initiatives (PFI) and contracting out. The former refers to private money being used to finance health care infrastructure that previously had been under government responsibility. So far, this technique has been mainly applied in the United Kingdom but is also spreading in many developing countries such as India, China, and Lebanon (see Section 4). The other approach of contracting out has met difficulties over the past 15 years. In Southern Africa researchers compared the operational cost per admission and per inpatient day between public rural district hospitals and subcontracted private for-profit hospitals. The few studies do not support the hypothesis that efficiency increases when care is subcontracted to private companies (McPake & Hongoro, 1995; Mills et al., 1997; Mills, 1998). These studies suggest that a similar quality of care can be achieved at a lower cost in the private sector, but at a total higher cost to the public authorities once private profit margins are included. The private providers' profit margins override the financial gains arising from improved cost-efficiency. The only positive outcomes were associated with buying care from NGOs, where there was no profit motive.

In addition, few studies have ever examined whether the pricing policy applied by the private sector is equitable and, to our knowledge, there has been no study to determine whether the private health sector in LIC improves patients' independence from professional care. However, the quest for gains that underpins the private sector is unlikely to favour solidarity or increase the patients' medical autonomy.

The strategy of developing hospital autonomy, publicly funded but managed according to principles of private provision, was expected to facilitate reinvestment and to improve staff motivation without drawing on the national budget. Managerial autonomy became a widespread policy in a number of LMICs. However, in practice, government hospitals were often granted managerial autonomy without defining their objectives or providing supervision. Health staff often managed 'autonomous' public hospitals as private facilities (Stefanini, 1997), enabling public hospitals to adapt a for-profit rationale while retaining public funds. This happened, for example, with Chinese state hospitals that depended on profit-making private services to break even (see Section 4, Chapter 10). This led to increased costs for users and to a reorientation of the bulk of hospital activities from secondary care to simple, first-line clinical services. Underpaid staff quickly understood that hospitalizing a rich person with bronchitis, for example, instead of a poor patient in need of a surgical intervention, generated income. Opportunistic cream skimming changed the case-mix. Neither the state nor communities were able to exert control. This managerial stance created obstacles for poor patients needing secondary care and favoured instead hospitalization of (middle class) primary cases. Similar processes can explain why private hospitals in Thailand had a shorter length of stay, a larger percentage of admissions of children and yet no increase in utilization of their operating theatre (Pannarunothai & Mills, 1997).

Lastly, staff motivation rarely went beyond an understandable eagerness to access hospital profits to supplement salaries, which in turn hampered reinvestment (Liu & Mills, 2003).

Evidence from national data: contracting out equals inefficiency, ineffectiveness and inequity

A comparison between Chile, Costa Rica and Colombia

(To access the detailed country case studies, see Section 3, Chapters 6–8).

Starfield demonstrated that health systems with a strong, comprehensive publicly oriented first-line provision obtained significantly better results in terms of health indicators and patient satisfaction in ten industrialized countries and in terms of overall costs (Starfield, 1991). Costa Rica, the Kerala State in India and Cuba appear to show the same tendency with their predominantly publicly oriented services (Ghai, 1999), especially when first-line services are run by general practitioners or family physicians.

Many international blue prints have advocated subcontracting care to the private sector in LICs, but few countries have been able to fully implement this. To some extent this is because most LMICs were unable to generate the required funds. Government finances were mainly earmarked for wages, leaving little latitude for contracting out. While in Western Europe government spending in 2001 represented more than 70% of total health expenditure, it was less than 40% in China, 30% in Vietnam, and 20% in India (World Health Organization, 2004). A few countries did, however, manage to subcontract to the private health sector, and we now briefly illustrate health care privatization in two of them – Colombia and Chile – contrasting them with Costa Rica, which maintained publicly oriented social insurance and health services.

In 1993, Colombia adopted a purchaser–provider split and contracting-out policy and committed resources to it (Law 100). The state largely freed itself from direct provision of services. The exceptions were disease-control activities and health care delivery for the non-insured and for pathologies not covered by health insurance – mainly in public hospitals.

Chile partly privatized its health insurance (ISAPRES, 1981) whilst keeping a large public health sector, through its public social insurance and its public health services. Private health insurance and care have never been more than a separate, marginal health system for the well off. But ISAPRES, private health care insurers set up during the period of the Chilean military dictatorship (1973–1989), never covered more than 25% of the population, and is now at less than 16% coverage. It is evident that the strong backbone of a public health system has not been broken by Pinochet, even though public health services financing was drastically reduced. Since 1989 a series of democratic governments have substantially increased public health expenditure.

In Costa Rica, at the end of the twentieth century, the average private health expenditure was only 25% of total health expenditure in contrast with 58% across Latin America (Molina et al., 2000). The Social Security Administration of Costa Rica (SSAC) is the single (and public) health insurer in Costa Rica (private health insurance exists but is marginal). It both purchases and provides care.

We contend that, unlike in Colombia, health systems' outputs in both Chile and Costa Rica are rated as very high. Also, Costa Rica was much more efficient than Chile in securing improving health status for its population. This situation, however, has been radically altered when Chile strengthened its public system and Costa Rica began privatizing its own.

The main success of the Colombian reform was progress in social insurance which almost doubled its coverage from 31% to 62% of the population between 1992 and 2004 (Acosta et al., 2005a) leading to an expansion in affiliation for some 18.5 million (from a target population of 22 million), with a remarkable acceleration of membership in 2004 and 2005, following its stagnation for several years (Ministerio de la protección social República de Colombia, 2006). However, some caution is warranted. The benefit package for the poor is still only half that for the contributing affiliates. Furthermore, before the reforms, on average a doctor would see some 61.7% of the population needing health care; this proportion however fell to 51.1% in 2000 (Ageel & Amin, 1997; Hsiao, 1995). Each year 6.26% of the population suffered catastrophic health expenditure, related debt and the poorest quintile had out-of-pocket payments four times higher than the richest (Castaño, 2004). Even more worrying, according to a periodical national survey, the proportion of people consulting in the month before the survey increased from 1993 to 1997 (from 7.5% to 23.8%), but then decreased dramatically in 2003 to 9.5%, meaning that theoretical high coverage by health insurance did not translate into higher utilization rates of health services, in spite of increased health expenditure (from 7 to 10% of GDP) (Acosta et al., 2005b).

In contrast, in Costa Rica, utilization of medical health services is high with acceptable, affordable and perceived good quality health care, compared to other developing countries. Only 0.12% of the Costa Rican households suffered from catastrophic health expenditure, 52 times less than in Colombia.

Given the inequity within both Chilean society and the health system's financing, one would expect accessibility to care by the poor to be limited. However, among those who declared having felt sick in the last month, 73.9% from the poorest quintile sought care compared to 79.7% from the richest (Ministerio de Planificación, 2003). Data on utilization rate also confirm this relatively equitable access with increases from 2.65 and 3.27 in 1990 to 3.85 and 4.12 in 1999, in FONASA, the public health fund of Chile, and ISAPRES, respectively (Rodríguez & Tokman, 2000). However, the utilization rates still differ between poor and rich municipalities: by a factor of 2.8 for PHC, 3.9 for emergencies and 2 for inpatient care (Pan American Health Organization, 2001).

The Infant Mortality Rate is known to reflect not solely access to medical care but the general social and economic conditions (Stefanini, 1997). However, child mortality due to acute respiratory infections and acute diarrhoeal diseases can be viewed as avoidable mortality and used as tracer pathologies for the quality of care (Hanson, 2004), including in less developed countries (Lönnroth et al., 2003). These rates have clearly increased in Colombia since 1997 (Broomberg & Mills, 1998). Perinatal mortality is also known to be an indicator for access to quality health care. It doubled from 1996 to 1997 and continues to rise (Broomberg & Mills, 1998). The same could be applied for maternal mortality, stable since 2000 at an unacceptably high level of about 100 deaths per 100,000 newborn (Así vamos en salud, 2009). By combining middle income with high human development since 1995 Costa Rica achieved a life expectancy at birth of 78 years (second only to Canada in the Americas), an infant mortality rate of 9/1,000, equivalent to a seven-fold reduction over the last 3 decades (equivalent data in Colombia is 19 with a four-fold reduction) and a tuberculosis prevalence of 19/100,000 (69 in Colombia). Several of these features are related to the social commitment of successive Costa

Rican governments (United Nations Development Programme, 2004). In particular public expenditure on health and education was 4.9 and 4.7% of GDP in 2001 compared with 3.6 and 4.4% in Colombia (United Nations Development Programme, 2004). However, the pivotal role of health services and policy played by Costa Rican human development should also be recognized. Numerous indicators suggest an impact directly attributable to health services:

1. A comparison of Infant Mortality Rates (IMR) and Maternal Mortality rates (MMR), with Chile and Colombia both at similar income levels, reveals the significant difference and advance of Costa Rica (see Table 2.1) until recently, when Chile outstripped Costa Rica in the level of resources it put into its public services;
2. Perinatal mortality rate dropped from 12.0/1,000 in 1972 to 5.4/1,000 in 2001 (Hiscock & Hojman, 1997), which suggests obstetric improvements;
3. Pneumonia-specific mortality in under ones dropped from 5.4/1,000 in 1972 to 0.3/1,000 in 2001 (Departamento de Información Estadística de los Servicios de Salud, 2003), which suggests improved and faster access to health services;
4. Tuberculosis-specific mortality dropped from 7.2/100,000 in 1972 to 4.4/100,000 in 2001 (Departamento de Información Estadística de los Servicios de Salud, 2003), despite increased incidence, which suggests a well-functioning programme.

Finally, in Chile, health indicators are good, with high life expectancy and very low infant mortality and maternal mortality.

These contrasting achievements were not, however, explained by the level of investments in health. Health expenditure had rocketed since the introduction of managed competition in Colombia, with an increase from 7% to almost 10% of GDP (Acosta et al., 2005b). In Costa Rica the high outputs were achieved at a moderate cost; one comparison for example summarized the Costa Rican health policy achievements: the country spends nine times less on health than the USA and scores better on life expectancy.

In Chile, the private ISAPRES spend three times more on administration per affiliated than public FONASA (about 20% vs. 6%). In 2000 the GDP share allocated to health was 7.3%, of which 3.1% was public and 4.2% private. Out-of-pocket expenditures were 27% of total health expenditure.

In recent years, Colombia's health policy has resulted in good health insurance coverage of the poor, but with a very limited benefit package, a reduction in real access and at a very high cost (almost 10% of GNP), due in part to the coexistence of supply and demand subsidies and to a generalized evasion of contributions to social health insurance.

Table 2.1. Infant and maternal mortality rates, Costa Rica, Chile and Colombia

	Infant mortality ratio[1]	Infant mortality ratio	Reduction in infant mortality ratio[2]	Maternal mortality ratio[3]
	1970	2001	1970–2001	1985–2001
Chile	78	10	8	23
Costa Rica	62	9	7	29
Colombia	69	19	4	80

Notes:
1 Probability of dying between birth and exactly 1 year of age, expressed per 1,000 live births.
2 Calculated from 1970 and 2001 figures.
3 Annual number of deaths of women from pregnancy-related causes per 100,000 live births (data refer to most recent year available during the period specified, adjusted for under-reporting and misclassification).

Source: United Nations Development Programme, 2003.

In Chile, the overall good demographic and epidemiologic records may in part be due to the sustained high economic growth rate, and the spectacular reduction in poverty: from 39% in 1990 to 21% in 2000, without precedent in Chile and also exceptional internationally (Arellano, 2004; Hiscock & Hojman, 1997). The good health indicators are due to this public system, good education levels and economic growth, and hardly to ISAPRES and private providers who attended the healthy, young, and urban well off. Instead the private care insurance and delivery can be blamed for the high cost of the Chilean health system, and for its lack of solidarity and equity.

In conclusion, the evidence of the three countries appears to contradict international recommendations to privatize health care in developing countries. The remarkable and sustained achievements of Costa Rica suggest the following:

1. A unified public health services system, in which government expenditure represents the bulk of total expenditure, permits integration.
2. Dominant, though non-monopolistic, publicly oriented services offer accessible health care.
3. Contracting in secures both management and production targets (as opposed to the much promoted contracting out).
4. A single, public insurer (private insurance being virtually non-existent), which contributes to solidarity and general access to care.
5. Users and communities can participate in publicly oriented health services management, as opposed to what the private for-profit sector permits.

Unmet conditions for contracting out: the mechanisms of a failure

The common cause of failure (both pilot and national) of contracting out in LMICs lies in a mix of technical and political features.

If we assume that contracting out guarantees access to good quality health care in Western Europe, why is it failing in LMICs? We would argue that the technical requirements for contracting out clash with political and administrative realities. Efficient subcontracting thrives on effective control and regulation, which does not occur in most LMICs and is also being exposed for its weaknesses in the higher income countries with the collapse of a large section of the financial sector and implications for the rest of the economies of most countries.

However, in terms of the health sector more generally in Europe, the government regulates and controls the private sector, draws up contracts for the provision of health care, checks whether these contracts are implemented and oversees reimbursement. This does not happen in the health sector of most LMICs, where the state apparatus to control patronage, biased decisions and elements of corruption at provider level and management at administrative level is weak. Furthermore, government doctors, who are generally underpaid, expect to have a parallel private practice; as such they are unlikely to cut off the branch they are sitting on by agreeing contracts favourable to the state. Large amounts of money, generated by contracting out, constitute a considerable temptation in the absence of adequate controls.

Administrative and regulatory structures were rarely in place in the social sector when most LMICs embarked upon neoliberal policies. This was a lethal situation, as 'Failure to develop such capacity and political conditions before or simultaneously with entering into contracting and demand-side financing reforms can have negative consequences to judge from experiences in India, Mexico, Papua New Guinea, South Africa and Zimbabwe.' (Ministerio de Planificación, 2003). 'Contracting out clinical services is particularly complex, even when limited to non-profit providers such as church hospitals in Ghana or the United Republic of Tanzania and Zimbabwe' (Ministerio de Planificación, 2003). Only established democratic governments with adequate regulatory resources can provide some guarantees of access to and quality of care, avoid fragmentation of the system, enforce a solidarity-based financing system, and keep NGOs and the private for-profit sector under control.

Figueras and Saltman note that the reform of the medical and health sector in Europe called on public health skills to estimate the needs, evaluate the interventions and the impact of the measures (Figueras & Saltman, 1998). As these skills are in short supply in LMICs, Brugha and Zwi notice 'major problems in service quality, especially in the private sector' and see the search for profit as responsible for the gap between health professionals' medical knowledge and its practice (Brugha & Zwi, 1998). Competent professionals from LMICs are numerous, but they are not in the right spot.

Impact of disease-specific programmes and privatization of health care on health systems in LMICs

Over the past 2 decades, health systems have largely collapsed in most LICs and fragile states (with an overall population of some 2.5 billion) – these being most of the same countries where international donor assistance has been most active. The role of donors in undermining health systems is now belatedly, but increasingly, recognized in numerous studies and research even though academia is often fearful of spelling out this fact. Even WHO has begun to recognize the problems of systematic undermining of both public provision and health systems. In a recent statement WHO Director General, M. Chan, provided what has been described as a 'withering critique of liberal economic governance and its impact on health' (Economic Governance for Health, 2009), which called for 'a fundamental reengineering of the international system, to give them a moral dimension and to invest them with social values – like equity, sustainability, community and social justice.' Chan has also argued that health systems needed to be strengthened if epidemiological objectives of the international cooperation were to be attained. The WHO thus identified six building blocks needing support: service delivery; workforce; medical products, vaccines, and technologies; financing; leadership and governance; and health information systems (World Health Organization, 2009).

This kind of critique was long overdue but was ignored when the doctrine of aid polices were being implemented under various guises of efficiency and effectiveness. Moreover, despite the flurry of activity aimed at strengthening health systems, this sort of analysis also needs to ask what is the nature of aid and the way it has been disbursed, and whether it has in effect, contributed to this collapse of the public health sector in LMICs?

This concern has been, partly at least, shared by the WHO Commission on Social Determinants of Health in 2008, which stated, 'There is … a danger that large new funding lines, running parallel to national budgeting, continue to distort national priorities for allocation of expenditure and action … While Global Health Initiatives have brought enormous new levels of funding to health care systems within LMICs (USD 8.9 billion in 2006 for HIV/AIDS alone), there is a concern that their vertically managed programmes have the potential to undermine the population health orientation of health care systems and as a result exacerbate health inequity' (Commission on Social Determinants of Health, 2008).

Nine key mechanisms through which neoliberal policies weakened LMIC health systems should be tackled by international health and aid policies if they are sincere in their desire to strengthen these systems:

1. Public hospitals were starved of resources.
2. Decentralization under the form of devolution promoted by WB and IMF segmented the public sector, which has had a largely negative effect (Grundy et al., 2003; Tang & Bloom, 2000).
3. Systems segmentation is also due to the wealth of DSPs (see above) and lack of responsiveness in government services, compelled to limit their activities to epidemiologically based interventions.
4. The large number of DSPs has dramatically increased transaction costs (and bureaucracy). For five neglected tropical diseases[5] it was estimated that by integrating their respective control programmes (through preventive chemotherapy), potential cost savings could be reached as high as 26–47%, or USD 58–81 million annually, versus USD 110 million for the five stand-alone programmes (Brady et al., 2006).
5. Managed care (e.g., pay-for-performance, management contracts or fixed capitation fees) (Gottlieb & Einhorn, 1997) was promoted in LMICs to limit health care costs. However, there is growing evidence that the problems generated by these policies overwhelm the intended benefits with regard to quality of care or cost, and often both (Friedenberg, 1999) (see Section 6, Chapter 18, Part 1).
6. The reduced status of public sector health professionals is a direct consequence of structural adjustment programmes and reductions in overall social-sector spending.
7. The loss of clinical skills among doctors, nurses and midwives has been aggravated by the weakening of academic clinical teaching and curricula and by the multiplication of commercial, unregulated, and uncontrolled medical schools in LMIC universities during the past 2 decades.
8. LICs have systematically failed to reduce the concentration of health staff in cities.
9. There is no evidence that accountability, problem number 1 in public services according to the WB, would be better assured in contracts with private for-profit providers.

Discussion

A signal of policy change has been sent by WHO. In an effort to diversify international aid to the health sector of developing countries this organization recommends the reconstruction of health systems to increase access to general, appropriate health care in the services, while at the same time developing disease control. The critical question is, how?

The commodification and privatization of services, with the public sector confined to deliver disease-control activities alongside a private sector increasingly taking over health care, constrains both disease-control programme performance and people's access to services. So why is neoliberal policy still actively promoted? Neoliberal health policies have aggravated the commodification and privatization of health care, but to attribute such sweeping changes to the 'imposition' of a doctrine by aid agencies would be to negate the complexity of this profoundly political process and the involvement of a set of actors that include economic

---

[5] Lymphatic filariasis, onchocerciasis, intestinal helminthiasis, schistosomiasis, and trachoma.

agents and political actors at the side of 'aid agencies,' the Bretton Woods Institutions, Western governments, the WHO and developing country governments, which have either actively promoted, or uncritically accepted, such policies (Section 4). The following vested interests have contributed to this position:

- The private medical sector in LMICs which lobbies for access to public funds;
- Local middle and upper classes that resist increased taxation to allow funding health care for the poor, since they can opt out for private health care;
- International health care companies based in industrial countries looking for opportunities to access the Asian and Latin American markets, through the GATS negotiation rounds;
- Pharmaceutical companies showing little interest in a public health care market that dispenses mostly generic and essential drugs and may not be very creditworthy. In contrast disease-control programmes financed by industrialized countries represent a market for the development of new products;
- European politicians supporting the control of infectious epidemics in LMICs that threaten the industrialized world (e.g., tuberculosis, AIDS, severe acute respiratory syndrom [SARS], avian flu) – hence the need to treat their control as a 'public good';
- Disease-control programmes enjoying potentially high political visibility and hence support through mechanisms such as PPPs;
- Civil servants in charge of disease-control programmes, enjoying privileged access to decision-makers in industrialized countries, see an emergent programme as a significant career opportunity.

These forces have systematically used recommendations of international aid agencies to promote national health policies in line with their interests. This explains the adoption of neoliberal health policies.

The GATS negotiations within the WTO (World Trade Organization, 2004) might further consolidate these results. GATS threatens to make illegal any public health care service that has not been privatized, based on the claim that the government should not offer subsidized services that the market also offers (Unger et al., 2004). An opt-out alternative exists in theory, but LMICs are unlikely to be in a strong bargaining position to use it through successive rounds of negotiation.

Neoliberal health policy promoted by international aid agencies in LMICs failed to control diseases successfully, nor did it improve access to care. Its results were, thus, out of step with majority public demand, as well as socio-political and economic realities, nor were they able to serve any humanitarian purpose.

We have argued that an alternative aid policy for LMIC health sectors is urgently needed if we genuinely aim to improve access to health care, controlling diseases and combating poverty.

References

Abouzahr C. & Wardlaw T. (2001). Maternal mortality at the end of a decade: Signs of progress? *Bulletin of the World Health Organization*, **79**(6), pp. 561–8.

Acosta O. L., Ramírez M., & Cañón C. I. (2005a). La viabilidad del sistema de salud. *Qué dicen los estudios*. Documento de trabajo 12. Bogotá, Colombia: Fundación Corona, Universidad del Rosario.

Acosta O. L., Ramírez M., & Cañón C. I. (2005b). Principales estudios sobre el equilibrio financiero del SGSS. In: Acosta O. L., et al. eds. La viabilidad del sistema de salud. *Qué dicen los estudios*. Bogotá: Universidad del Rosario, pp. 35–60.

Ageel A. R. & Amin M. A. (1997). Integration of schistosomiasis-control activities into the primary health care system in the Gizan region, Saudi Arabia. *Annals of Tropical Medicine and Parasitology*, **91**(8), pp. 907–15.

Arellano J. P. M. (2004). Políticas sociales para el crecimiento con equidad Chile 1990–2002. *Santiago de Chile: Plataforma Universidad de Chile*. report n°26. Series Estudios Socio/ Económicos.

Así vamos en salud. (2009). Estado de salud de la población. *Así Vamos en Salud – Seguimiento al sector salud en Colombia*. 2009.

Bossyns P. (1997). Big programmes, big errors? *Lancet*, **350**(9093), pp. 1783–4.

Brady M. A., Hooper P. J., & Ottesen E. A. (2006). Projected benefits from integrating NTD programs in sub-Saharan Africa. *Trends in Parasitology*, **22**(7), pp. 285–91.

Broomberg J. & Mills A. (1998). To purchase or provide. *Insights Issue* 26, pp. 1–3. 1998.

Brugha R. & Zwi A. (1998). Improving the quality of private sector delivery of public health services: Challenges and strategies. *Health Policy and Planning*, **13**(2), pp. 107–20.

Castaño R. (2004). *Elementos fundamentales del equilibrio financiero del sistema general de seguridad social en salud, que inciden en las decisiones de ajuste del POS y/o de la UPC*. Bogotá – Colombia: Fundación Corona.

Commission on Social Determinants of Health. (2008). *Closing the Gap in a Generation: Health Equity Through Action on the Social Determinants of Health. Final Report of the Commission on Social Determinants of Health*. Geneva: World Health Organization.

Criel B., De Brouwere V., & Dugas S. (1997). *Integration of Vertical Programmes in Multi-Function Health Services*. Antwerp: ITG Press.

Departamento de Información Estadística de los Servicios de Salud. (2003). Cambios en la morbilidad y mortalidad por edad y sexo, Costa Rica, 1987, 1992, 1997 y 2002. San José, Costa Rica: Caja Costarricense de Seguro Social, Gerencia de División Médica, Dirección Técnica de Servicios de Salud. Serie Estadísticas de la Salud No. 8C.

Economic Governance for Health. (2009). Economic Governance for Health Newsletter 5, 10th May 09. http://www.eg4health.org/20 09/05/11/1052/#more-1052.

England R., De Lay P., Greener R., & Izazola J. A. (2007). Are we spending too much on HIV? *British Medical Journal*, **334**(7589), pp. 344–5.

Figueras J. & Saltman R. B. (1998). Building upon comparative experience in health system reform. *European Journal of Public Health*, **8**, pp. 99–101.

Friedenberg R. M. (1999). The primary care physician's view of managed care in 1998. *Radiology*, **210**(2), pp. 297–300.

George S. & Gould E. (2000). *Organisation Mondiale du Commerce. Libéraliser, sans avoir l'air d'y toucher*. Paris: Le Monde Diplomatique.

Ghai D. (1999). Social Development and Public Policy. *A Study of Some Successful Experiences*. Basingstoke: United Nations Research Institute UNRISD.

Gottlieb S. & Einhorn T. A. (1997). Current concepts review – managed care: Form, function, and evolution. *Journal of Bone and Joint Surgery*, **79**(1), pp. 125–36.

Grundy J., Healy V., Gorgelon L., & Sandig E. (2003). Overview of devolution of health services in the Philippines. *Rural and Remote Health*, **3**(online) (2003), p. 220.

Gupta S., Verhoeven M., & Tiongson E. R. (2003). Public spending on health care and the poor. *Health Economics*, **12**(8), pp. 685–96.

Hanson K. (2004). Public and private roles in malaria control: The contributions of economic analysis. *American Journal of Tropical Medicine and Hygiene*, **71**(Supplement 2), pp. 168–73.

Hiscock J. & Hojman D. (1997). Social policy in a fast growing economy: The case of Chile. *Social Policy and Administration*, **31**(4), pp. 354–70.

Hsiao W. C. (1995). The Chinese health care system: Lessons for other nations. *Social Science & Medicine*, **41**(8), pp. 1047–55.

Kavalier F. (1998). Uganda: Death is always just around the corner. *Lancet*, **352**(9122), pp. 141–2.

Kotloff K. L., Winickoff J. P., Ivanoff B., et al. (1999). Global burden of Shigella infections: Implications for vaccine development and implementation of control strategies. *Bulletin of the World Health Organization*, **77**(8), pp. 651–66.

Liu X. & Mills A. (2003). The influence of bonus payments to doctors on hospital revenue: Results of a quasi-experimental study. *Applied Health Economics and Health Policy*, **2**(2), pp. 91–8.

Lönnroth K., Thuong L. M., Lambregts K., Quy H. T., & Diwan V. K. (2003). Private tuberculosis care provision associated with poor treatment outcome: Comparative study of a semi-private lung clinic and the NTP in two urban districts in Ho Chi Minh City, Vietnam. *International Journal of Tuberculosis and Lung Disease*, **7**(2), pp. 165–71.

Lönnroth K., Uplekar M., Arora V. K., et al. (2004). Public–private mix for DOTS implementation: What makes it work? *Bulletin of the World Health Organization*, **82**(8), pp. 580–6.

Loretti A. (1989). Leprosy control: The rationale of integration. *Leprosy Review*, **60**(4), pp. 306–16.

MacKellar L. (2005). Priorities in global assistance for health, AIDS, and population. *Population and Development Review*, **31**(2), pp. 293–312.

McCoy D., Bennett S., Witter S., et al. (2008). Salaries and incomes of health workers in sub-Saharan Africa. *Lancet*, **371**(9613), pp. 675–81.

McPake B. & Hongoro C. (1995). Contracting out of clinical services in Zimbabwe. *Social Science & Medicine*, **41**(1), pp. 13–24.

Mills A. (1998). To contract or not to contract? Issues for low and middle income countries. *Health Policy and Planning*, **13**(1), pp. 32–40.

Mills A., Hongoro C., & Broomberg J. (1997). Improving the efficiency of district hospitals: Is contracting an option? *Tropical Medicine & International Health*, **2**(2), pp. 116–26.

Ministerio de la protección social República de Colombia. (2006). Sigue creciendo cobertura en régimen subsidiado. *Boletín de Prensa*, N°28 de 2006.

Ministerio de Planificación. (2003). *Encuesta de caracterización socioeconómico nacional 2004*. Mideplan. Ministerio de Planificación, Gobierno de Chile. Encuesta de Caracterización Socioeconómica Nacional CASEN.

Mintzberg H. (1989). *Mintzberg on Management: Inside Our Strange World of Organisations*. New York: The Free Press.

Moerman F., Lengeler C., Chimumbwa J., et al. (2003). The contribution of health care services to a sound and sustainable malaria-control policy. *Lancet Infectious Diseases*, **3**(2), pp. 99–102.

Molina R., Pinto M., Henderson P., & Vieira C. (2000). Gasto y financiamiento en salud: Situación y tendencias. *Revista Panamerica de Salud Publica*, **8**(1–2), pp. 71–83.

Molyneux D. H. & Nantulya V. M. (2004). Linking disease control programmes in rural Africa: A pro-poor strategy to reach Abuja targets and millennium development goals. *British Medical Journal*, **328**(7448), pp. 1129–32.

Norad. (2008). The global health landscape and innovative international financing for health systems: trends and issues. Oslo: Norwegion Agency for Development Cooperation.

Pan American Health Organization. (2001). *Información para la equidad en salud en Chile*. Santiago de Chile: Organización Panamericana de la Salud.

Pannarunothai S. & Mills A. (1997). Characteristics of public and private health care providers in a Thai urban setting. In: Bennett S., et al. eds. *Private Health Providers in Developing Countries: Serving the Public Interest?* London: Zed Books, p. 67.

Potter J. E., Berquo E., Perpetuo I. H., et al. (2001). Unwanted caesarean sections among public and private patients in Brazil: Prospective study. *British Medical Journal*, **323**(7322), pp. 1155–8.

Rodríguez C. & Tokman M. R. (2000). *Resultados y rendimiento del gasto en el sector público de salud en Chile 1990–1999*. Report n°106. Serie Financiamiento del Desarrollo. Santiago de Chile: Comisión Económica para América Latina y el Caribe (CEPAL).

Shiffman J. (2006). Donor funding priorities for communicable disease control in the developing world. *Health Policy and Planning*, **21**(6), pp. 411–20.

Shiffman J., Beer T., & Wu Y. (2002). The emergence of global disease control priorities. *Health Policy and Planning*, **17**(3), pp. 225–34.

Sridhar D. & Batniji R. (2008). Misfinancing global health: A case for transparency in disbursements and decision making. *Lancet*, **372**(9644), pp. 1185–91.

Starfield B. (1991). Primary care and health. A cross-national comparison. *Journal of the American Medical Association*, **266**(16), pp. 2268–71.

Stefanini A. (1997). The hospital as an enterprise: Management strategies. *Tropical Medicine & International Health*, **2**(3), pp. 278–83.

Stocker K., Waitzkin H., & Iriart C. (1999). The exportation of managed care to Latin America. *New England Journal of Medicine*, **340**(14), pp. 1131–6.

Stratton L., O'Neill M. S., Kruk M. E., & Bell M. L. (2008). The persistent problem of malaria: Addressing the fundamental causes of a global killer. *Social Science & Medicine*, **67**(5), pp. 854–62.

Tang S. & Bloom G. (2000). Decentralizing rural health services: A case study in China. *International Journal of Health Planning and Management*, **15**(3), pp. 189–200.

Taylor R. & Blair S. (2002). *Public Hospitals: Options for Reform Through Public–private Partnerships*. Washington: World Bank.

Tulloch J. (1999). Integrated approach to child health in developing countries. *Lancet*, **354**(Supplement 2), p. SII16–SII20.

UNAIDS. (2008). *2008 Report on the Global AIDS Epidemic*. Geneva: UNAIDS. UNAIDS/08.25E / JC1510E.

Unger J. P., De Paepe P., Ghilbert P., & De Groote T. (2004). Public health implications of world trade negotiations. *Lancet*, **363**(9402), p. 83.

Unger J. P., De Paepe P., & Green A. (2003). A code of best practice for disease control programmes to avoid damaging health care services in developing countries. *International Journal of Health Planning and Management*, 18(Supplement 1), pp. 27–39.

Unger J. P., Van Dessel P., Sen K., & De Paepe P. (2009). International health policy and stagnating maternal mortality: Is there a causal link? *Reproductive Health Matters*, **17**(33), pp. 91–104.

United Nations Development Programme. (2003). Human development report 2003.

Millennium Development Goals: A Compact Among Nations to End Human Poverty. New York, NY: UNDP

United Nations Development Programme. (2004). *Human Development Report 2004: Cultural Liberty in Today's Diverse World*. New York, NY: UNDP.

Walgate R. (2002). Crisis in East European health systems – 'Europe's best kept secret.' *Bulletin of the World Health Organization*, **80**(5), p. 421.

Wilkinson D. (1999). Tuberculosis and health sector reform: Experience of integrating tuberculosis services into the district health system in rural South Africa. *International Journal of Tuberculosis and Lung Disease*, 3(10), pp. 938–43.

World Health Organization. (2000). *Medicines Strategy: Framework for Action in Essential Drugs and Medicines Policy 2002-2003*. Geneva: World Health Organization.

World Health Organization. (2004). *World Health Report 2004 Statistical Annex. Annex Table 5: Selected National Health Account Indicators: Measured Levels of Expenditure on Health, 1997-2001*. Geneva: World Health Organization.

World Health Organization. (2006). Malaria deaths are the hardest to count. *Bulletin of the World Health Organization*, **84**(3), pp. 165–9.

World Health Organization. (2007a). Fact Sheet N°104: Tuberculosis. http://www.who.int/mediacentre/factsheets/fs104/en/.

World Health Organization. (2007b). Maternal Mortality Ratio Falling Too Slowly to Meet Goal. http://www.who.int/mediacentre/news/releases/2007/pr56/en/print.html.

World Health Organization. (2009). Health Systems Building Blocks. http://www.who.int/healthsystems/topics/en/.

World Health Organization. (2008). *World Health Statistics 2008*. Geneva: World Health Organisation.

World Trade Organization. (2004). Agreement establishing the World Trade Organization. *Annexe 1B: General Agreement on Trade in Services, article 1, 3, C*. Geneva: World Trade Organization.

The failure of the aid paradigm: poor disease control in developing countries

Introduction to Section 2

We have seen in Section 1 that international health and aid policy failed on its own paradigm – disease control in LMICs. This failure encompasses the conditions addressed by the MDGs and the so-called neglected diseases – with a few, minor successes in some places. The chronic degenerative diseases (cancers, cerebro- and cardiovascular diseases, diabetes) were not even tackled by these programmes.

In this section, we demonstrate why disease-specific programmes should be redesigned since their current format has yielded poor results, for example:

- on the one hand, these programmes need to access a pool of patients in the services where they do deliver their specialized care (which is demonstrated in Section 2, Chapter 3);
- on the other hand, they strain the delivery of polyvalent health care (Section 2, Chapter 4).

Within the prevailing international juridical and policy frame, the only conceptual solution to this inextricable situation would have been to privatize both polyvalent, curative health care and disease-specific interventions. But the initial results of contracting out these activities in domains as different as tuberculosis control (Section 2, Chapter 5) and maternal health (Unger et al., 2009) are nothing less than unpromising. We argue that disease prioritization and exclusion of polyvalent curative care from public services portfolio is not a policy that is tenable. Consequently, no company should be entitled to sue a government on the grounds, of GATS,[1] Free Trade Agreement (in the Americas) or other such covenant for subsidizing its hospitals and first-line services. Rather, those who promote the inclusion of health care in bi- and multilateral trade agreements should be held responsible for the avoidable deaths in LMICs related to the this policy.

References

Unger J. P., Van Dessel P., Sen K., & De Paepe P. (2009). International health policy and stagnating maternal mortality: is there a causal link? *Reproductive Health Matters*, **17**(33), pp. 91–104.

---

[1] The GATS is a multilateral agreement held under the WTO. Amongst others, it deals with social, health and education sectors.

**Section 2
Chapter**

3

The failure of the aid paradigm: poor disease control in developing countries

Why do disease-control programmes require patients in health services to succeed in delivering? The case of malaria control in Mali

Adapted from: Unger J.-P., d'Alessandro U., De Paepe P., Green A. Can malaria be controlled where basic health services are not used? Tropical Medicine and International Health 2006; 11(3): 314–322.

Introduction

In this chapter, we aim to demonstrate that successful implementation of disease-control programmes requires health facilities that are being used by patients. Intuitively these patients, presenting with various symptoms, represent a pool of users that the programmes require for early case detection and adequate follow-up. We assess the potential of integrating malaria control interventions in basic health services with low levels of utilization of curative care. To do so we examined the expected malaria cure rate with a predictive model that includes parameters influencing access to anti-malarial treatment at home and in health facilities. The parametric values were selected from published African programmes that gave the best results. They were applied to the population in a district in Mali (Yanfolila), where the health-seeking behaviour of mothers/guardians with children with a fever had been quantified over a period in time.

One important component of the malaria control strategy promoted by WHO (Brugha et al., 2002; World Health Organization, 2003) is that of having adequate case management (early diagnosis and prompt and effective treatment). The cost-effectiveness of improvement in case management has been estimated around USD 1–8 per disease-adjusted life years averted. It compares favourably with other interventions, such as provision of insecticide-treated bed nets (USD 19–85, USD 4–10 for the re-impregnation of bednets), residual spraying (USD 32–58), chemoprophylaxis for children (USD 3–12), and intermittent preventive treatment during pregnancy (USD 4–29) (Font et al., 2001; Goodman et al., 1999). There has been some controversy over an increasing resistance to chloroquine and sulfadoxine-pyrimethamine (Attaran et al., 2004), but while the introduction of Artemesinine Combination Therapy (ACT) might change these cost-effectiveness ratios (Belsky et al., 2004; Coleman et al., 2004; Webb et al., 2004), it would not alter the importance of relying on case management (Moerman et al., 2003), both in countries where chloroquine remains temporarily the primary drug, such as Mali, and in countries where more complex and expensive protocols require the availability of laboratory tests and of skilled professionals.

Theoretically, case management can be promoted and implemented using both formal public and private health services and through the informal sector by shopkeepers (Brugha & Zwi, 1998). Nevertheless, the latter might not be entirely practical in developing countries. The shift to more complex therapeutic protocols, encompassing combined anti-malarial drugs,

„might be more difficult to implement through unofficial routes than a chloroquine mono-therapy, and poor-quality drugs are more likely to be found in this sector. Within the official sector, private professional practitioners could provide another channel for malaria control interventions, but they are scarce in rural African, where 66% of the population lives. In addition they are frequently reluctant to implement national health policy guidelines or to refer their patients to public health facilities (Lönnroth et al., 1999).

This strongly suggests that the public-interest sector (NGOs, denominational, city, community, social security, and government services) is often the appropriate outlet to deliver adequate case management (World Bank, 1997; World Health Organization, 1999). Unfortunately, in Africa these services, and more particularly government health facilities, are underutilized. They were already 12 years ago. In Mali, for example, there were 0.15 new cases per inhabitant per year, in Ivory Coast 0.12, in Benin 0.24, and in Guinea 0.34 (Levy-Bruhl et al., 1997).

The present study aims to discover whether malaria case management is bound to fail in such settings. If this hypothesis is verified, it could reasonably apply to any disease-control programme in which case management is an important component. The recent call of WHO Director General to strengthen health systems (Jong-wook, 2003) could then be seen as a call to increase access to general curative health care in the services that deliver disease-control case management. This requires technical and financial support to such basic health services.

Methods

We reviewed the literature on malaria case management in Africa with the Piot operational model, which proved useful in the assessment of disease-control programmes for tuberculosis (Piot, 1967), malaria (Mumba et al., 2003), sleeping sickness (Robays et al., 2004), and sexually transmitted diseases (Buvé et al., 2001). This 'operational analysis' model aims at estimating (1) treatment rates, the numbers of cases correctly treated over the number of symptomatic cases in the population; and (2) cure rates, the number of cases clinically cured over the number of symptomatic cases in the population.

It encompasses different steps between illness onset and completion of treatment, such as patients' awareness and motivation; treatment in the home setting or in public health facilities; correctness of diagnosis and treatment; compliance with (Mumba et al., 2003), and sensitivity to drugs. Figure 3.1 outlines the application of the Piot model to malaria.

As the quality of professional decision making was not known, we first re-analyzed cure rate data from the Yanfolila health district to determine the effectiveness of detection and treatment in home settings, together with a fictitious 100% cure rate in patients using professional health services.

Data were collected in a study conducted in November 1998, when no specific malaria control programme was being implemented. The method employed and the results have been reported elsewhere (Thera et al., 2000). Firstly, a structured questionnaire about health-seeking behaviour was administered to randomly selected mothers/guardians. Parasitaemia and body temperature were determined in every child whose mother thought that he/she was sick at the time of interview, and the sensitivity and specificity of the mothers' diagnoses of uncomplicated malaria were assessed. For children who, according to their mothers' definition and perception, had had malaria in the previous rainy season, the

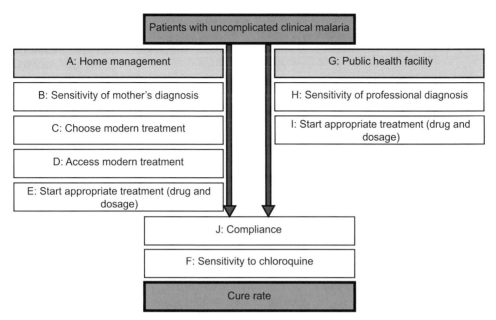

Figure 3.1. Operational model of malaria case management to determine the clinical cure rate.

optimal dose of chloroquine was calculated on the basis of age and then compared with the dose given by the mother.

Secondly, we used the results derived from studies in other African countries, where malaria control programmes were more effective and/or new interventions were tested, to assess their potential impact on malaria cure rates where health service use is low. To do so we entered data into the model from settings where the 'best' results had been published. These settings were:

- Tanzanian first-line services (Font et al., 2001), where the programme aimed at increasing the proportion of appropriate treatment in patients with malaria symptoms;
- Ghana, where a (quasi-experimental design) study tested the impact of a combination of improved information provision to patients and drug labelling on compliance to recommended oral chloroquine regimens, for the outpatient management of acute uncomplicated malaria (Agyepong et al., 2002);
- Uganda, where professional sensitivity was relatively high because professionals tend to treat most feverish patients with chloroquine (plus other treatment if necessary) (Lubanga et al., 1997);
- Kenya, where shopkeepers were trained in malaria case management (Marsh et al., 1999).

Thirdly, we looked at the impact of achieving a service use rate of 0.95 new cases per inhabitant per year, as in Namibia in 1996 (el Obeid et al., 2001; Stryckman, 1996), compared with only 0.17 new cases per inhabitant per year in Yanfolila. In 2003, 50% of malaria patients in Namibia were treated in official health services (Oxfam, 2003). We examined the potential impact of higher service use rates in Yanfolila, together with the results for the best interventions targeting health professionals.

Tests for proportion were calculated for each parametric value to determine its confidence interval, if not provided by the original article referred to. Maximum error rates of the model were then computed while using a two-step procedure. Firstly, they were computed for home treatment and professional treatment groups using the formula $SD(A + B) = \sqrt{A^2 SD^2(B) + B^2 SD^2(A)}$. Secondly, their sum's standard deviation was established using the formula $SD(A + B) = \sqrt{A^2 SD^2(A) + B^2 SD^2(B)}$ where co-variance is equal to zero, assuming that the terms are independent.

Results

Table 3.1 provides data derived from Yanfolila and other African settings. Table 3.2 provides cure rates under different parametric assumptions. Both tables present results using different parameters from A to J, as explained in Figure 3.1. In Yanfolila without any specific malaria control interventions, the cure rate in home settings was 8.4 ± 2.3% (a), corresponding with a 9.56% population cure rate at 88 ± 3.2% of treatment at home. A further 6.1% of malaria patients could be cured through professional settings (b) assuming a treatment rate of 100% in professional settings; 7.6% of Yanfolila malaria patients seeking care in professional services; and 80% chloroquine efficacy (as in Mali). Adding (a) to (b), the total population cure rate in Yanfolila would be an unsatisfactory 14.5% under these assumptions.

Table 3.1. Parameters derived from African countries

Country	Data set	A (% ±CI)	B (% ±CI)	C (% ±CI)	D (% ±CI)	E (% ±CI)
Yanfolila (Mali)	1	88 ± 3.2	39.9 ± 0.49	82.1 ± 6.4	56.5 ± 9	64.6 ± 11.6
Tanzania	2					
Ghana	3					
Uganda	4		37.4 ± 5.7			
Kenya	5				82.2 ± 3.6	72.9 ± 5.1
Namibia	6	33				

Notes: A: Home management; B: Sensitivity of mother's diagnosis; C: Choose modern treatment; D: Access modern treatment; E: Start an appropriate treatment at home

Table 3.1. continued. Parameters derived from African countries

Country	Data set	K (% ±CI)	G (% ±CI)	H (% ±CI)	I (% ±CI)	J (% ±CI)
Yanfolila (Mali)	1	80.0	7.6 ± 2			
Tanzania	2				65 ± 2.3	
Ghana	3					83.5 ± 6.6
Uganda	4			97.8 ± 1.8		
Kenya	5					
Namibia	6		50			

Notes: K: Sensitivity to chloroquine; G: Attend public health facility; H: Sensitivity of professional diagnosis; I: Start appropriate treatment in public facility; J: Compliance.

Table 3.2. Cure rates under different parametric assumptions

Cure rates in different settings	Formula	Home cure rates (%)	Professional cure rates (%)	Total cure rates (%)
Cure rate in Yanfolila home setting	$B1 \times C1 \times D1 \times E1 \times F1$	9.6		
Population cure rate in Yanfolila home setting	$A1 \times B1 \times C1 \times D1 \times E1 \times F1$	8.4		
Cure rate in Yanfolila population through professional treatment assuming that treatment rate is 100% treatment	$G1 \times 100\% \times F1$		6.1	
Total cure rate in Yanfolila, assuming 100% treatment rate through professional management	$(A1 \times B1 \times C1 \times D1 \times E1 \times F1) + (G1 \times 100\% \times F1)$			14.5 (8.4 + 6.1)
Cure rate through professional management applying Uganda/Tanzania/Ghana interventions	$G1 \times H4 \times I2 \times J3 \times F1$		3.2	
Total cure rate in Yanfolila assuming that Uganda/Tanzania/Ghana interventions are applied in Yanfolila professional setting	$(B1 \times C1 \times D1 \times E1 \times F1) + (G1 \times H4 \times I2 \times J3 \times F1)$			11.6 (8.4 + 3.2)
Cure rate in home-setting with Kenya shopkeepers intervention	$A1 \times B1 \times C1 \times D5 \times E5 \times F1$	13.0		
Total cure rate applying Kenya shopkeepers intervention in home setting and Uganda/Tanzania/Ghana interventions in professional settings	$(A1 \times B1 \times C1 \times D5 \times E5 \times F1) + (G1 \times H4 \times I2 \times J3 \times F1)$			15.2 (13 + 3.2)
Cure rate in professional setting applying Namibia services utilization rates and Tanzania/Ghana/Uganda interventions	$G6 \times H4 \times I2 \times J3 \times F1$		2.6	
Total cure rate applying Namibia services utilization rates and Tanzania/Ghana/Uganda interventions	$(A6 \times B1 \times C1 \times D1 \times E1 \times F1) + (G6 \times H4 \times I2 \times J3 \times F1)$	4.9		26.1 (21.2 + 4.9)

Notes: For parameters A–J, see Figure 3.1. The number following the parameter letter relates to the data set, see Table 3.1.

As a 100% treatment rate is impossible to achieve, we applied the following estimates to assess the likely impact of malaria control interventions designed to improve malaria case management in a professional environment: using Tanzanian data, $65 \pm 2.3\%$ of patients with malaria symptoms were assumed to receive appropriate treatment. As in a Ghanaian study the maximum post-intervention proportion of minimum daily adherence to chloroquine tablets (preferred to syrup) was put at $83.5 \pm 6.6\%$ (Agyepong et al., 2002). Based on the Ugandan study, sensitivity of professional diagnosis was put at $97.8 \pm 1.8\%$. A combination of these best practice interventions suggests a cure rate of $3.2 \pm 0.9\%$ in professional services.

In the home treatment group, training shopkeepers in Kenya resulted in an increase in appropriate use of over-the-counter chloroquine by at least 61.5%. The Kenya experiment also resulted in a sales increase of 45% in purchased anti-malarial drugs. Applying these figures to the Yanfolila home case management data would increase the access to modern treatment from 56.9% to $82.2 \pm 3.6\%$, and to $72.9 \pm 5.1\%$ of people receiving appropriate drug and dosage, instead of $64.6 \pm 11.6\%$. This approach would increase the cure rate by 18% in the self-treatment group – from 11.7% to 13% of total patients. Combining the Uganda/Tanzania/Ghana results in a professional setting, patients with an intervention similar to that in Kenya might experience a total cure rate in the general population of 16.2%.

A hypothetical increase in the health service user rate from to 0.95 new cases/inhabitant/year applied to the Yanfolila setting could, as in Namibia in 2003, result in 50% of patients with malaria attending professional health services, a more than six-fold increase from current values. This service use rate, together with the interventions in the professional setting set out above, could result in a cure rate in the total population of 26.1%, $4.9 \pm 0.9\%$ for home treatment and $21.2 \pm 1.8\%$ for professional treatment.

Discussion

Yanfolila is representative of other West African countries in terms of population structure (median age is 16.3 years in Mali, 16.4 in Benin and 17.7 in Guinea), density (15.5 inhabitants/km^2 in Sikasso district, 57 in Benin and 30 in Guinea), epidemiology (low HIVprevalence, tuberculosis prevalence rate around 200 per 100,000 inhabitants), health system inputs (a small part of government budget for health and high dependency on external resources for health), and limited access to health care, resulting in a low use rate of public services.

In Yanfolila, where use of public health services was low (0.17 new cases/inhabitant/year), the proportion of malaria patients seeking professional treatment was only 7.6%. Even a hypothetical professional treatment rate of 100% would not raise the total cure rate beyond 11.2%. In this context the combination of best-published programmes in home and professional settings (including shopkeepers' training) could only increase the total population cure rate to 16.2%. Instead an adequate use rate as in Namibia, together with the interventions in the professional setting, permits a 2.2-fold increase with a $26.1 \pm 2.1\%$ cure rate in the total population.

This assumption is conservative, as health service attendance may motivate some users of traditional medicine to use professional treatment. We also assumed that, applying Namibia's utilization rate, 50% of malarial patients would be treated in the health services in Yanfolila and that an increase in symptomatic malaria patients attending health services (+42.4%, concretely from 7.6% to 50%) would result in a similar reduction in home care frequency (−42.4%, namely from 75.8% to 33.4%).

The Ugandan approach is part of the Integrated Management of Childhood Illnesses programme. It minimizes false negative cases, particularly among patients associating malaria with other aetiology of fever, particularly acute lower respiratory infection among children, but leads to a high false positive rate. Access to laboratory equipment is poor in most developing countries and, consequently, high sensitivity and specificity is difficult to achieve. Our sensitivity of diagnosis rate of 98%, with low specificity, achieved by malaria treatment given to all febrile patients, is undesirable in view of its poor efficiency and contribution to drug resistance. This strategy may be acceptable with cheap treatment as in Mali, but not in chloroquine-resistant countries where new high-cost treatment combinations are introduced. Improvement in the diagnosis process is needed (through staff training and better criteria), but financial considerations will inevitably reduce professional sensitivity.

Training informal providers (shopkeepers) permits a 54.7% gain in cure rate in the self-treatment group, but would lift the total cure rate to only 16.2%. Moreover, this hypothesis overestimates the impact of activities directed to the self-treatment group because: (1) drug intake considerations have not been included in the model. In the Ghanaian study compliance data (83%) can be considered as drug intake data. Where shopkeepers are trained, an increase in purchased drugs does not guarantee correct drug intake; when symptoms disappear, people often stop their medication and drugs are saved for future episodes or are given to family members. This intake is probably better in professional rather than in home treatment groups, as malaria control programmes begin to rely on direct observation of treatment for single dose regimens and health education advice may be more adequately given by health professionals. (2) Treatment delay is an important factor of prognosis deterioration. Experience suggests that patient delay tends to be high when use rates are low. In Burkina Faso low overall effectiveness of malaria management was largely because of low use of health services (Krause & Sauerborn, 2000). Early detection of severe cases and timely hospital referral is more frequent in the professional group, but this factor was not taken into account.

Furthermore, several factors impair the scaling-up of pilot projects focusing on shopkeepers: one factor is that training shopkeepers to prescribe rationally for multiple diseases is not realistic, although it led to positive results for sexually transmitted infections (Jacobs et al., 2003), family planning (Agha et al., 1997), and malaria in Kenya. Another factor is that professional organizations may resist approval of less-qualified providers, which reduces the feasibility of this approach. Also, the practice of many private providers is determined by biased information from pharmaceutical companies. A fourth factor is described by numerous studies that highlight the inadequacy of interventions directed solely at enhancing provider knowledge, even to professional providers (Paredes et al., 1996), who are theoretically at least motivated by a strong ethical code. Lastly, in other contexts such as Uganda, the sensitivity of the mothers' diagnosis of malaria was found to be only 37% (Lubanga et al., 1997). In that setting training of shopkeepers will have an even smaller impact than in Yanfolila.

Finally, the parameters used may not be independent from one another, although this is an assumption of the Piot model. For instance, sensitivity of the mother's diagnosis, access to modern treatment or choice of modern treatment and then the start of treatment in a public health facility may be correlated. This simplification, if confirmed, would lead to overestimating the impact of the best African programmes in Yanfolila and strengthen further our hypothesis.

Standardized malaria case management is usually integrated in not-for-profit, publicly oriented services. Until convincing evidence shows that the private for-profit sector can be reached by the entire population and efficiently undertake disease-control activities, these services will need to increase their generally low use rates to achieve more satisfactory malaria cure rates. Complementary strategies are required and include the following elements.

Some conditions for effective integration of disease-specific integration within health care delivery services:

- Access to essential drugs in health services; in-service training and service reorganization, which are needed to increase service accessibility, acceptability to patients and to introduce patient-centred, bio-psychosocial care (Unger et al., 2002).
- Support of human resource policy. No health policy can succeed without skilled staff. Health professionals need decent salaries, a merit-based selection process (for instance based on in-service examination), an appropriate training programme and job security. Consideration should be given to recruiting experienced staff and offering them posts in district health management teams, with a joint responsibility to improve health care services, whilst implementing disease-control programmes.
- Support to district and regional hospitals. These are indispensable. They are complementary components of first-line health care. Public hospitals need to be bolstered by greater investments, a reliable operating budget and a management that aims to integrate resources and structures into a system. Such a process can be led both by health district teams and/or networks of committed professionals.

Conclusion

Together with other components of malaria control, such as impregnated bed nets, interventions aiming at improving use rates of general health services, combined with improvement in professional malaria case management, will have a much deeper impact on malaria cure rates than malaria control interventions on their own. The number of existing vertical disease-control programmes and candidate diseases for new programmes jeopardizes the feasibility of their joint implementation.[1] These two factors bear several consequences for international health policies.

Firstly, the requirement of more patients attending public-oriented services amounts to a plea for competition for general health care delivery between subsidized services delivering disease-control programmes and the others.

Secondly, disease-control initiatives need to be embedded into general strategies to revitalize those services in which disease-control programmes are implemented. Aid funds should be directed to public-oriented services, characterized by specific management and care delivery (Unger et al., 2003). Subsidized disease-control programmes should not be entitled to interfere with the polyvalent health care delivery in services where they are implemented. The Global Fund to fight AIDS, Tuberculosis and Malaria, for instance, should use

---

[1] For instance, the so-called neglected diseases (soil transmitted helminths and schistosomiasis, lymphatic filariasis, leprosy, visceral leishmaniasis, Guinea worm, trypanosomiasis, trachoma, cholera, and rabies); in other communicable pathologies as shigellosis and salmonellosis; and in non-communicable diseases which increase with the demographic transition.

its resources not only to control these diseases, but also to strengthen national health services, and this should be reflected in actual disbursements to applying countries (The Global Fund, 2003).

Which research priorities could be designed to maximize Piot model terms? Because of its resistance status, Mali is one of the last places in the world where chloroquine can be used. New drugs, such as artemesinine combinations, will be more effective than the values used in our model. Their cost will probably make a diagnostic test mandatory, resulting in an undetermined amount of false negatives and positives. Operational research will thus be needed to develop clinical decision trees according to local values of malaria incidence, finances and availability of diagnostic tests and treatments; evaluate home-based treatment of malaria with new drugs; and implement in practice molecular markers of resistance to these new drugs. Meanwhile, we must monitor resistance to chloroquine at a regional level in West African countries where chloroquine is still in use.

References

Agha S., Squire C., & Ahmed R. (1997). *Evaluation of the Green Star Pilot Project.* Washington, DC: Population Services International.

Agyepong I. A., Ansah E., Gyapong M., Adjei S., Barnish G., & Evans D. (2002). Strategies to improve adherence to recommended chloroquine treatment regimes: A quasi-experiment in the context of integrated primary health care delivery in Ghana. *Social Science & Medicine,* 55(12), pp. 2215–26.

Attaran A., Barnes K. I., Curtis C., et al. (2004). WHO, the Global Fund, and medical malpractice in malaria treatment. *Lancet,* 363(9404), pp. 237–40.

Belsky L., Lie R., Mattoo A., Emanuel E. J., & Sreenivasan G. (2004). The general agreement on trade in services: Implications for health policy makers. *Health Affairs (Millwood),* 23(3), pp. 137–45.

Brugha R., Starling M., & Walt G. (2002). GAVI, the first steps: Lessons for the Global Fund. *Lancet,* 359, pp. 435–8.

Brugha R. & Zwi A. (1998). Improving the quality of private sector delivery of public health services: Challenges and strategies. *Health Policy and Planning,* 13(2), pp. 107–20.

Buvé A., Changalucha J., Mayaud P., et al. (2001). How many patients with a sexually transmitted infection are cured by health services? A study from Mwanza region, Tanzania. *Tropical Medicine & International Health,* 6(12), pp. 971–9.

Coleman P. G., Morel C., Shillcutt S., Goodman C., & Mills A. J. (2004). A threshold analysis of the cost-effectiveness of artemisinin-based combination therapies in sub-saharan Africa. *The American Journal of Tropical Medicine and Hygiene,* 71(Supplement), pp. 196–204.

el Obeid S., Mendelsohn J., Lejars M., Forster N., & Brulé G. (2001). *Health in Namibia: Progress and challenges.* Windhoek, Namibia: Research and Information Services of Namibia.

Font F., Alonso G. M., Nathan R., et al. (2001). Diagnostic accuracy and case management of clinical malaria in the primary health services of a rural area in south-eastern Tanzania. *Tropical Medicine & International Health,* 6(6), pp. 423–8.

Goodman C. A., Coleman P. G., & Mills A. J. (1999). Cost-effectiveness of malaria control in sub-Saharan Africa. *Lancet,* 354, pp. 378–85.

Jacobs B., Kambugu F. S. K., Whitworth J. A. G., et al. (2003). Social marketing of pre-packaged treatment for men with urethral discharge (Clear Seven) in Uganda. *International Journal of STD AIDS*, **14**(3), pp. 216–21.

Jong-wook L. (2003). Global health improvement and WHO: Shaping the future. *Lancet*, **362**(9401), pp. 2083–8.

Krause G. & Sauerborn R. (2000). Comprehensive community effectiveness of health care. A study of malaria treatment in children and adults in rural Burkina Faso. *Annals of Tropical Paediatrics*, **20**(4), pp. 273–82.

Levy-Bruhl D., Soucat A., Osseni R., et al. (1997). The Bamako Initiative in Benin and Guinea: Improving the effectiveness of primary health care. *International Journal of Health Planning and Management*, **12**(Supplement 1), pp. S49–S79.

Lönnroth K., Thuong L. M., Linh P. D., & Diwan V. K. (1999). Delay and discontinuity – a survey of TB patients' search of a diagnosis in a diversified health care system. *International Journal of Tuberculosis and Lung Disease*, **3**(11), pp. 992–1000.

Lubanga R. G., Norman S., Ewbank D., & Karamagi C. (1997). Maternal diagnosis and treatment of children's fever in an endemic malaria zone of Uganda: Implications for the malaria control programme. *Acta Tropica*, **68**(1), pp. 53–64.

Marsh V. M., Mutemi W. M., Muturi J., et al. (1999). Changing home treatment of childhood fevers by training shop keepers in rural Kenya. *Tropical Medicine & International Health*, **4**(5), pp. 383–9.

Moerman F., Lengeler C., Chimumbwa J., et al. (2003). The contribution of health care services to a sound and sustainable malaria-control policy. *Lancet Infectious Diseases*, **3**(2), pp. 99–102.

Mumba M., Visschedijk J., van Cleeff M., & Hausman B. (2003). A Piot model to analyse case management in malaria control programmes. *Tropical Medicine & International Health*, **8**(6), pp. 544–51.

Oxfam. (2003). *False hope or new start? The Global Fund to fight HIV/AIDS, TB and Malaria.* Rome: Oxfam International.

Paredes P., de la Peña M., Flores-Guerra E., Diaz J., & Trostle J. (1996). Factors influencing physicians' prescribing behaviour in the treatment of childhood diarrhoea: Knowledge may not be the clue. *Social Science & Medicine*, **42**(8), pp. 1141–53.

Piot M. A. (1967). *A Simulation Model of Case Finding and Treatment in Tuberculosis Control Programmes. TECHNICAL INFORMATION.* Geneva: World Health Organization.

Robays J., Bilengue M. M. C., Van der Stuyft P., & Boelaert M. (2004). The effectiveness of active population screening and treatment for sleeping sickness control in the Democratic Republic of Congo. *Tropical Medicine and International Health*, **9**(5), pp. 542–50.

Stryckman B. (1996). *Comparative analysis of cost, resource use, and financing of district health services in sub-Saharan Africa and Asia.* New York: UNICEF.

The Global Fund. (2003). *Scaling up the fight against HIV/AIDS, TB and Malaria in Namibia. Section IV: Detailed Information on Malaria (Goal 3) Component of the Proposal.* Geneva: The Global Fund.

Thera M. A., d'Alessandro U., Thiero M., et al. (2000). Child malaria treatment practices among mothers in the district of Yanfolila, Sikasso region, *Mali. Tropical Medicine & International Health*, **5**(12), pp. 876–81.

Unger J. P., Marchal B., & Green A. (2003). Quality standards for health care delivery and management in publicly oriented health services. *International Journal of Health Planning and Management*, **18** p. S79–S88.

Unger J. P., Van Dormael M., Criel B., Van der Vennet J., & De Munck P. (2002). A plea for an initiative to strengthen family medicine in public health care services of developing countries.

International Journal of Health Services,
32(4), pp. 799–815.

Webb D., D'Alessandro C., Bull N., & Sainz T.
(2004). *Meeting the Challenge? A
Comprehensive Review of the First Three
Funding Rounds of the Global Fund to Fight
AIDS, Tuberculosis and Malaria.* London:
Save the Children.

World Bank. (1997). *Health, Nutrition,
and Population Sector Strategy.*

pp. *1–112.* World Bank. Part of the
Health, Nutrition, and Population Series
(HNP).

World Health Organization. (1999). *The
World Health Report 1999: Making a
Difference.* Geneva: World Health
Organization.

World Health Organization. (2003). *Roll Back
Malaria Technical Strategies.* Geneva:
World Health Organization.

4 How do disease-control programmes damage health care delivery in developing countries?

Adapted from: Unger J.-P., De Paepe P., Green A. A code of best practice for disease control programmes to avoid damaging health care services in developing countries. Int J Health Planning and Management 2003; 18: S27-S39.

Introduction

In 2002 already, Oxfam had demanded 'programmes which are designed for and imple-mented to strengthen existing health systems, in order to ensure effectiveness and sustainable impact' (Oxfam, 2003). The dilemma of picking up the pieces of decades of neglect and in some cases of devastation remains. Thus the question facing us now is how? To answer this, we re-examined the several possibilities starting from a managerial perspective in order to try and gauge the feasibility of effective integration.

To do this, based on a review of the literature, we first examined mechanisms whereby integrated disease-control activities can jeopardize accessibility and acceptability of general health care delivery, resulting in low service utilization and low programme target detection rates. We then put disease-control programmes into three categories and assessed the impact of each on local health care facilities. Finally, we suggest a series of measures designed to help aid agencies and national governments support local health care infrastructures or, at least, to avoid damaging them (details are given in Section 5, Chapter 16).

In this chapter, integration is defined as a process where disease-control activities are functionally merged or tightly coordinated with polyvalent health care delivery. However, another definition is sometimes used in the technical literature. This makes reference to a situation where different disease-control interventions are delivered simultaneously, in the absence of any form of 'patient-centred' care.

In industrialized countries, family medicine has espoused a 'patient-centred' model of doctor–patient interaction (Engel, 1977), whereby the doctor actively seeks the patient's point of view. This approach has been shown to result in greater patient compliance and satisfaction (Stewart, 1984). Key elements of patient-centred care are described in Section 6, Chapter 17.

In HICs, such patient-centred care is led by general practitioners (GPs), while in many LICs this role may be undertaken by nurses or auxiliaries who are often the first-line pro-viders of general health care. The principles of patient-centred care still apply, however, irrespective of the type of practitioner. Specific managerial strategies are available to pro-gressively overcome obstacles such as lack of skills (e.g., coaching, peer exchange of experi-ence, in-service training), lack of time (e.g., through task delegation, redesign of patient flow, reprogramming of personnel time, use of family files, etc.), or lack of privacy in health facilities (such as booking special appointments). In an appropriate organization GPs and nurses can direct their patients whose health status requires it to appropriate disease-specific programmes.

This raises the question of whether, in developing countries, disease-control programmes should be integrated among themselves, such as in UNICEF's Growth monitoring, Oral rehydration, Breast-feeding and Immunisation (GOBI) programme or with the general health care services.

For decades, echoing tensions on whether health care delivery in public services should or should not be limited to disease-control interventions (Section 1, Chapter 1), the debate around the pros and cons of vertical versus horizontal health care organization modes has divided the public health community. In the 1950s and 1960s pharmaceutical and vector control breakthroughs were translated straightforwardly in malaria, smallpox and other disease-control programmes (Mills, 1983). In 1978 the Alma Ata Declaration expressed an international will to promote CPHC and community participation in health. One year later, Walsh and Warren proposed SPHC as an alternative to CPHC (Walsh and Warren, 1979). SPHC focused on provision of a few programmes selected on the grounds of cost-effectiveness. This concept is quite close to: WHO's definition in 1996 of 'integrated health services' or 'integrated programmes' (WHO Study Group, 1996); WB's definition of the 'minimal package of activities' (Shaw & Elmendorf, 1994), otherwise called 'benefit packages,' and 'priority programmes'; strategies designed by UNICEF and WHO to deliver combined interventions, such as GOBI or later Integrated Management of Childhood Illness.

The features distinguishing these strategies from comprehensive approaches to first-line health care include not seeing health improvement as part of a long-term development process (Rifkin & Walt, 1986) and the lack of preoccupation for holistic patient and family-centred care (see Section 6, Chapter 17).

During the 1990s, international policies began to recommend disease-control prioritization within the public sector, together with increasing privatization of curative care on the grounds of (supposed) higher efficiency of the for-profit sector (European Commission, 2002; World Bank, 1997; World Health Organization, 2000).

This debate is far from theoretical. On the ground, as will be seen, disease-control programmes may seriously hamper broader health care delivery, which in turn could limit the effectiveness of the disease-control programmes. To avoid such a negative feedback loop this book proposes a code of best practice for disease-control programmes to avoid damaging health care services in developing countries (see summary at the end of this chapter and details in Section 5, Chapter 16).

Possible use of our proposed code of good practice for disease-control programmes:

- health professionals and planners can follow it when designing or reforming programmes;
- international organizations could pledge to respect such a code;
- research workers can find in this code a source of benchmarks to evaluate public health strategies;
- members of parliament, political parties and activists could use it to interrogate health sector aid and exert democratic control on governmental and international interventions.

A typology of disease-control programmes

Coherent sets of activities, know-how, and resources designed to control a single or a limited number of related disease(s), are termed disease-control programmes (DCP) (Cairncross et al., 1997). The sponsors of a DCP intend that health professionals use it to meet standards set

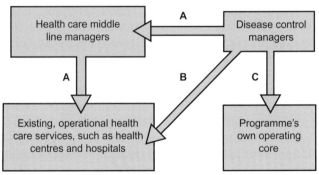

Figure 4.1. Organizational templates in disease control.

A: Integrated programme (operational and administrative integration)
B: Indirect programme (operational integration alone)
C: Vertical Programme (no integration at all)

by specialists involved in the programme. Outputs are usually measured in terms of rational clinical decision making, coverage, detection or cure rates.

Two key criteria may be used to distinguish between types of DCP:

- in health services, where these programmes are delivered, they may, or may not, attempt to attract and treat patients suffering from conditions outside of the programmes' remit – that is to deliver general, patient-centred care. Accordingly, such programmes will be deemed either to be, or not to be, operationally integrated with general health care delivery;
- DCP middle management may or may not be integrated with the middle management of (public) health care services – typified by district management teams. Such programmes will be deemed either administratively integrated, or not, with local health care administrations according to whether or not local health care managers make decisions about programme implementation.

Based on these two criteria, three main types of programmes can be delineated (see Figure 4.1) – though in reality all programmes fall somewhere along a spectrum between being free standing (vertical) at one end and administratively integrated at the other.

Vertical programmes

In theory, these programmes supply environmental interventions and clinical resources in parallel with local health care providers. Vertical programmes operate outside the existing general health care structure. They may also operate separately from local health care structures. For example, the substantial funds available through several private foundations are often channelled through public/private, independently governed structures separate from public health services (Brugha et al., 2002; Yamey, 2002).

Some of the achievements of vertical programmes must be acknowledged, of which the best known is smallpox eradication – a success that has not yet been repeated (poliomyelitis could be the next candidate).

In fact, there are clear indications for vertical programmes such as: vector control; the control of diseases too rare for general health professionals to maintain the necessary specialist skills; outreach to specific risk groups such as commercial sex workers and drug addicts; the control of some epidemics and emergencies; and providing health services for which there is no demand, such as epidemiological surveillance (Criel et al., 1997). Where an epidemic places a considerable strain on health services, temporary solutions can be adopted. For example, AIDS community home-based care programmes are justified in Eastern and Southern Africa because of the overwhelming workload AIDS puts on first-line facilities. In addition there are prerequisites for successful integration – principally, a functioning health service, a functioning middle management, adequate resources and useable facilities (Hanson, 2000). Where these do not exist, efforts must be made to build up this capacity for integration as soon as possible.

There are, however, disadvantages to vertical programmes. They usually address only a fraction of the demand, or need, for health care. Patients are likely to demand a range of treatments from curative care, relief from suffering, reassurance, to prevention and advice on use of health services – not just the control of one single cause of ill health. In contrast vertical programmes focus on restricted objectives, largely ignoring patient demand for access to wider health care. Thus dialogue between 'programme' professional and patient is limited to matters of education and information – one-way communication – to promote aims of the campaign.

A report prepared for the Swiss Agency for Development and Cooperation (SDC) identifies other disadvantages of vertical programmes. They create duplication (each single disease-control programme requires its own bureaucracy), lead to inefficient facility utilization by recipients, they may lead to gaps in care, are incompatible with decentralized health care delivery, and where they are funded externally, they undermine the government's ability to provide services by reducing the responsibility of the state to improve its own health care (Brown, 2001).

Since vertical programmes are seldom created to meet local demand, patients may be unwilling to pay for these initiatives, which means they are rarely co-financed by users. However, the reassuring sense of control available to the sponsoring organization, the capacity to record results directly, and the ability to set targets and measure results, mean that vertical programmes are frequently supported by donors, even when not appropriate.

Integrated programmes

Integrated programmes are fully integrated disease-control activities, often conceived at high levels but organized by middle, health care managers in their own area. The managers can set priorities and targets and decide on resource allocation and coverage. Disease-control specialists function as technical advisors.

Integrated programmes have some disadvantages. They lack close financial control and need a longer development phase. They experience difficulties in monitoring outputs, often show a loss of technical effectiveness (a generalist will never have the technical competence of a specialist in a specific disease), and they may be slower to build coverage.

It has been argued that the data are not available to justify disease-control integration. In the early 1980s Mills reviewed a number of cost-effectiveness studies to establish exactly what information was available on the way in which individual programmes, such as malaria control and immunization activities, were structured so as to maximize their cost-effectiveness (Mills, 1983). She concluded that detailed cost–benefit analysis was urgently needed. More recently, the Cochrane Collaboration examined the effects of primary medical care integration in LMICs, on performance, costs and patient outcomes (Briggs et al., 2001). It concluded that, despite the mass of work supporting such integration, there has been no systematic assessment of the published research to determine whether integration strategies improve health service performance or health outcomes. One could argue, however, that collecting sufficient quantitative information to decide whether integration is or is not desirable leads to 'paralysis by analysis,' since optimal solutions are context-dependent.

Many authors have stressed the need to integrate disease-specific programmes into local health facilities in order to achieve a reasonable prospect of successful disease control (Ageel and Amin, 1997; Tulloch, 1999; Wilkinson, 1997). Admittedly, they did so in papers which did not meet the inclusion criteria for an evidence-based literature review. Methodological problems may help to explain why, after decades of debate on the pros and cons of integration, controlled studies on this issue remain so scarce. The obstacles are, in fact, similar to those met in clinical practice when trying to accommodate evidence-based medicine directives: real life situations do not revolve around the management of DCPs taken in isolation, whilst their cost-effectiveness depends on the configuration of their individual mix (Goodman, 1999; Naylor, 1995).

In this paper, we argue that integration should be, in principle, more effective and efficient and should be the main template for health service organization. Three management arguments can be marshalled to support our case.

Firstly, case management is sometimes the only practical control procedure (for example in tuberculosis control). Furthermore, in practice, virtually all control strategies require clinical services to achieve any prospect of success. Even those that used to rely on environmental interventions such as for onchocerciasis, lymphatic filariasis, schistosomiasis, and helminthiasis, are now largely based on 'morbidity control' through the administration of drugs to individuals and entire groups or communities. In general patients consult for the relief of (generally non-specific) symptoms, not for a diagnosis, because they are usually unaware of the aetiology of their condition (Redwood-Campbell & Plumb, 2002). These patients represent a pool of users that DCP can target for early case detection. Clinical services that incorporate disease-control interventions – be they provided by MoH, municipal or non-governmental organizations – need thus to attract general care users through the offer of comprehensive, quality care and an array of services flexible enough to adapt to local needs. Patient-centred care also permits professional–patient dialogue and provides measures tailored to ensure continuity of care, thus discouraging patients from 'falling-out' of health care programmes. These conditions are a prerequisite for high detection rates, continuity of care, high cure rates and improved prognosis.

Secondly, 'organizational structures requiring independent staff for each disease programme are extremely expensive and difficult to sustain.' By contrast, services which provide a full spectrum of health care can improve operating efficiency through the integration of separate sources of finance and real resources including, and most importantly, staff. Even if we were to accept that vertical programmes are more cost-effective in terms of controlling the specific diseases they target – and this remains to be proved – higher efficiency thresholds could not be achieved since the high costs of sustaining parallel disease-control administrations could not be financed in developing countries. This would rule out the template considered by the Cochrane Collaboration. This is why Narayan (Narayan, 2001), who performed an in-depth analysis of externally aided projects that received a great deal of aid in Karnataka, India, could conclude that 'there is an urgent need to integrate health with family welfare, PHC and the population agenda with each other to avoid not only duplication by compartmentalization but also to reach the community and tackle the health problems of people especially the poor in a more integrated way.'

Thirdly, resources, new skills and techniques introduced as part of a DCP greatly increase the scope of the conditions that can be tackled by health professionals. This is the process by which integration helps to enhance the credibility of existing structures by increasing the range and scope of health care problems that can be treated by health centres and hospitals.

Maintaining the possibility of integration has two policy consequences:

- public health services should be tailored to deliver general, clinical care – not exclusively to patients targeted by disease-control programmes;
- the rationale of those international aid policies, which tend to restrict public service operations to disease control and a few maternal and child programmes, should be questioned (European Commission, 2002; World Bank, 1997; World Health Organization, 2000). This approach is integral also to the MDGs and remains questionable since it reinforces the need for disease-specific regimens.

Indirect programmes

These are operationally integrated (but administratively vertical) programmes. The health care staff reports to the programme manager for each programme, rather than to a health service manager (a district medical officer, for example). Operationally integrated/administratively autonomous programmes are popular with donor agencies on the grounds that they overcome bottlenecks in health care bureaucracies and achieve rapid results. In addition indirect programmes by-pass some of the problems (previously described) of integrated systems and can offer significant financial savings to donors through the use of resources provided by the recipient state.

According to a WB technical paper: 'Successful control programmes are largely centralised in formulating strategy and decentralised in operations (tactics). No single structural pattern applies universally, but the tendency is toward decentralised, and categorical or partially integrated organisations' (Liese et al., 1991).

A number of authors (Bachmann and Makan, 1997; Gish, 1992; Lush et al., 1999; Tulloch 1999; Unger, 1991) have expressed concern that, in practice, integrated programmes place considerable strain on PHC workers. In fact they were highlighting drawbacks of 'indirect' DCPs. Throughout the 1980s and 1990s health professionals in developing countries were encouraged to participate in prevention programmes and standard therapy plans such as the use of oral rehydration and tuberculostatics. These programmes were frequently based upon 'management by objective.' Such management, together with the under-resourcing of non-programme activities, distorted the balance of health care in first-line services. Only in exceptional cases did these health professionals implement preventive programmes at a local level that were not part of a national plan. In general they found it almost impossible to introduce prevention tailored to individual patient needs. With an armamentarium of perhaps two or three disease-specific programmes, and maybe not many more curative treatments, the principle of patient-centred medicine was no longer relevant. All that was required was a small number of parameters to enable health professionals to channel the patient into the appropriate programme: does the woman want to postpone the next pregnancy? Is the child vaccinated? In fact, the main – perhaps the only – communication skill required was the ability to recruit patients and ensure their compliance. Over-simplification of the professional role contributed to a fall in self-esteem and low morale among the health care staff.

These factors, along with funding cuts, seriously reduced access to public health care in developing countries. This in turn, together with the introduction of user fees, has resulted in reduced utilization of public facilities. Completing the circle, low utilization levels created problems for disease-control programmes themselves by reducing detection, continuity and cure rates.

How could this happen?

- pressure exerted by disease-control administrations, whether governments or international aid agencies (Gish, 1992);
- multiplication of disease-specific divisions in international and national health administrations;
- setting ill-defined priorities and increasing opportunity costs (Gish, 1992);
- strains which arise from inadequate budgets, financial overruns and unrealistic costing (Tulloch, 1999);
- failure to make clear the lines of command (Lush et al., 1999);
- tension between health care professionals over income disparity, treatment discrepancies, and opportunity costs (Bachmann & Makan, 1997), and problems with sustainability (Unger, 1991).

These problems are all linked to the nature of highly autonomous administrations. Indirect programmes multiply conflicting lines of command, competing for the attention of health care providers. Each programme supervisor will try to maximize his/her specific programme results. Health professionals will tend to bias their activities towards those that yield most revenue, and well-funded programmes will divert attention away from holistic bio-psychosocial treatment – or patient-centred care. These factors, in combination, will undermine care delivery and discourage patients from using health facilities.

A 'code of best practice'

In order to take advantage of suitable methods of integration and prevent DCP from damaging general care delivery, we propose the development of a 'code of best practice' for governments and international aid organizations, in order to protect health care in facilities where DCPs are delivered. This would be a voluntary code, but non-compliance might be used to lobby governments and donor agencies to reconsider their funding plans.

These principles are exposed in Section 5, Chapter 16. They can be summarized as follows:

1. Disease-control activities should generally be integrated, with the exception of certain well-defined situations. They should be integrated in health centres which offer patient-centred care;
2. Disease-specific programmes should be integrated in not-for-profit health services;
3. Disease-control programmes should plan to avoid conflict with polyvalent health care delivery (e.g., family medicine or general practice, possibly delegated, 'shifted' to nurses).

Conclusions

Although some vertical programmes should not be integrated, two conditions are essential to the integration of others:

- disease control needs to be integrated with general health care delivery and in particular patient-centred care;
- integration of both operational and administrative aspects should take place simultaneously.

We have attempted to draw attention to the negative impact on health care delivery that could arise from any tendency of DCPs becoming the cornerstone of public health centres. By drafting a 'code of best practice' for programme sponsors we will suggest ways in which fragmentation in health care delivery can be minimized. If implemented, this code would assist DCPs both to achieve their own objectives and to support and strengthen PHC services in developing countries.

References

Ageel A. R. & Amin M. A. (1997). Integration of schistosomiasis-control activities into the primary health care system in the Gizan region, Saudi Arabia. *Annals of Tropical Medicine and Parasitology,* **91**(8), pp. 907–15.

Bachmann M. O. & Makan B. (1997). Salary inequality and primary care integration in South Africa. *Social Science & Medicine,* **45**(5), pp. 723–9.

Briggs C. J., Capdegelle P., & Garner P. (2001). Strategies for integrating primary health services in middle-and low-income countries: Effects on performance, costs and patient outcomes. *Cochrane Database of Systematic Reviews,* (4), CD003318.

Brown A. (2001). *Integrating Vertical Health Programmes Into Sector Wide Approaches: Experiences and Lessons. Swiss Agency for Development and Co-operation.* London, UK: Institute for Health Sector Development.

Brugha R., Starling M., & Walt G. (2002). GAVI, the first steps: Lessons for the Global Fund. *Lancet,* **359**, pp. 435–8.

Cairncross S., Periés H., & Cutts F. (1997). Vertical health programs. *Lancet,* **349**(Supplement III), pp. 20–2.

Criel B., De Brouwere V., & Dugas S. (1997). *Integration of Vertical Programmes in Multi-Function Health Services.* Antwerp: ITG Press.

Engel G. L. (1977). The need for a new medical model: A challenge for biomedicine. *Science,* **196**(4286), pp. 129–36.

European Commission. (2002). *Communication From the Commission to the Council and the European Parliament Health and Poverty Reduction in Developing Countries.* Brussels, Belgium: European Commission. COM/2002/0129.

Gish O. (1992). Malaria eradication and the selective approach to health care: Some lessons from Ethiopia. *International Journal of Health Services,* **22**(1), pp. 179–92.

Goodman S. N. (1999). Probability at the bedside. The knowing of chances or the chances of knowing? *Annals of Internal Medicine,* **130**(7), pp. 604–6.

Hanson S. (2000). Health sector reform and STD/SIDS control in resource poor settings: The case of Tanzania. *International Journal of Health Planning and Management,* **15**(4), pp. 341–50.

Liese B., Sachdeva P., & Lochrane D. (1991). *Organising & Managing Tropical Disease Control Programs. Lessons of Success.* WB technical paper. Washington, DC: The World Bank.

Lush L., Cleland J., Walt G., & Mayhew S. (1999). Integrating reproductive health: Myth and ideology. *Bulletin of the World Health Organization,* **77**(9), pp. 771–7.

Mills A. (1983). Vertical vs horizontal health programmes in Africa: Idealism, pragmatism, resources and efficiency. *Social Science & Medicine.* **17**(24), pp. 1971–81.

Narayan R. (2001). *Review of externally aided projects in the context of their integration into the health service delivery in Karnataka.* CMH Working Paper Series. Geneva: World Health Organization.

Naylor C. D. (1995). Grey zones of clinical practice: Some limits to evidence-based medicine. *Lancet,* **345**, pp. 840–2.

Oxfam. (2003). *False Hope or New Start? The Global Fund to Fight HIV/AIDS, TB and Malaria.* Rome: Oxfam International.

Redwood-Campbell L. & Plumb J. (2002). The syndromic approach to treatment of sexually transmitted diseases in low-income countries: Issues, challenges and future directions. *Journal of Obstetrics and Gynaecology Canada,* **24**(5), pp. 417–24.

Rifkin S. B. & Walt G. (1986). Why health improves: Defining the issues concerning 'comprehensive primary health care' and 'selective primary health care.' *Social Science & Medicine,* **23**(6), pp. 559–66.

Shaw R. P. & Elmendorf A. E. (1994). Better Health in Africa. *Experience and lessons learned*. Washington, DC: World Bank.

Stewart M. A. (1984). What is a successful doctor-patient interview? A study of interactions and outcomes. *Social Science & Medicine*, **19**(2), pp. 167–75.

Tulloch J. (1999). Integrated approach to child health in developing countries. *Lancet*, **354**(Supplement 2), p. SII16–SII20.

Unger J. P. (1991). Can intensive campaigns dynamise front line health services? The evaluation of an immunisation campaign in Thies health district, Senegal. *Social Science & Medicine*, **32**(3), pp. 249–59.

Walsh J. A. & Warren K. S. (1979). Selective primary health care: An interim strategy for disease control in developing countries. *New England Journal of Medicine*. **301**, pp. 967–74.

WHO Study Group. (1996). *Integration of Health Care Delivery*. Geneva: World Health Organization.

Wilkinson R. G. (1997). Socioeconomic determinants of health - health inequalities. Relative or absolute material standards. *British Medical Journal*, **314**(7080), pp. 591–5.

World Bank & Chibber A. (1997). World Development Report 1997. *The State in a Changing World*. New York: Oxford University Press.

World Health Organization. (2000). *World Health Report 2000. Health Systems, Improving Performance*. Geneva: World Health Organization.

Yamey G. (2002). Why does the world still need WHO? *British Medical Journal*, **325**, pp. 1294–8.

**Section 2
Chapter**

5

The failure of the aid paradigm: poor disease control in developing countries

Privatization (PPM-DOTS) strategy for tuberculosis control: how evidence-based is it?

Jean-Pierre Unger, Pierre De Paepe, Patricia Ghilbert, Walter Zocchi, Patrick van Dessel, Imrana Qadeer and Kasturi Sen

Summary

The Public-Private Mix for Directly Observed Treatment, Short Course (PPM-DOTS) programme has been hailed as a success story in international cooperation. However, the evidence emerging from a range of sources suggests that this confidence may be motivated more by a desire to eulogize participation by private providers per se rather than on evidence of impact in terms of the cases treated.

This review of literature has therefore been triggered by the need for a sober assessment of the progress of the strategy of PPM-DOTS to date, and queries the extent to which tuberculosis control is embedded in sustainable national tuberculosis control programmes.

Our concerns over PPM-DOTS relate to three factors:

Firstly, there is growing doubt about the stewardship role of the state in LICs to adequately supervise the private for-profit sector. There is evidence from some regions that the current arrangements further weaken what remains of the public health system.

Secondly, the nature of the private for-profit sector, which in most settings is highly diverse, requires a coherent national health system absent in many cases; this fragments tuberculosis control, and undermines the long-term sustainability of PPM-DOTS.

Thirdly, the complex nature of partnerships and the frequent lack of adequate public sector supervision are leading to a rise in multidrug resistance as reported from many regions.

Introduction

In May 1991, the World Health Assembly set two global targets for tuberculosis control for the year 2000: at least 70% of estimated infectious cases detected and at least 85% successfully treated. In 1993, WHO declared tuberculosis a global emergency. It introduced a new framework for effective tuberculosis control, namely the internationally recommended DOTS strategy. By the year 2000 the global targets were unmet, especially with regard to case detection. That same year, WHO established the Stop TB Partnership.

> The Partnership is a coordinated network of over 500 committed international organizations, countries, donors from the public and private sectors, governmental and non-governmental organizations and individuals.

The expected outputs of PPM-DOTS are four-fold:
* To increase case detection rate or increase quality in tuberculosis case management;
* To increase equity in access to quality tuberculosis care especially for the poor and vulnerable;

- To achieve cost-effectiveness in PPM-DOTS implementation, with a reduced cost for tuberculosis patients;
- To strengthen health systems.

In the following sections we will examine each of these expected outputs against the emerging literature.

Methodology / search strategy and selection criteria

Data for this paper were identified by searches in Google scholar™ (during the first half of the year 2007) and snowball references from relevant articles. Search terms were: PPM-DOTS, tuberculosis, private providers, PPP and Stop TB partnership. Only English-language papers were reviewed.

Results

Increasing the case detection rate?

PPM-DOTS strategy promised an increasing detection rate and an improved access to good quality tuberculosis care, especially for the poor and vulnerable. However this takes for granted that a percentage of people, with symptoms of tuberculosis, will first contact a private practitioner in tuberculosis high-burden countries (Alubo, 2001; Auer et al., 2000; Government of India, 2002; Lönnroth et al., 2006; World Health Organization, 2006b). Pilot projects of PPM-DOTS show that there was an increase in the case detection rate by improving case notification through different types of private for-profit providers (Malmborg et al., 2006). Lönnroth reported increases in case detection rates of 10% to 36% in 8 of 15 PPM-DOTS pilot projects involving private practitioners in national tuberculosis programmes (Lönnroth et al., 2006).

However, it is also clear that, in all the mentioned PPM-DOTS projects, national tuberculosis programme managers were pivotal in training, motivating and monitoring participant private practitioners. Many of these initiatives have also involved NGOs as intermediaries between national tuberculosis programmes and private practitioners. All these varied and complex relations contributed to increasing the detection rate. There is concern about their reproducibility when scaling up PPM-DOTS in different contexts, unless these have been set within the framework of a strong national tuberculosis control programme (Lönnroth et al., 2004).

An increased official detection rate does not imply per se an increase in case finding. It might just reflect the fact that private practitioners now notify cases they previously treated without notifying.

There are also problems related to the varied mix of private practitioners in most developing countries. Malmborg et al. reported to the WHO that, for PPM-DOTS to achieve its targets, the selection of private practitioners is important in order to ensure meeting needs of high risk groups, and also the need for more evidence to gauge exactly which groups are being reached under PPM-DOTS (Malmborg et al., 2006). The chain of reporting and referral under varied conditions as well as the quality of national reporting systems are problematic and need further scrutiny (Dye et al., 2003).

Improving equity in access to tuberculosis care?

What of improved access for patients with tuberculosis? Some 30% of the world's population lives on less than USD 1 a day and 2.7 billion struggle to survive on less than USD 2 a day (UNF-PA, 2005; World Health Organization, 2004). These populations were exposed to structural adjustment programmes which resulted in reduced access to public health sector provision, a legacy that remains (Deshpande et al., 2004; Nunn et al., 2005). One result is that the poor would now spend an even greater proportion of their income on paying for healthcare (Khe et al., 2002). It has been noted that poor patients with tuberculosis are unlikely to get much benefit from PPM-DOTS since many already face barriers to care prior to DOTS and have access often only to unqualified practitioners (Jeffery & Jeffery, 2008).

There is insufficient information about the case holding of vulnerable patients with tuberculosis by private practitioners (Zhang et al., 2007). The huge heterogeneity in PPM-DOTS implementation methodologies, and the often inconsistent pilot results, make it difficult to perform a sound evaluation of the proportion of poor and vulnerable who may have been actually referred by private practitioners to a national tuberculosis programme (Sykes et al., 2003).

There is urgent need therefore to determine the proportion of poor and vulnerable among tuberculosis patient cohorts, since these are the highest risk groups. Evidence suggests that some of the poorest patients with tuberculosis are deliberately excluded from DOTS in some public programmes, in order to report a good treatment rate (Auer et al., 2000; Balasubramanian et al., 2000; Singh et al., 2002). Instead the presence of employed, educated and – possibly – health insured people in urban and florid rural settings has always been found to improve demand, providing support for a flourishing private for-profit sector (Hanson & Berman, 1998). In a PPM-DOTS project in Delhi more than 95% of tuberculosis cases notified by private practitioners belonged to the middle income group (Arora et al., 2003).

Qualified private practitioners tend to perform near these settings, where their income will be guaranteed. Less trained or unqualified private practitioners, on the other hand, set up practices near urban slums or in more remote rural areas (Deshpande et al., 2004), which is also the case in sub-Saharan African countries (Alubo, 2001). Neither are likely to extend their coverage just because of PPM-DOTS, since this programme cannot compensate related opportunity costs incurred with poor clientele.

A study by Zhang on health-seeking behaviour of 400,000 households in China shows that one-third of tuberculosis suspects who did not seek any professional care were those on low incomes (Zhang et al., 2007).

Will private practitioners manage tuberculosis cases as well as national tuberculosis programmes?

Quality tuberculosis case management is defined according to the following parameters (Selvam et al., 2007):

- Diagnostic quality: at least 65% of all registered pulmonary cases should be sputum smear-positive;
- Case management quality: 100% of registered cases should be treated with a national tuberculosis programme recommended regimen under direct observation at least in the intensive phase;
- Treatment outcome: success rate for new smear-positive cases should be 85% or higher.

PPM-DOTS advocates ad hoc training and supervision of private practitioners by national tuberculosis programme managers or not-for-profit organizations to improve tuberculosis case management. The effectiveness of tuberculosis control by private practitioners in the absence of interaction with strong public health institutions is known to be generally low (Baru & Nundy, 2008; Selvam et al., 2007; Thakur et al., 2006). In many LICs there exists tremendous variation in private practitioners' expertise as they often act without any form of regulation (Deshpande et al., 2004). In such settings it is found that private practitioners deliver substandard health care and public health facilities actually perform better (Barber, 2006; Nshuti et al., 2001). Poor diagnostic and treatment practices in the private sector have been widely reported for tuberculosis, increasing disease transmission and drug resistance (Auer et al., 2006; Newell, 2002; Portero & Rubio, 2003; Shimeles et al., 2006; Uplekar et al., 1998; Uplekar et al., 2001). Moreover, a key issue here is that unsuccessful initiatives are less likely to be evaluated and reported (Lönnroth et al., 2006).

> Many patients with tuberculosis approach private practitioners to maintain privacy and prevent social stigma around the disease. Convenient timings and easy access to private practitioners are another such factor.

As is the case for tuberculosis case detection, valuable treatment results achieved in some of the PPM-DOTS pilot projects relied mainly on strong commitment of solid national tuberculosis programmes and intermediary NGOs (Lönnroth et al., 2004). Often interacting on a one-to-one basis with private practitioners, they provided information, training and support in order to upgrade private practitioners' technical competence. In other projects, despite efforts to improve diagnostic and treatment practices, some of the private practitioners continued to apply costly, useless and dangerous diagnostic tests and to offer erratic treatment (Rao et al., 2008).

Furthermore, PPM-DOTS pilot projects do not systematically evaluate opportunity costs incurred by private practitioners, should they provide reliable information on free tuberculosis tests and treatment in public health facilities, monitor proper drug intake and retrieve defaulters.

> Cases reported from Kerala show that a coherent national tuberculosis programme at state level was an important factor in monitoring and implementation of PPM-DOTS (Baru & Nundy, 2008).

It is clear that sustainability of any PPM-DOTS model depends on the commitment, ability, cooperation and communication of public health staff (Nunn et al., 2005). Countries with a weakened public sector and health staff shortage often find it difficult to replicate the PPM-DOTS model at national scale (Baltussen et al., 2005; Malmborg et al., 2006). Only the best-performing national tuberculosis programmes have also been able to increase staff. Long-lasting and successful efforts to influence private providers have been identified, but sanctions for bad treatment practices encountered strong opposition from powerful professional groups (Mills et al., 2002). The question would not be whether private practitioners could perform well in PPM-DOTS pilot projects with strong involvement of international donors and local organizations, but whether this improvement in tuberculosis case management would be sustainable in the long run, in non-pilot situations at national level.

Efficient PPM-DOTS?

To our knowledge, only one published study compared the cost-effectiveness of PPM-DOTS by private practitioners with DOTS programmes in the public sector (Floyd et al., 2006). Another study compared the cost-effectiveness of tuberculosis management in national tuberculosis programmes with cost-effectiveness of tuberculosis management by an NGO or by major mining companies but none with private practitioners (Sinanovic & Kumaranayake, 2006). A third was more comprehensive but designed to estimate only median rather than the mean costs of treating a patient through PPM-DOTS (Karki et al., 2007). The study by Floyd et al. (Floyd et al., 2006) suggested that cost-effectiveness of PPM-DOTS pilot projects was similar to that of public DOTS programmes. As expected cost-effectiveness of non-DOTS treatment in the private sector was lower than PPM-DOTS programmes in the public sector, because of high patient expenditure on unsubsidized drugs and lower cure rates. In this study the cost to the public sector per treated tuberculosis was lower in PPM-DOTS (USD 24–33) than in public DOTS programmes (USD 63). However, the difference was related to the large voluntary contribution made by private practitioners: premises, staff time and project management were provided at no cost, and valued at USD 30–40 per patient. Including these costs the cost-effectiveness of the PPM-DOTS project levelled with public health sector performance.

A major dilemma with costing the above PPM-DOTS programmes is that the study conditions were rather exceptional and its results may not be reproducible in other contexts; private practitioners would, in our view, be unlikely to offer their premises and time for free, as they did in the projects evaluated. The huge variability of PPM-DOTS systems under different conditions does, therefore, not allow making definitive conclusions about the real cost-effectiveness of PPM-DOTS programmes.

Efficiency in most cases studied in India related to the level of engagement with national tuberculosis programmes, in particular supervision and monitoring to ensure application of guidelines without which the risk of adding to cases of multidrug resistance increases (Thakur et al., 2006).

Chronic diseases and long-term treatments often need repeated patient-provider interaction: for tuberculosis, between 40 and 50 contacts are required for a complete DOTS treatment. The opportunity costs for private practitioners under these circumstances could be unsustainable, if they continued to act on a voluntary base. However, if 'fee-for-service' were introduced while scaling-up PPM-DOTS and incentives were provided to private practitioners for tuberculosis management, costs for the public sector would increase quite significantly.

Reduced costs for patients?

The claim of 'reduced costs for patients' relies on the assumption that, in developing countries, MoHs are capable of regulating and controlling the health sector, public or private. This assumption, however, is more than debatable and especially in the tuberculosis high-burden countries; for example in China's 'public sector' hospitals, financial barriers are recognized as a major cause of limited access for poor patients with tuberculosis (Zhang et al., 2007). Most of the expenditure in China is related to unnecessary treatment in public health facilities: useless hospitalizations, extra diagnostic tests and inappropriate prescriptions of additional drugs (Meng et al., 2004).

These practices may provide additional revenue for health staff, but are the cause of delayed cure, increased transmission and drug resistance. The market incentive structure appears to have had a strong regressive effect, with doctors adapting to new incentive structures and finding ways of keeping revenue at old levels at the expense of patients with tuberculosis (Xu et al., 2006).

The cases from China may be replicated in India where bribes can take account of any regulatory force to control private providers in general (Baru, 1998; Chakraborty & Frick, 2002; Jesani, 2003).

In the Hyderabad project private practitioners continued to obtain chest radiographs (for which they often receive a financial incentive) on at least 80% of patients prior to referral. This continued despite the training private practitioners received before their engagement in the PPM-DOTS programme (Murthy et al., 2001).

Strengthening health systems?

Tuberculosis cannot be controlled simply by expanding DOTS coverage. It is acknowledged that the lack of political will, poor financial support, poor organization of health services, shortage of trained staff and irregular drug supply inhibit the expansion of quality DOTS. These factors are also the main causes of poor accessibility to decent health care for the vast majority of the poor (Nunn et al., 2002; World Health Organization, 2005).

PPM-DOTS advocates state that it will 'contribute to health system strengthening and actively participate in efforts to improve system-wide policy, human resources, financing, management, service delivery, and information systems' (World Health Organization, 2006b). To do so it strongly promotes private sector involvement in tuberculosis control. Paradoxically, at the same time WHO highlights 'the risk that the role of the government sector is played down as a result of a new focus on the involvement of the private sector' (World Health Organization, 2006b).

In 2007, only 3 of the 22 tuberculosis high-burden countries received any funds to strengthen their health systems (World Health Organization, 2007). Funds are shifted away from strengthening of public health systems, with national tuberculosis programmes confined to 'stewardship,' and very few additional resources to undertake public functions including those related to PPM-DOTS.

Discussion

PPM-DOTS is the first PPP dealing with diseases of public health interest. WHO states that other diseases such as HIV/AIDS and malaria are eligible to be managed by the private health sector under the stewardship of government institutions (Conway, 2006). So PPM-malaria and PPM-HIV-AIDS are in the pipeline. In order for this to work the current imbalance in investment between public and private providers needs to alter radically to ensure that public providers are able to continue to provide the coordinating role for the current strategy. The past three decades have witnessed systematic disinvestment in public health systems as well as creeping privatization of large elements of it. The involvement of the private sector in tuberculosis control may be a highly pragmatic approach in the face of its prominent role as a provider of health care. However, the aim of many private practitioners is underwritten by a profit motive, and not a public health one. This review shows that claims made by advocates of PPM-DOTS rest on conflicting rather than consistent evidence. It suggests that an imbalanced partnership can also create further confusion and a greater weakening of national tuberculosis programmes and, hence, the need for much more caution with plans for scaling up PPM-DOTS. More follow-up studies of PPM-DOTS initiatives are needed to prove that they are not counterproductive for the whole tuberculosis control programmes.

PPM-DOTS was based on prima facie acceptance that the public health system was not delivering, but without a careful understanding of political, economic and historical factors. Instead it was simply assumed that a change in tuberculosis control strategy was needed. The new strategy of involving the private health sector in the tuberculosis control programme relies too much on this assumption. Our evidence suggests that the public sector, given adequate resources and political support, can be effective and efficient. For the year 2005, 26 countries in the world achieved both tuberculosis detection and treatment success rate targets. Another 67 achieved at least 70% case detection. Finally, 57 countries reported treatment success rates of 85% or more (World Health Organization, 2007). The way tuberculosis epidemiology and health systems organization are present in these countries differs widely. However, the feature they all have in common is their strategy: they achieved remarkable results in tuberculosis control mainly through public health services.

Conclusion

The DOTS Expansion Working Group states: a PPM-DOTS programme is suitable in a context with a strong formal private for-profit sector and a mature national tuberculosis programme 'that should not only have demonstrated how DOTS can be successfully implemented, but should also have additional capacity to set up and support a sustainable partnership' (World Health Organization, 2006a).

Thus, governments and international agencies are not mobilizing resources to adequately finance public health care systems while being aware that DOTS expansion without general health services strengthening is not sustainable. Publicly oriented health services should be sustained to not just compete with the private for-profit health sector, but to support and guide them through the adoption of organizational and behavioural attitudes attractive to patients. User-friendly public services should be geographically accessible, offer acceptable opening times, adopt flexibility by giving patients some degree of choice in the form of treatment management most suited to their daily life, ensure confidentiality and a patient-centred approach (Macq et al., 2003). And all this is possible only when these systems of services come out of the 'client' and 'stewardship' roles imposed upon them.

References

Alubo O. (2001). The promise and limits of private medicine: Health policy dilemmas in Nigeria. *Health Policy and Planning*, **16**(3), pp. 313–21.

Arora V. K., Sarin R., & Lönnroth K. (2003). Feasibility and effectiveness of a public–private mix project for improved TB control in Delhi, India. *International Journal of Tuberculosis and Lung Disease*, 7(12), pp. 1131–8.

Auer C., Lagahid J. Y., Tanner M., & Weiss M. G. (2006). Diagnosis and management of tuberculosis by private practitioners in Manila, Philippines. *Health Policy*, 77(2), pp. 172–81.

Auer C., Sarol J., Tanner M., & Weiss M. (2000). Health seeking and perceived causes of tuberculosis among patients in Manila, Philippines. *Tropical Medicine & International Health*, 5(9), pp. 648–56.

Balasubramanian V. N., Oommen K., & Samuel R. (2000). DOT or not? Direct observation of anti-tuberculosis treatment and patient outcomes, Kerala State, India. *International Journal of Tuberculosis and Lung Disease*, **4**(5), pp. 409–13.

Baltussen R., Floyd K., & Dye C. (2005). Achieving the millennium development goals for health – Cost effectiveness analysis of strategies for tuberculosis control in developing countries. *British Medical Journal*, **331**(7529), pp. 1364–8.

Barber S. L. (2006). Public and private prenatal care providers in urban Mexico: How does their quality compare? *International Journal for Quality in Health Care*, **18**(4), pp. 306–13.

Baru R. V. (1998). *Private Health Care in India: Social Characteristics and Trends*. New Delhi: Sage Publications.

Baru R. V. & Nundy M. (2008). Blurring of boundaries-public private partnerships in health services in India. *Economic and Political Weekly*, pp. 62–71.

Chakraborty S. & Frick K. (2002). Factors influencing private health providers' technical quality of care for acute respiratory infections among under-five children in rural West Bengal, India. *Social Science & Medicine*, **55**(9), pp. 1579–87.

Conway S. (2006). *Public– Private Mix for HIV (PPM-HIV)*. London, UK: HLSP Institute.

Deshpande K., RavishankarDiwan, V. K., Lönnroth K., Mahadik V. K., & Chandorkar R. K. (2004). Spatial pattern of private health care provision in Ujjain, India: A provider survey processed and analysed with a Geographical Information System. *Health Policy*, **68**, pp. 211–22.

Dye C., Watt C. J., Bleed D. M., & Williams B. G. (2003). What is the limit to case detection under the DOTS strategy for tuberculosis control? *Tuberculosis*, **83**(1–3), pp. 35–43.

Floyd K., Arora V. K., Murthy K. J. R., et al. (2006). Cost and cost-effectiveness of PPM-DOTS for tuberculosis control: Evidence from India. *Bulletin of the World Health Organization*, **84**(6), pp. 437–45.

Government of India. (2002). *National Health Policy – 2002*. http://mohfw.nic.in/np2002.htm.

Hanson K. & Berman P. (1998). Private health care provision in developing countries: A preliminary analysis of levels and composition. *Health Policy and Planning*, **13**(3), pp. 195–211.

Jeffery P. & Jeffery R. (2008). 'Money itself discriminates': Obstetric emergencies in the time of liberalisation. *Contributions to Indian Sociology*, **42**(1), pp. 59–91.

Jesani A. (2003). Social objectives of health care services: Regulating the private sector. In: Prabhu K. S. & Sudarshan R., eds. *Reforming India's Social Sector; Poverty, Nutrition, Health and Education*. New Delhi: Social Science Press, pp. 205–20.

Karki D. K., Mirzoev T. N., Green A., Newell J., & Baral S. C. (2007). Costs of a succesful public–private partnership for TB control in an urban setting in Nepal. *BMC Public Health*, 7, p. 84.

Khe N. D., Toan N. V., Xuan L. T. T., Eriksson B., Höjer B., & Diwan V. K. (2002). Primary health concept revisited: Where do people seek health care in a rural area of Vietnam? *Health Policy*, **61**(1), pp. 95–109.

Lönnroth K., Uplekar M., Arora V. K., et al. (2004). Public–private mix for DOTS implementation: What makes it work? *Bulletin of the World Health Organization*, **82**(8), pp. 580–6.

Lönnroth K., Uplekar M., & Blanc L. J. (2006). Hard gains through soft contracts: Productive engagement of private providers in tuberculosis control. *Bulletin of the World Health Organization*, **84**, pp. 876–83.

Macq J. C., Theobald S., Dick J., & Dembele M. (2003). An exploration of the concept of directly observed treatment (DOT) for tuberculosis patients: From a uniform to a customised approach. *International Journal of Tuberculosis and Lung Disease*, 7(2), pp. 103–9.

Malmborg R., Mann G., Thomson R., & Squire S. B. (2006). Can public–private collaboration promote tuberculosis case detection among the poor and vulnerable?

Bulletin of the World Health Organization, **84**(9), pp. 752–8.

Meng Q., Li R., Cheng G., & Blas E. (2004). Provision and financial burden of TB services in a financially decentralised system: A case study from Shandong, China. *Intetnational Journal of Health Planning and Management,* 19(Supplement 1), p. S45–S62.

Mills A., Brugha R., Hanson K., & McPake B. (2002). What can be done about the private health sector in low-income countries? *Bulletin of the World Health Organization,* **80**(4), pp. 325–30.

Murthy K. J., Frieden T. R., Yazdani A., & Hreshikesh P. (2001). Public–private partnership in tuberculosis control: Experience in Hyderabad, India. *International Journal of Tuberculosis and Lung Disease,* 5(4), pp. 354–9.

Newell J. (2002). The implications for TB control of the growth in numbers of private practitioners in developing countries. *Bulletin of the World Health Organization,* **80**(10), pp. 836–7.

Nshuti L., Neuhauser D., Johnson J. L., & Whalen C. C. (2001). Public and private providers' quality of care for tuberculosis patients in Kampala, Uganda. *International Journal of Tuberculosis and Lung Disease,* 5(11), pp. 1006–12.

Nunn P., Harries A., Godfrey-Faussett P., Gupta R., Maher D., & Raviglione M. C. (2002). The research agenda for improving health policy, systems performance, and service delivery for tuberculosis control: A WHO perspective. *Bulletin of the World Health Organization,* **80**, pp. 471–6.

Nunn P., Williams B., Floyd K., Dye C., Elzinga G., & Raviglione M. C. (2005). Tuberculosis control in the era of HIV. *Nature Reviews Immunology,* 5, pp. 819–26.

Portero J. L. & Rubio M. (2003). Private practitioners and tuberculosis control in the Philippines: Strangers when they meet? *Tropical Medicine & International Health,* 8(4), pp. 329–35.

Rao S. N., Mookerjee A. L., Obasanjo O. O., & Chaisson R. E. (2008). Errors in the treatment of tuberculosis in Baltimore. *Chest,* **117**, pp. 734–7.

Selvam J. M., Wares F., Perumal M., et al. (2007). Health-seeking behaviour of new smear-positive TB patients under a DOTS programme in Tamil Nadu, India, 2003. *International Journal of Tuberculosis and Lung Disease,* **11**(2), pp. 161–7.

Shimeles E., Aseffa A., Yamuah L., Tilahun H., & Engers H. (2006). Knowledge and practice of private practitioners in TB control in Addis Ababa. *International Journal of Tuberculosis and Lung Disease,* **10**(10), pp. 1172–7.

Sinanovic E. & Kumaranayake L. (2006). Financing and cost-effectiveness analysis of public–private partnerships: Provision of tuberculosis treatment in South Africa. *Cost Effectiveness and Resource Allocation,* **4**(1), p. 11.

Singh V., Jaiswal A., Porter J. D. H., et al. (2002). TB control, poverty, and vulnerability in Delhi, India. *Tropical Medicine and International Health,* 7(8), pp. 693–700.

Sykes M., Tolhurst R., & Squire S. B. (2003). *Vulnerable Patients and the Public–private Mix in Tuberculosis. EQUI-TB Knowledge Programme.* Liverpool, UK: Liverpool School of Tropical Medicine.

Thakur J. S., Kar S. S., Sehgal A., & Kumar R. (2006). Private sector involvement in tuberculosis control in Chandigarh. *Indian Journal of Tuberculosis,* **53**(3), pp. 149–53.

UNFPA. (2005). *Reducing Poverty and Achieving Sustainable Development.* New York: UNFPA.

Uplekar M., Juvekar S., Morankar S., Rangan S., & Nunn P. (1998). Tuberculosis patients and practitioners in private clinics in India. *International Journal of Tuberculosis and Lung Disease,* 2(4), pp. 324–9.

Uplekar M., Pathania V., & Raviglione M. (2001). Private practitioners and public health: Weak links in tuberculosis control. *Lancet,* **358**(9285), pp. 912–6.

World Health Organization. (2004). *DOTS in the African Region. A framework for engaging private health care providers.* Geneva: World Health Organization.

World Health Organization. (2005). *Addressing Poverty in TB Control: Options for National TB Control Programmes*. Geneva: World Health Organization.

World Health Organization. (2006a). *Engaging All Health Care Providers in TB Control. Guidance on Implementing Public–private Mix Approaches*. Geneva: World Health Organization. WHO/HTM/TB/2006.360.

World Health Organization. (2006b). *The Stop TB Strategy. Building on and Enhancing DOTS to Meet the TB-related Millennium Development Goals*. Geneva: World Health Organization. WHO/HTM/TB/2006.368.

World Health Organization. (2007). *Global Tuberculosis Control: Surveillance, Planning, Financing*. WHO Report 2007. Geneva: World Health Organization. WHO/HTM/TB/2007.376.

Xu B., Dong H. J., Zhao Q., & Bogg L. (2006). DOTS in China: Removing barriers or moving barriers? *Health Policy and Planning*, **21**(5), pp. 365–72.

Zhang T., Tang S. L., Jun G., & Whitehead M. (2007). Persistent problems of access to appropriate, affordable TB services in rural China: Experiences of different socio-economic groups. *BMC Public Health*, 7, p. 19.

Section 3

Impact of international health policies on access to health in middle-income countries: some experiences from Latin America

Introduction to Section 3

In this section we question why markets in health care have been so compelling to policy makers, globally and nationally, and scrutinize the evidences to commodify health care delivery in MICs such as those covered in this section. Thus the experience of health sector reforms in three Latin American countries has been presented here in order to understand the nature of the reforms and their variance in impact on health care. This section focuses on primary and secondary data on national health systems, hospitals and first-line health services. We illustrate how global policies shaped both health services and systems, in addition to the pressures placed upon countries to adopt them and explore the extent to which these functioned to serve health needs and demand for access to health care.

Health policies in Costa Rica (Section 3, Chapter 6) have followed the principles of equity and solidarity to strengthen access to care through public services and universal health insurance. The role of the for-profit sector has been limited. Boosted by the robust performance of the public health system, Costa Rica has achieved health status comparable to the most developed countries. Compared to this, in Columbia the health sector was privatized in line with the internationally advocated paradigm (Section 3, Chapter 7). Even following 15 years of implementation the reforms could not deliver the declared goals of universal coverage and equitable access to high quality care, despite an explosion in both public and private expenditures. Furthermore, most key health indicators have deteriorated. In Chile during the regime of Pinochet rampant neoliberal reforms were adopted with very negative consequences. Public expenditure was severely cut back whilst private insurance was promoted, resulting in an overall deterioration of health indicators. The democratic coalition that came into power in the early 1990s tried to reinvigorate the public sector, without discarding the core parts of health reforms. We argue that, using Chile as a model of health sector reforms (as is the case with the likes of the IMF and the

WB), one could easily gloss over the fact that it was the limited application of neoliberal reforms rather than its success that resulted in relatively better health care provision in Chile (Section 3, Chapter 8). The three country experiences discussed here can provide some meaningful conclusions for the countries that are preparing to embark upon health sector reforms based on a neoliberal doctrine in the years to come.

Section 3
Chapter

6

Impact of international health policies on access to
health in middle-income countries: some experiences
from Latin America

Costa Rica: achievements of a heterodox health policy

Adapted from: Unger JP, De Paepe P, Buitrón R, Soors W. Costa Rica: Achievements of a
heterodox health policy. American Journal of Public Health 2008; 98(4): 636–643.

Introduction

Costa Rica is a MIC with a strong governmental emphasis on human development. For more
than half a century, its health policies have applied the principles of equity and solidarity to
strengthen access to care through public services and universal social health insurance.

Costa Rica's population measures of health service coverage, health service use, and health
status are excellent, and in the Americas, life expectancy in Costa Rica is second only to that
in Canada. Many of these outcomes can be linked to the performance of the public health care
system.

However, the current emphasis of international aid organizations on privatization of
health services threatens the accomplishments and universality of the Costa Rican health
care system.

For several years, international development agencies, including the WB and the IMF,
have promoted the role of for-profit health care facilities and programmes in the delivery
of health care services in developing countries while narrowing the role of the not-for-profit
sector in disease control (World Bank, 1993). Using as an example the experience of Costa
Rica, we question the privatization of health care policy promoted by international aid
agencies.

During a 2001 press conference, former WB president James D. Wolfensohn recognized Cuba for having done a 'terrific job' in the area of health (World Bank, 2001). His
laudatory comments were remarkable given that Cuba is well known for evading WB and
IMF recommendations. Jo Ritzen, the WB's vice president for development policy at the
time, provided a clue to Wolfensohn's lack of hesitation in acknowledging Cuba by suggesting that the Cuban experience might not be replicable in other countries (Lobe, 2001).
We would say that the Cuban policy was not exportable, at least not without its authoritar-
ian regime.

What would WB senior officers have said about Costa Rica, which is a benchmark democracy by international standards (Freedom House, 2004)? Its health policy also differs radically
from the health policies of international loaning agencies. Despite resisting the recommendations of the WB and IMF, Costa Rica has accomplished a great deal in the health arena;
for example, compared with all the countries in the Americas, Costa Rica's life expectancy
is second only to Canada's (United Nations Development Programme, 2003). Although the
country's per capita income is approximately the same as that of Mexico and one-fourth that
of the United States, total health expenditures in Costa Rica are one-ninth those of the United

Table 6.1. Health and equity indicators for Costa Rica, the United States and Mexico

	Costa Rica	United States	Mexico
GDP per capita, USD[1]	6,460	34,320	8,430
Health expenditure per capita, USD	562	4887	544
Infant mortality[2]	9	7	24
Life expectancy at birth[3]	78.0	77.0	73.3
Gini index[4]	46.5	40.8	54.6

Notes: GDP = Gross Domestic Product. All data are for 2001 with the exception of the Gini index, which reflects 2000 figures.
1 Purchasing power parity.
2 Probability of dying between birth and 1 year of age, expressed per 1,000 live births.
3 Number of years a newborn infant would live if prevailing patterns of age-specific mortality at the time of the infant's birth were to stay the same throughout his or her life.
4 Measurement of inequality in the distribution of income or consumption within a country, expressed as a percentage. A value of 0 represents perfect equality and a value of 100 represents perfect inequality.

Source: UNICEF et al., 1997; United Nations Development Programme, 2003.

States. Moreover, other health and equity indicators in Costa Rica rank close to the United States and well above Mexico (Table 6.1).

Certainly Costa Rica's achievements are not simply the product of good health services. Indeed the country maintained annual growth rates (gross domestic product [GDP] per capita) of 1.2% between 1975 and 2001 and 2.8% between 1995 and 2001, even though it never rose to the high-income category (GDP per capita of USD 9,206 or more in 2001) (United Nations Development Programme, 2003). Since 1995 Costa Rica has occupied a stable position among countries with high scores (0.80 or above) on the human development index (which measures average achievement in three basic dimensions of human development: quality of life, knowledge, and standard of living) (United Nations Development Programme, 2003).

Despite the potential contributions of economic development to health outcomes, it would be unfair to credit the health achievements in Costa Rica mainly to rapid income growth, as the World Development Report did in its spotlight on Costa Rica and Cuba in 2004 (World Bank, 2004a). Such an attribution overlooks the sensitivity to health service performance of indicators such as infant and maternal mortality. In the case of both indicators Costa Rica has shown equal or better performance than its Latin American neighbours Chile (World Bank, 1993), Venezuela, Panama, Colombia and Mexico, countries in the same income group and with comparable health care expenditures (Table 6.2).

From 1970 on Costa Rica needed less than one-third of the Chilean economic growth rate to achieve reductions in infant mortality similar to those achieved in Chile (Homedes & Ugalde, 2002). With economic growth rates similar to Colombia, Costa Rica had twice the reduction in infant mortality. Costa Rica also achieved twice the reduction in infant mortality rates as Mexico with similar economic growth rates and health care expenditures.

In the 1970s, Costa Rica departed from the Latin American pattern of stagnation and closed the gap with the industrialized world in terms of infant mortality. According to Rosero-Bixby (Rosero-Bixby, 1986; Seligson et al., 1997) only one-fifth of the country's spectacular infant mortality reduction can be accounted for by economic growth, whereas three-fourths can be attributed to improvements in public health services. Such

Table 6.2. Infant and maternal mortality, health expenditure and economic growth in selected years: Costa Rica, Chile, Venezuela, Panama, Colombia and Mexico

	Infant mortality[1]		Reduction in infant mortality[2]	Maternal mortality[3]	Health expenditure per capita[4]	GDP per capita[4]	GDP per capita annual growth rate
	1970	2001	1970–2001	1985–2001	2001, USD	2001, USD	1975–2001, %
Costa Rica	62	9	7	29	562	9460	1.2
Chile	78	10	8	23	792	9190	4.1
Venezuela	47	19	2	60	386	5670	0.9
Panama	46	19	2	70	458	5750	0.8
Colombia	69	19	4	80	356	7040	1.5
Mexico	79	26	3	55	544	8430	0.9

Notes: GDP = Gross Domestic Product.
1 Probability of dying between birth and exactly 1 year of age, expressed per 1,000 live births.
2 Calculated from 1970 and 2001 figures.
3 Annual number of deaths of women from pregnancy-related causes per 100,000 live births (data refer to most recent year available during the period specified, adjusted for underreporting and misclassification).
4 Purchasing power parity.

Source: UNICEF et al., 1997; UNICEF, 2002; United Nations Development Programme, 2003; World Bank, 2004b.

impressive achievements in themselves make the Costa Rican health system worthy of study.

However, the results of a MEDLINE search we conducted for the period 1975 to 2004 suggested a lack of interest among the scientific community in the Costa Rican experience, with only 122 papers published on Costa Rica as compared with 249 for Colombia and 424 for Chile. The Costa Rican health policy experience has also been largely ignored by international decision makers. We sought to address this knowledge gap and to derive important implications from the Costa Rican experience for international aid agencies and health policies.

Methodology

We complemented our MEDLINE search with reports and evaluations of the Costa Rican government and publications on health policy and Latin America in general. We made field visits to the two existing hospitals and a representative selection of primary care centres (n=10) in the eight health zones (secondary division of regions in Costa Rica) of Costa Rica's Atlantic region (Huetar Atlántica) in August 2004, October 2005 and March 2006. Also, we visited health centres in the central and southern Pacific regions.

We conducted three focus group discussions (n=47) with health care providers, as well as key informant interviews with all available providers in the health structures we visited (n=32) and with decision makers and administrative staff at the regional and national levels (n=14). Our data synthesis relied on systematic triangulation of the findings from our literature review, field visits, and stakeholder discussions and interviews, framed in a model of the different variables addressed. Our model of the relationships among Costa Rican developmental achievements, health service outputs (utilization and coverage rates), health service characteristics and observed health policy features is shown in figure 6.1.

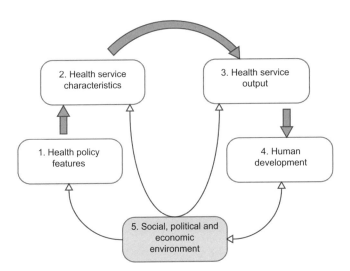

Figure 6.1. Relationships between the variables addressed.

Findings

Health policy features

Until 1940, health care delivery in Costa Rica was based in hospitals and other facilities of the MoH, public charities, and banana companies. Since the creation of Costa Rica's Social Security Administration (CCSS; Caja Costarricense de Seguro Social) in 1941 the country has had a social security system for wage-earning workers in place, with coverage gradually being extended to dependents (Homedes & Ugalde, 2002).

In 1973 the CCSS assumed control over the MoH and charitable health facilities with the exception of first-line health service facilities (i.e., facilities providing a first means of contact for health care users from an ascribed target population), which would be added some years later. The CCSS became the sole delivery institution of public hospital care, with 29 hospitals (23.9% of total health expenditures were devoted to public hospitals, as compared with 2% for private hospitals). This dominant quasi-monopolistic position of public hospitals was in contrast to the promotion by international aid agencies of multiple, competing providers, largely in the private sector. Because its health care system was unified from the outset, Costa Rica avoided the social insurance stratification typical of other Latin American countries and achieved a high degree of integration of its health care facilities.

Also in 1973, 5 years before the Alma Alta conference on PHC, Costa Rica launched its Rural Health Program (Programa de Salud Rural) to extend comprehensive primary care services to rural areas (Seligson et al., 1997). In 1976 the Community Health Program (Programa de Salud Comunitaria) was established, and this programme applied the same principles of improving access to primary care services to suburban neighbourhoods. A few years later, the two programmes merged into a single PHC department.

During the 1978 to 1982 government of Rodrigo Carazo, community participation was made the centrepiece of the social agenda. Health committees were activated in rural health posts under the Unit for People's Participation (Unidad de Participación Popular), a newly created programme division in the MoH. Meanwhile, the international context was changing. The

Alma Ata concept of CPHC, which stressed community participation, was challenged by the so-called strategy of SPHC, a package of low-cost technical interventions designed to address the primary disease problems of poor countries (Cueto, 2004; Walsh & Warren, 1979).

When UNICEF and the WHO abandoned the notion of CPHC for SPHC, Carazo's successor and political opponent Luis Alberto Monge suspended the budget of the Unit for People's Participation and renamed the unit the Community Promotion and Fomentation Program (Programa de Pro-moción y Fomento de la Comunidad). The unit was quietly dismantled in 1985 (Morgan, 1990).

With the health system still lacking democratization, the plea for users' and communities' participation in the management of health facilities gained strength and was reinforced by the 1993 Deconcentration Law (Ley de Desconcentración Hospitalaria). At the peripheral level users were now represented by elected health boards, together with social security representatives, employers and social organizations. Although participation did not reach its full potential, a civil audit on the quality of the country's democratic processes assigned a high ranking to health care provision as a result of its contribution to the population's well-being (Estado de la Nación, 1999; Estado de la Nación, 2001).

The employment drop of the 1980s was followed by an attempt on the part of the country to ensure that social security benefits were accessible to self-employed individuals and the state-subsidized poor. By the year 2000 social health insurance coverage was available to 82% of the Costa Rican population (Saenz Madrigal & Ulate, 2002).

The number of PHC clinics (EBAIS; Equipos Básicos de Atención Integral en Salud) in the country began to increase in 1994. Health committees occasionally co-manage these clinics. In theory there is 1 health committee (Junta de Salud y Seguridad Social) for each of the 83 administrative cantons of Costa Rica (cantons are not identical to the health subdivisions of areas and zones), but not all health committees are functional. The EBAIS share the market of first-line health services with the private sector (15.7% of total health expenditures are devoted to public first-line services, as compared with 14.4% for private first-line services).

After a failed pilot experiment with a capitation system in the 1980s under President Óscar Arias (Martínez-Franzoni, 2006), contracting within the country's publicly oriented services (hereafter 'contracting in') became the cornerstone of the Costa Rican health policy. As part of a WB project the CCSS introduced performance agreements (United Nations, 2006) in 1996. Outputs of five priority programmes for chronic and preventive care were defined on a negotiated basis by central and local decision makers. Failure to comply would prevent health services from gaining 'budget bonuses.' However, in contradiction to international agencies' policies, Costa Rica contracted with private for-profit services only on a limited scale (e.g., as a means of reducing waiting lists or accessing expensive technology).

The government has provided the lion's share of total health expenditures in Costa Rica. During the 1990s, approximately 7% of the GDP was allocated to the health sector, more than 70% of which was in the form of public funds and less than 30% in the form of private funds (Pan American Health Organization, 2003). Such a high percentage of public funds was unusual during that period. In most developing countries with more orthodox policies, including Colombia, total health expenditures grew mainly when the bulk of the budget was targeted toward the private for-profit sector (De Groote et al., 2005).

It is interesting to compare the Costa Rican share of public health expenditures with that of HICs: Costa Rica is in line with Canada (71% of public funds in 2000), lags behind New Zealand and Sweden (78% and 85%, respectively) and fares far better than the United States (44%) (Organisation for Economic Co-operation and Development, 2004). These figures demonstrate the high degree of solidarity of the Costa Rican health system.

Similarly, public insurance coverage illustrates the system's equity. As an example public health insurance coverage in 2000 was universal in Canada, New Zealand, and Sweden; in that same year, the coverage rate in Costa Rica was 82%, as compared with approximately 25% in the United States (Organisation for Economic Co-operation and Development, 2003).

By and large, Costa Rica's health policies differ substantially from international aid recommendations. First, the CCSS is, in essence, the single insurer in Costa Rica; private insurance is virtually non-existent. The WB is ambiguous on this issue. On the one hand, it warns against private health insurance, which is subject to market imperfections as a result of information asymmetries and is prone to risk selection (Preker, 1997). On the other hand, privatized health insurance promotes competition between insurers, as in Chile and Colombia.

Second, the CCSS both purchases and provides care services, and the MoH remains external to these processes. Consequently, no purchaser–provider split occurs in the public sector. This situation explains the low administrative cost (the proportion of the budget related to but not included in service provision or salaries) of between 3% and 4% since 1990 (Rodríguez Herrera, 2006), in sharp contrast with double-digit numbers among competing private insurers in Chile and Colombia.

Finally, the country's contracting-in strategy, introduced in 1996, is not sustained by real contracts. Rather, it consists of a yearly negotiation between a CCSS central body (the purchasing directorate) and CCSS area medical officers on a list of performance indicators and targets for a series of programmes. Targets are set according to resource availability, population size and density, and historical results. They are used merely to monitor coverage progress; their attainment does not influence health professionals' incomes, and it influences only marginally their professional resources.

As suggested by the deviations of Costa Rica's health policies from international aid agency recommendations described here, relations with international agencies have often been strained. When José María Figueres Olsen became president in 1994, he opposed recommendations for privatization of the IMF, instead favouring greater government intervention in the economy. The WB subsequently withheld USD 100 million in financing to the country (Mkandawire, 2006).

More recently, in 2003, Costa Rica temporarily abandoned the Central American Free Trade Agreement (CAFTA) discussions. In the best interest of its citizens the Costa Rican government hesitated in accepting the US condition of opening up the insurance market (Homedes & Ugalde, 2005). Costa Rica resumed negotiations in 2004, and Óscar Arias made joining CAFTA an essential part of his 2006 election platform. Now elected president for a second term, Arias faces considerable opposition of his plan, and the decision of whether to enrol in CAFTA will be decided by an upcoming referendum.

Health service characteristics

The CCSS's publicly oriented outpatient facilities include the EBAISs (approximately 1 per 5,000 inhabitants), which comprise health centres with a general practitioner, an assistant nurse, a clerk, a pharmacy assistant, and a primary health technician, and second-line clinics (clinics providing first-referral care in the context of a multi-tiered health care system) located in proximity to the CCSS's area headquarters. Physical facilities are in remarkably good condition. Individuals knowledgeable about the state of public facilities in most Latin American countries would view the quality, extent and maintenance of Costa Rica's hospital equipment as being at surprisingly high levels.

Outpatient facilities are attached to administrative areas (a total of 98 in the country). Both areas and hospitals are attached to medical regions (a total of seven). Several types of hospitals are operated by the CCSS, including 5 specialty national hospitals, 3 general national hospitals, seven regional hospitals, 13 peripheral hospitals, and 10 major clinics serving as referral centres for the EBAISs. Public expenditures appear to have increased the share of the EBAISs (from 38% to 40% between 1997 and 2001), compared with hospitals (whose share decreased from 62% to 60% in the same time span (Pan American Health Organization, 2003)). Since the 1993 reforms these first-line facilities have delivered individual bio-psychosocial care services, although to varying degrees (Rosero-Bixby, 2004). They also offer family and community medical services as well as promotion and prevention programmes.

The Costa Rican system promotes limited private care. Public facilities may refer patients to the private sector when they are overloaded, or patients may choose to see a private physician to avoid waiting lists. Patients must then pay their full consultation expenditure, but the CCSS reimburses drug and laboratory costs incurred during the private consultation. A similar system exists for corporate businesses, and in 1992, a system of free medical choice (i.e., no referral is needed) was established for consultations with certain specialists (Mesa-Lago, 2005).

The CCSS system has contracted with health cooperatives since 1988. Groups of physicians have been engaged to offer outpatient care; their budgets are determined by the CCSS, which also maintains property rights over infrastructure and equipment. The use of health cooperatives has been limited to the San José capital area, with four cooperatives having been organized to date. There are no plans to expand the model. An evaluation of the cooperatives by Gauri et al. (Gauri et al., 2004) suggested that the overall cost to the state was the same and changes in the quality of care delivered still had to be assessed. According to Homedes and Ugalde (Homedes & Ugalde, 2005), the overall cost to the state increased as a result of unnecessary referrals, without evidence of improved quality.

Finally, the CCSS has signed contracting agreements with the University of Costa Rica and with ASeMeCo (Asociación de Servicios Médicos Costarricense), a private partner, for delivery of outpatient care in three areas of San José. The former agreement was evaluated and found to benefit the university more than it did the CCSS (Villalobos Solano et al., 2004).

All in all, the Costa Rican health system is rational. Its functioning is effective and efficient. It 'trains' doctors and nurses by structuring their job and providing the necessary resources. The system's organization permits and favours individualized, rather than one-size-fits-all, clinical activities. Medical schools offer in-service training within CCSS services. Unlike the case in many developing countries, continuing medical education is based not on seminars but on clinical rotations in well-functioning facilities. Area medical officers involve themselves in clinical medicine and use this experience to provide technical assistance to first-line physicians. Teamwork has been introduced and is practiced by many of the health teams. In fact the limitations in competition between providers favour cooperation among them. Evaluation is part of the medical culture and is promoted by the system.

Costa Rican health professionals generally display strong motivation for their work and a high level of identification with their health system as a result of several factors, including the following:

- Incomes are adequate, and there is a high degree of social prestige associated with their work.

- The organizational structure leaves room for creative decision making.

- Managers below the regional level are appointed on technical merit, after a selection procedure that includes an examination.
- The system is explicitly based on solidarity and equity, which may satisfy the political identities of certain professionals.

Health service output

In terms of health service output, although improvements are still needed, use and coverage rates are excellent. Use of medical health services in Costa Rica is high in comparison with other developing countries: there were 0.58 new general practitioner consultations and 0.33 new specialist consultations per capita during 2002, for example, and a hospital admission rate of 8.1% (Departamento de Información Estadística de los Servicios de Salud, 2003b). However, there are problems with accessibility, as suggested by the changing share of emergency consultations, which increased from 16% of all medical consultations in 1980 to 38% in 2002. Still, the overall high use rates observed are compatible with a level of acceptable, affordable and quality health care.

The coverage rates achieved by various types of programmes are high. In 2002, for example, 96% of Costa Rican women used some form of contraception (Maine et al., 1997), and antenatal care services were provided to 87% of all pregnant women (Departamento de Información Estadística de los Servicios de Salud, 2003b). Well-baby clinics were accessible to virtually all children aged under 1 year, and the immunization coverage rate was above 91% for all antigens (Departamento de Información Estadística de los Servicios de Salud, 2003b; Maine et al., 1997). Coverage rates among chronic patients in first-line facilities were 73% for hypertensive disorders and 61% for diabetes (Departamento de Información Estadística de los Servicios de Salud, 2003b; Maine et al., 1997).

There has been effective integration between disease-control programmes and health care delivery services since the initiation of the 'integrated care' system established by the 1993 reforms. Up until that time, CCSS units had delivered health care services and MoH units had provided disease-control interventions, hampering integration of these entities (Unidad de Estadística del Ministerio de Salud, 2003). This more recent integration process, although still not completed, partly explains the disease-control successes achieved in Costa Rica, such as a low malaria incidence of 48 per 100,000 in 2000 and no reported cases of measles in 2002.

Integration of care between the EBAISs (on the first line) and hospitals (as referral structures) can be improved. A referral–counter-referral system, although available in theory, is not well used. Significant numbers of primary care consultations occur in hospital emergency rooms, resulting in poor, non-integrated, non-holistic care. Part of this phenomenon can be seen in the administrative structure of the CCSS: the EBAISs have no administrative links with hospitals, area medical officers have no authority over hospitals and budget allocations take into account past workloads, resulting in EBAISs and hospitals competing for the same patients instead of performing complementary functions.

The ways in which promotion and prevention are implemented also lead to patients being pushed to emergency departments. For example, it is perhaps the case that prevention at the PHC level is overly standardized. The existence of strong mandatory preventive programmes in the EBAISs leads doctors to neglect non-standard prevention activities during consultations (i.e., activities not included in their established performance agreements, for instance addressing obesity, depression, tobacco, and drug addiction).

In addition, certain disease-control programmes (especially those focusing on chronic conditions such as diabetes and hypertension) and care services targeting high-risk groups (pregnant women, children younger than 5 years, adolescents and elderly) overstretch the performance agreements of the EBAISs. As a consequence the general practitioners in these primary care facilities see their availability for curative services reduced, with hospital emergency departments filling the gap.

An additional explanation for hospitals' large share of primary care services is that emergency departments are particularly attractive to non-contributors (who are responsible for up to one of every three hospital consultations) such as migrants and citizens not covered by social insurance (Departamento de Información Estadística de los Servicios de Salud, 2003b). There is also room to improve overall health care efficiency, as suggested by the following: (1) EBAISs (as described) do not function particularly well as gatekeepers; (2) between 1997 and 2002, the number of laboratory tests increased by 45% and prescription drug consumption by 24% (or more, given that data from private providers might not be included in these figures) (Departamento de Información Estadística de los Servicios de Salud, 2003b); (3) average lengths of stay are 3 days or less in some peripheral hospitals (Departamento de Información Estadística de los Servicios de Salud, 2003b), possibly as a result of avoidable admissions; and (4) the caesarean section rate was close to 22% in 2002 (UNICEF and WHO guidelines say the maximum acceptable level is 15%) (Departamento de Información Estadística de los Servicios de Salud, 2003b; Maine et al., 1997).

Effects on human development

With its combination of a middle-income population and a policy emphasis on human development, Costa Rica is an exceptional developing country. With 40% of its population still living in rural areas, the following achievements of Costa Rica in 2002 are even more remarkable (Maine et al., 1997):

- Only 9.5% of the population was below the USD 2 per day income poverty level and only 2.0% below USD 1 per day (vs. 22.6% and 8.2%, respectively, in Colombia and 26.3% and 9.9% in Mexico).
- Ninety-five percent and 93% of the population had sustainable access to drinking water and sanitation, respectively (vs. 91% and 86% in Colombia and 88% and 74% in Mexico).
- The literacy rate was 95.8% (vs. 92.1% in Colombia and 90.5% in Mexico).
- The Gini index, a measurement of inequality in the distribution of income or consumption within a country, expressed as a percentage, with 0 representing perfect equality and 100 representing perfect inequality, was 46.5 (vs. 57.6 in Colombia and 54.6 in Mexico).
- The country's gender-empowerment initiatives were superior to those of all other Latin American countries.
- Life expectancy at birth was 78 years (second only to Canada in the Americas).
- The infant mortality rate was 9 per 1000, representing a seven-times reduction over a 3-decade span (vs. 19 per 1000 and a four-times reduction in Colombia and 24 per 1000 and a three-times reduction in Mexico).
- The tuberculosis prevalence rate was 19 per 100,000 population (vs. 69 in Colombia and 44 in Mexico).

Several of these features are related to the social commitments of successive Costa Rican governments. The absence of armed forces, one of the country's unique features, allowed for strong social investments, with public expenditures on health and education, respectively, of 4.9% and 4.7% of GDP in 2001 (as compared with 3.6% and 4.4% in Colombia and 2.7% and 5.1% in MexicoMexico) (United Nations Development Programme, 2004).

Numerous indicators suggest effects directly attributable to health services. For example, comparisons of infant and maternal mortality reductions with countries in the same region at similar income levels reveal that Costa Rica has made significant advances (Table 6.2). Also, the perinatal mortality rate dropped from 12.0 per 1000 in 1972 to 5.4 per 1000 in 2001 (Departamento de Información Estadística de los Servicios de Salud, 2003a), which suggests obstetric improvements. Finally, pneumonia-specific mortality among infants aged younger than 1 year dropped from 5.4 per 1000 in 1972 to 0.3 per 1000 in 2001 (Departamento de Información Estadística de los Servicios de Salud, 2003a), suggesting improved and faster access to health services, and tuberculosis-specific mortality in the general population decreased from 7.2 per 100,000 in 1972 to 4.4 per 100,000 in 2001 (United Nations Development Programme, 2004) despite increased incidence levels, suggesting effective interventions.

Public policies in support of Costa Rica's health services help explain these high development standards and health status indicators. Whereas the average percentage of private health expenditures at the end of the twentieth century was 58% among Latin American countries as a whole, it was only 25% in Costa Rica (Molina et al., 2000), and only 0.12% of Costa Rican households had suffered a catastrophic health expenditure (in sharp contrast with Colombia, for instance, where 6.26% of households incurred such an expenditure) (Xu et al., 2003). In addition Costa Rican public health expenditures have focused on equity, with 29% targeting the poorest income quintile and 11% targeting the richest (Trejos, 2002), in 2000. This situation differs markedly from that of Ecuador, for example, where the richest quintile accounted for 30% of public health expenditures in 2000.

The Costa Rican approach reduced health inequities between 1980 and 2000 as well; potential years of life lost were reduced by 48% in the poorest quintile of the population and by 39% in the richest. Public health expenditures were found to be the most equitable component of social investment (Trejos, 2002), with the poorest families receiving the largest proportion of resources. This investment is progressive in that it reduces income inequality. However, those groups that contribute most to social insurance (i.e., the upper income quintiles) are the ones that use its services the least, given their tendency to seek services from private ambulatory providers. This situation may result in reductions in solidarity and support for the CCSS among members of the higher classes.

Not everything in Costa Rica is positive. For example, before showing a reverse trend in 2002, income inequality rose between 1997 and 2001, with households in the richest quintile earning 8 times more than households in the poorest quintile in 1997 and 11 times more in 2001 (Programa Estado de la Nación, 2004). A similar pattern was evident in the human development index, which decreased from 0.889 in 1997 to 0.797 in 2000 and then rose from 0.821 in 2001 to 0.834 in 2004. Public health expenditures decreased from 77% to 71% between 1991 and 2001 (Pan American Health Organization, 2003). The major component of the increase in private expenditures was household-level out-of-pocket payments.

The CCSS has continued to contract out more diagnosis and treatment procedures to the private sector as well. As a result more patients are using private services, in which over prescription is a common practice. For instance, between 1997 and 2002, the number of x-rays requested by private doctors and paid for by the CCSS increased by 41% (Departamento de Información Estadística de los Servicios de Salud, 2003b). Of equal concern is that, as the share of private health expenditures has increased, total expenditures on health care have risen steeply (Pan American Health Organization, 2003).

All in all, Costa Rica's health policy during the past 30 years has been effective and equitable. The country's health system basically comprises a form of compulsory social health insurance, with 50% of contributions from households (25% direct contributions to social insurance and 25% out of pocket), 40% from employers, 5% from the state and a very small percentage from international loans. Several political and social elements have allowed this relative equity in the dimensions of financing, access and health outcomes. For example:

Intelligent decision makers have been involved in policy making, some of them educated in Europe (for instance, Calderón Guardia, considered the 'father' of Costa Rican social insurance, observed and appreciated the Belgian social security system during his training in that country).

Middle-class groups with a vision and strong trade unions had an impact as well. Moreover, given that the middle classes still use CCSS services, they provide indispensable political support. A certain degree of inequity in use of public expenditures may be the necessary price to pay for a public sector with a high level of political support.

Recently, several factors have jeopardized the Costa Rican political and health systems. Firstly, some of the executive staff of the CCSS have come under attack by the press, leading to the resignation of a CEO and several top executives. Moreover, various former heads of state and one ex-president of the CCSS are under investigation. Painful as these events may seem, they may actually lead to an institutional strengthening of Costa Rica, where the vast majority of citizens proudly express confidence in their political and judicial structures (Seligson, 2000). Secondly, for more than 10 years, CCSS executive officers have been selected through a political process. The institution has generally overcome this drawback through the strength of its organization at the operational and middle administration levels.

Thirdly, there is an oversupply of physicians because of increases in private medical faculties. This group could represent a future, powerful lobby for the privatization of PHC services. Finally, the most worrying phenomenon is the continuing external pressure (Homedes & Ugalde, 2005), with clear economic interests, to privatize large sectors of the health delivery system, including primary care. Until now, a majority of health professionals and the Costa Rican population have resisted such threats.

Conclusions

The impressive advances made by the Costa Rican health system have been the result of an intelligent social and democratic long-term policy and the establishment of a public compulsory social health insurance system. Such coherence in policy might be equally or more important than financing, as highlighted by the poor improvements in the health status of populations in other comparable Latin American countries.

Necessary improvements in the system could target relatively minor issues. Bio-psychosocial and patient-centred care could be promoted in PHC services, reducing the bureaucratic burden generated by disease-control and prevention programmes. In-service training and mentoring could be introduced, as well as action research and evaluation applied to health programmes. Together these measures could optimize time management among first-line health professionals, increase efficiency, and reduce waiting lists.

In addition, coordination of primary and hospital care and continuity of care could be improved with the organization of local health systems. Hospital costs could be cut without hampering the quality of health care (for instance, by avoiding unnecessary admissions). The MoH (in a true role of stewardship) should control the proliferation of private medical schools to avoid a contingent of second-rate professionals. Finally, the CCSS should re-evaluate its overstretched contracting-in mechanism (consisting of performance agreements) and carefully analyze its limited experiences in contracting with private for-profit services.

International entities should pay particular attention to several successful policy features of Costa Rica's health system:

- The unique, unified public system facilitates integration;
- Publicly oriented services function as the dominant (but not monopolistic) means of care delivery;
- Contracting in is a cornerstone of the national health policy (as opposed to the practice of contracting with private for-profit services);
- Both users and communities participate in health service management (in contrast to the situation in the private for-profit sector);
- Government expenditures represent the bulk of overall health expenditures;
- There is, for the most part, no purchaser–provider split or hospital managerial autonomy;
- There is a single public insurer (private insurance being virtually non-existent).

In view of the remarkable and long-lasting achievements of the heterodox Costa Rican social and democratic approach, we believe Costa Rica should become a benchmark for international donors and decision makers. In fact orthodox health policy axioms may need to be reassessed.

Acknowledgements

We are indebted to the Belgian Directorate-General of Development Cooperation for the funding of the research and to Rocío Saenz, MD, ex-minister of health of Costa Rica, for pivotal comments on this chapter.

Note: The authors are solely responsible for any errors present in this article.

References

Cueto M. (2004). The origins of primary health care and selective primary health care. *American Journal of Public Health*, **94**(11), pp. 1864–74.

De Groote T., De Paepe P., & Unger J. P. (2005). Colombia: In vivo test of health sector privatization in the developing world. *International Journal of Health Services*, 35(1), pp. 125–41.

Departamento de Información Estadística de los Servicios de Salud. (2003a). *Cambios en la morbilidad y mortalidad por edad y sexo, Costa Rica, 1987, 1992, 1997 y 2002*. San José, Costa Rica: Caja Costarricense de Seguro Social, Gerencia de División Médica, Dirección Técnica de Servicios de Salud. Serie Estadísticas de la Salud No. 8C.

Departamento de Información Estadística de los Servicios de Salud. (2003b). *Estadísticas generales de los servicios de atención de la salud, 1980–2002*. San José, Costa Rica: Caja Costarricense de Seguro Social, Gerencia de División Médica, Dirección Técnica de Servicios de Salud. Serie Estadísticas de la Salud No. 5–1.

Estado de la Nación. (1999). Programa Estado de la Nación en Desarrollo Humano Sostenible. Equidad e integración social. In: Forastelli M. R., et al., eds. *Quinto Informe Sobre El Estado De La Nación*. San José, Costa Rica: Estado de la Nación. http://www.estadonacion.or.cr/Info99/nacion5/cap1–98b.html.

Estado de la Nación. (2001). *Programa Estado de la Nación en Desarrollo Humano Sostenible. Informe de la auditoria ciudadana sobre la calidad de la democracia en Costa Rica. Programa de Estado de la Nación*. San José, Costa Rica: Estado de la Nación.

Freedom House. (2004). *Annual Freedom in the World Country Scores, 1973 Through 2007*. Washington, DC: Freedom House.

Gauri V., Cercone J., & Briceno R. (2004). Separating financing from provision: Evidence from 10 years of partnership with health cooperatives in Costa Rica. *Health Policy and Planning*, **19**(5), pp. 292–301.

Homedes N. & Ugalde A. (2002). Privatización de los servicios de salud: las experiencias de Chile y Costa Rica. *GAC Sanit*, **16**(1), pp. 54–62.

Homedes N. & Ugalde A. (2005). Why neoliberal health reforms have failed in Latin America. *Health Policy*, **71**(1), pp. 83–96.

Lobe J. (2001). *Learn from Cuba, says World Bank*. Washington, DC: Inter Press Service.

Maine D., Wardlaw T. M., Ward V. M., McCarthy J., Akalin M. Z., & Brown J. E. (1997). *Guidelines for Monitoring the Availability and Use of Obstetric Services*. New York: United Nations Children's Fund.

Martínez-Franzoni J. (2006). ¿Presión o legitimación? Poder y alternativas en el diseño y adopción de la reforma de salud en Costa Rica, 1988–1998. *História, Ciências, Saúde – Manguinhos*, **13**(3), pp. 591–622.

Mesa-Lago C. (2005). *Las Reformas De Salud En América Latina y El Caribe: Su Impacto En Los Principios De La Seguridad Social., LC/W.63 edn*. Santiago de Chile: Naciones Unidas.

Mkandawire T. (2006). *Disempowering New Democracies and the Persistence of Poverty*. Geneva: United Nations Research Institute for Social Development.

Molina R., Pinto M., Henderson P., & Vieira C. (2000). Gasto y financiamiento en salud: situación y tendencias. *Revista Panamerica de Salud Publica*, **8**(1–2), pp. 71–83.

Morgan L. M. (1990). International politics and primary health care in Costa Rica. *Social Science & Medicine*, **30**(2), pp. 211–9.

Organisation for Economic Co-operation and Development. (2003). *OECD Health Data 2003: A Comparative Analysis of 30 Countries*. Paris: Organisation for Economic Co-operation and Development.

Organisation for Economic Co-operation and Development. (2004). *OECD Health Data 2004: A Comparative Analysis of 30 Countries*. Paris: Organisation for Economic Co-operation and Development.

Pan American Health Organization (2003). *Gasto y financiamiento de la salud en Costa Rica: situación actual, tendencias y retos*. San José, Costa Rica: Organización Panamericana de la Salud, Ministerio de Salud, Caja Costarricense de Seguro Social.

Preker A. S. (1997). *Health, Nutrition and Population Strategy Paper*. Washington, DC: The World Bank.

Programa Estado de la Nación. (2004). *Compendio estadístico*. San José, Costa Rica: Estado de la Nación.

Rodríguez Herrera A. (2006). La reforma de salud en Costa Rica. Santiago de Chile: Naciones Unidas, Comisión Económica para América Latina y el Caribe (CEPAL), *Unidad de Estudios Especiales*. 173.

Rosero-Bixby L. (1986). Infant mortality in Costa Rica: Explaining the recent decline. *Studies in Family Planning*, **17**(2), pp. 57–65.

Rosero-Bixby L. (2004). Spatial access to health care in Costa Rica and its equity: A GIS-based study. *Social Science & Medicine*, **58**(7), pp. 1271–84.

Saenz Madrigal R. & Ulate E. A. (2002). *Análisis sectorial de salud Costa Rica 2002*. San José, Costa Rica: Ministerio de Salud.

Seligson M. A. (2000). *Toward a model of democratic stability: Political culture in Central America. Estudios Interdisciplinarios de América Latina y el Caribe (EIAL)*. Tel Aviv, Israel: Tel Aviv University.

Seligson M. A., Martínez J., & Trejos J. D. (1997). Reducción de la pobreza en Costa Rica: el impacto de las políticas públicas. In: Zevallos J. V., ed. *Estrategias Para Reducir La Pobreza En América Latina y El Caribe. Proyecto 'Mitgación de la Pobreza y Desarrollo Social' edn*. Quito, Ecuador: Programa de Naciones Unidas para el Desarrollo, pp. 105–92.

Trejos J. D. (2002). *La equidad de la inversión social en el 2000. Octavo informe sobre el Estado de la Nación en desarrollo humano sostenible*. San José, Costa Rica: Estado de la Nación.

UNICEF. (2002). *The State of the World's Children 2003*. New York: UNICEF.

UNICEF, World Health Organization, & United Nations Population Fund. (1997). *Guidelines for Monitoring the Availability and Use of Obstetric Services*. WA 310 97GU. Geneva: World Health Organization.

Unidad de Estadística del Ministerio de Salud. (2003). *Indicadores básicos: situación de salud en Costa Rica 2003*. San José, Costa Rica: Ministerio de Salud, Organización Panamericane de la Salud / Organización Mundial de la Salud.

United Nations Development Programme. (2003). *Human Development Report 2003. Millennium Development Goals: A Compact Among Nations to End Human Poverty*. New York: UNDP.

United Nations Development Programme (2004). *Human Development Report 2004: Cultural Liberty in Today's Diverse World*. New York: UNDP.

United Nations. (2006). *Shaping the Future of Social Protection: Access, Financing and SOLIDARITY*. Montevideo, Uruguay: United Nations – Economic Commission for Latin America and the Caribbean (ECLAC). LC/G.2294(SES.31/3)/I.

Villalobos Solano L. B., Chamizo García H., Piedra González M., Navarro Vargas A.,

Carballo Rosabal M., & Vargas Fuentes M. (2004). *¿Es la contratación gubernamental de servicios de salud privados en el primer nivel de atención en Centroamérica una opción para asegurar una atención eficiente, equitativa y sostenible?* San José, Costa Rica: Programa Investigación en Políticas de Salud, Escuela de Salud Pública, Universidad de Costa Rica.

Walsh J. A. & Warren K. S. (1979). Selective primary health care: An interim strategy for disease control in developing countries. *New England Journal of Medicine*, **301**(18), pp. 967–74.

World Bank (1993). *World Development Report 1993: Investing in Health*. London: Oxford University Press.

World Bank. (2001). *Development Committee Press Conference*. Washington, DC: World Bank.

World Bank. (2004a). *Spotlight on Costa Rica and Cuba*. Washington, DC: World Bank.

World Bank. (2004b). *World Development Indicators 2001*. Washington, DC: World Bank.

Xu K., Evans D. B., Kawabata K., Zeramdini R., Klavus J., & Murray C. J. L. (2003). Household catastrophic health expenditure: A multicountry analysis. *Lancet*, **362**(9378), pp. 111–7.

**Section 3
Chapter**

7

Impact of international health policies on access to health in middle-income countries: some experiences from Latin America

Colombia: in vivo test of health sector privatization in the developing world

Adapted from: De Groote T., De Paepe P., & Unger J.-P. (2005). Colombia: In vivo test of health sector privatization in the developing world. *International Journal of Health Services*, **35**(1), pp. 125–41.

Introduction

The reform of the Colombian health sector in 1993 was founded on the internationally promoted paradigm of privatization of health care delivery. Taking into account the lack of empirical evidence for the applicability of this concept to developing countries and the documented experience of failures in other countries, Colombia tried to overcome these problems by a theoretically sound, but complex, model. Some 10 years after the implementation of 'Law 100,' a review of the literature shows that the proposed goals of universal coverage and equitable access to high-quality care have not been reached. Despite an explosion in costs and a considerable increase in public and private health expenditure, more than 40% of the population is still not covered by health insurance, and access to health care proves increasingly difficult. Furthermore, key health indicators and disease-control programmes have deteriorated. These findings confirm the results in other LMICs. The authors suggest the explanation lies in the inefficiency of contracting out; the weak economic, technical and political capacity of the Colombian Government for regulation and control; and the absence of real participation of the poor in decision making on (health) policies.

Privatization of health care delivery in developing countries received support from virtually all international aid agencies (European Commission, 2002; World Bank, 1997; World Health Organization, 2000). Expressions such as 'stewardship' and 'steering rather than rowing,' used in policy documents on the global agenda for health sector reform from the WB and WHO (Human Development Network, 1993; World Health Organization, 1999), allude to the desired characteristics of this new PPP. The recommendation that clinical care delivery be contracted out to private for-profit organizations, while MoH first-line facilities limit their field of operations to disease control, changes the role of the public sector to provide less and control more. Article 1.3(c) of the WTO GATS could even be interpreted as prohibiting the provision of health care services that are not related to disease-control programmes within subsidized government health services. The current wave of sector reforms is underpinned by seductive theoretical arguments (Preker et al., 1999). However, there is a lack of empirical evidence that in developing countries, private for-profit health care companies and providers can deliver high-quality care that covers entire populations (Sen & Koivusalo, 1998).

Colombia is probably one of the rare developing countries that has adopted contracting out as the key paradigm of its national health care policy and committed a sufficient budget to health care, with an increase in national budget allocated to health from 3.5% of GDP in 1993 to 5.5% in 1999 (Departamento Nacional de Planeación et al., 2001). This article examines evidence in the published and the 'grey' literature to assess whether health care privatization in Colombia has managed to (a) improve insurance coverage, (b) improve access to and utilization of health services, (c) improve the health status of the population, and (d) control health expenditures growth. It goes on to look at the mechanisms involved and relates these findings to the country's health policy.

Features of Colombia's reform

Reform of the health sector in Colombia started in the 1980s with a process of political, fiscal and administrative decentralization. This was followed by the implementation of Law 100 in 1993, which resulted in a general system of social health security with two main features: purchaser–provider split and contracting out. The individual effects of decentralization as against those of Law 100 are sometimes difficult to distinguish because 'at times they are synergic and at other times antagonistic' (Yepes & Sánchez, 2000). Nevertheless, correlation over time can give an inkling of the causal effect of one or other of these reform processes.

Law 100 provided the legal framework for the creation of a decentralized social health insurance with universal coverage, based on the principles of equity, solidarity, efficiency, quality and community participation. This ambitious proposal was made possible by petroleum discovery, providing the financial capacity to introduce a 'Big R' reform (Berman & Bossert, 2000). Two systems were created:

- The contributory system for those who can afford it, mainly the formally employed, who contribute 12% of their salary for health insurance. The Health Promoting Enterprises (HPE) (Empresas Promotores de Salud, EPS) receive a premium per capita, adjusted according to age, sex and geographic location. The Obligatory Health Plan (OHP), managed by the HPE, covers a complete package of health interventions.
- The subsidized system, which covers the rest of the population. Funding is obtained from the contributory system and by government subsidies. The capitation fee, and the accompanying package of services offered, was arbitrarily fixed at 50% of the value of the contributory system. Subsidized System Administrators (SSA) (Administradores de Regimen Subsidiado, ARS) are responsible for the management of this scheme.

It was expected that by 2001 the benefits in the subsidized scheme would equal those of the obligatory plan of the contributory system (El Congreso de Colombia, 1993).

A national survey (Sistema de Selección de Beneficiarios a Programas Sociales del gobierno, SISBEN) assessed the socio-economic status of the population and categorized it in six strata (1 being the poorest, 6 the richest). Those belonging to strata 3 to 6 would join the contributory system, and the subsidized system accommodated strata 1 and 2. This was the theory. In practice 13.7% of the non-poor were in the subsidized system and 10.7% of the poor population were registered in the contributory system (Pan American Health Organization, 2002). Health care delivery institutions (HCDI) (Instituciones Prestadores de Servicios de Salud; IPS) and the autonomous former public hospitals and health centres (Empresas Sociales del Estado; ESE) were contracted by the insurance entities for health service delivery. HPE, SSA, and HCDI could be public or private or mixed, and for-profit or not-for-profit.

The state assumed a steering role of policy formulation, monitoring and evaluation, freeing itself quasi-completely from directly offering services. Exceptions were activities with high externalities (mainly disease-control programmes) and health care delivery for the uninsured (the vinculados). Managed competition between public and private providers of care, with free choice of insurer by the population, would safeguard the quality and efficiency of health care. In practice the provider was chosen by the insurer, limiting people's freedom to choose a provider to an indirect option.

Insurance coverage

Two achievements were claimed to illustrate the success of the Colombian health reform:

- A considerable advance in social insurance coverage following health sector reform: health insurance almost doubled between 1992 and 1997, from 26% to 52% of the population (Colombia Country Management Unit & PREM Sector Management Unit, 2002) (Figure 7.1).
- A growth in health insurance coverage that was highest among the poor: coverage in the poorest 10% of the population rose from 4 to 41% between 1992 and 1997, a 10-fold increase, whereas the increase among the richest 10% was from 65 to 80% (Colombia Country Management Unit & PREM Sector Management Unit, 2002)[1](Riveros, 2004).

Let us assess these claims. Firstly, although before the reform 69% of the population did not have any form of insurance, this does not imply that they did not receive medical treatment. The reform entailed a shift from a supply-oriented model (without the need to register) to a demand-oriented model (Organización Mundial de la Salud et al., 2001). According to the National Household Survey (NHS) (Encuesta Nacional de Hogares; ENH) of 1992, dating from before the reform, 81% of the population claimed to have access to health services (Organización Mundial de la Salud et al., 2001).

Another issue is equity in insurance coverage. Most poor people were not covered by the pre-reform health insurance, which was mainly for the officially employed. The 10-fold increase in coverage for the poorest 10% of the population differs greatly from the progress among the richest 10% (from 65% to 80%), but insurance coverage among the poor is still only half that of the rich. Furthermore, only one-quarter of the newly insured entered the subsidized system, while the rest enrolled in the contributory scheme (Colombia Country

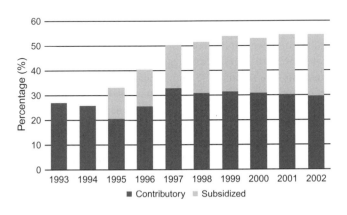

Figure 7.1. Evolution of health insurance coverage, 1993–2002. *Source:* Rivero, G. Ministerio de Salud de Colombia. Pan American Health Organization. Diez años de la reforma a la seguridad social de salud en Colombia (1993–2003). Powerpoint Presentation at http://www.isapre.cl/seminarios/SeminarioColombia/Dr_Riveros.ppt

---

[1] Most information is derived from two national surveys: the National Household Survey (Encuesta Nacional de Hogares) of 1992 with data from the pre-reform period, and the National Quality of Life Survey of 1997, conducted 3 years after implementation of the reform. Much of our discussion therefore compares the 1992 and 1997 situations.

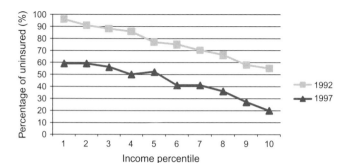

Figure 7.2. Percentage of uninsured (vinculados) as function of income percentile, 1992 and 1997. *Source:* Colombia Country Management Unit, PREM Sector Management Unit. Latin America and the Caribbean Region Colombia Poverty Report. World Bank, 2002.

Management Unit & PREM Sector Management Unit, 2002). The largest share of expansion of enrolment in the contributory system was due to incorporation of family members and dependents of those previously covered by the social security regime – an increase in family coverage from 18% of members to 100% (Almeida et al., 2000). This increase was thus not accompanied by an increase in revenues from contributions, as these still consisted of 12% of the salary of those officially employed.

In fact, the curve depicting the evolution of the percentage of people enrolled shows a stagnating trend over several years (see Figure 7.1). More than 40% of the population remains without health insurance – more than 16 million people. These vinculados receive treatment in public hospitals against a payment of 30% of the actual cost, as a continuation of the pre-reform supply-oriented model. Most of these people are in the lower income groups. Figure 7.2 shows the distribution of these vinculados over the different income groups. This distribution casts doubt on the process of equity, as the difference in improvement between the lowest and highest income groups is less impressive and the coverage increase is similar across income percentiles. For example, in income percentile 1, the percentage of uninsured diminished 37%, and in percentile 10 dropped 35% (Jaramillo, 2002). The largest proportion of uninsured population – the challenge to achieving universal coverage – remains in the lowest income groups.

The number of persons enrolled in a health insurance scheme has stagnated at around 55% since 1998 (Figure 7.1). Twenty-five percent of the two richest deciles remain outside these schemes, because they have the means to opt for private insurance, thus avoiding responsibility for solidarity. Furthermore, two-thirds of those eligible have not enrolled in the subsidized system, although their enrolment is free. The lack of information available to the poor, the prime target group of the reform mechanisms, has sometimes been invoked to explain this (Plaza et al., 2001). But 10 years after implementation of Law 100, this is unlikely. Even if the government and insurance companies were not duly informing people information would have spread by word of mouth if the health services were providing effective, affordable care. Rather, the failure to interest the poorest Colombians could be rooted in the reform process itself.

While Law 100, Article 153, states that 'the General Social Health Insurance System will gradually provide health services of equal quality to all the inhabitants of Colombia, independent of their capacity to pay,' the creation of two different systems runs counter to this objective. Insufficient solidarity between rich and poor, reflected in the financing schemes, results in a package of services for the subsidized system that is generally only half of a reference standard of what is possible and necessary in Colombia – that is, the package of the contributory scheme (Félix et al., 2002). For instance, hospitalization in an internal medicine ward or follow-up for chronic diseases – which typify the epidemiological transition – are excluded from the subsidized package (such as diabetes; cardiovascular diseases other than hypertension). The reluctance of those in the poorest percentiles to enrol in the subsidized system might reflect a refusal of such a package – even if fashioned along a cost-effectiveness rationale. An additional explanation – cream-skimming (risk selection) – could be invoked if data on insurance coverage of the poor by private companies were available (we did not have access to such data).

It has been argued that only those with full insurance coverage should be counted when determining enrolment rate (Félix et al., 2002). Those with half the package (in the subsidized system) cannot really be considered insured, as they are entitled only to essential clinical services, some surgical interventions and the treatment of catastrophic diseases (Organización Mundial de la Salud et al., 2001). This is important, as the law foresaw an equal health plan for all. In practice the health plan of the subsidized system has never exceeded 70% of the contributory system package (Hernández, 2002).

Finally, insurance coverage was overestimated because of multiple enrolments. In a survey in March 2000, 2.3% of the population (500,000 people) declared that they held more than one insurance card. People enrol with different insurance companies with a futile expectation of getting better care – although all companies offer the same legal package. Further distortion of insurance estimates may be related to the fact that some names are not immediately erased from an insurance list while the individuals are changing insurer or losing their job (Organización Mundial de la Salud et al., 2001). This frequent practice permits insurers to obtain the full capitation fee while providing a fraction of the required care.

Access to and use of health services

What does 'enrolment in a health insurance plan' really mean? Basically, it means nothing more than a person holding an insurance card. Indeed several obstacles keep cardholders from accessing health care services (Plaza et al., 2001):

- Some insurance companies have declared persons or families, especially the poor, to be registered for their scheme without issuing an insurance card, thus collecting premiums without providing service.
- The poor are frequently unaware of their rights. They do not know how to use their insurance card, and they continue to pay for the services they receive.
- Sometimes, they simply do not use the services because of a lack of psychological, intra-institutional, financial (see below), or geographic accessibility.
- Investigations about enrolment are abundant because data are easy to obtain, but evidence on actual access to care is rare, and data on real utilization of the health services even more so.
- A comparison of pre-reform 1992 national household survey with 1997 National Quality of Life Survey (NQLS) data suggests an improvement in access to care in absolute numbers. However, when converted to the percentage of population covered by health insurance who report receiving treatment when sick, the comparison reveals a reduction of 3% (Colombia Country Management Unit & PREM Sector Management Unit, 2002). This lower treatment rate may in part be attributable to the larger demands placed on the system.

Other proxies permit one to indirectly assess access to care:

- High percentages of death without diagnosis are typical of poor municipalities with a high prevalence of unsatisfied basic needs. In Colombia institutionally certified mortality is higher in the richer municipalities: 50.5% for stratum 6, according to unsatisfied basic needs, versus 28.6% for stratum 1 (Pan American Health Organization, 2002).

- Yearly doctor utilization rate: before the reform, 61.7% of people needing health care were actually seen by a doctor. In 2000 this proportion had fallen to 51.1% (Colombia Country Management Unit & PREM Sector Management Unit, 2002; Yepes; 2003).
- Co-payments – meant to put a limit on demand related to moral hazard – can also limit access to health care (Manning et al., 1987). Admittedly, in 1992, 51% of patients did not consult a doctor because they lacked the money to do so (1992 national household survey), versus 41% in 1997 (Plaza et al., 2001). But this is certainly not an impressive gain, even if the data are reliable despite different methodologies in the two surveys. Moreover, national rates erase significant geographic fluctuations, ranging from 29.1% in Bogota to 62.2% in the poor Atlantic region (Profamilia Colombia, 2000). In the population without health insurance finances remained the first obstacle to consulting a doctor, and for insured persons was the second – perceived lack of seriousness of the illness was the first (Almeida et al., 2000).

Disease control and heath indicators

In the decades preceding reform, Colombia, like most developing countries, underwent a decrease in most morbidity and mortality indicators. This trend changed direction in the second half of the 1990s.

Infant mortality rate is known to reflect general social and economic conditions, not just access to medical care (Van Lerberghe & De Brouwere, 1989). However, child mortality due to acute respiratory infections and acute diarrhoeal diseases can be considered avoidable mortality and these deaths can be used as tracer pathologies for quality of care (Rutstein et al., 1976), also in less developed countries (Westerling, 2001). These deaths are clearly on the rise since 1997 (Pan American Health Organization, 2002). Disorders of the perinatal period, including perinatal mortality, are also known to be an indicator for access to quality health care. The rate doubled from 1996 to 1997 and continues to rise (Pan American Health Organization, 2002).

A decline of vaccination coverage was documented both at local (Ayala & Kroeger, 2002) and national levels (Profamilia Colombia, 2000). Between 1990 and 2000, the national coverage for total vaccination of children below 1 year of age dropped from 67.5 to 52% (Yepes, 2003), even more in rural areas (Málaga et al., 2001). This deterioration could be related to excessive emphasis on programmes that adhere to an explicit demand (Jaramillo, 1997), difficulties in accessing vaccination services, excessive procedures and documentation requested by the insurers (Ayala & Kroeger, 2002) and decreased budgets (Málaga et al., 2001).

Malaria and tuberculosis control and the Extended Program on Immunisation (EPI) are vertical disease-control programmes in Colombia. They form an important part of the public health functions assumed by the government. Malaria transmission was on the increase, and the magnitude of the rise cannot be explained just by better diagnosis and by environmental conditions (El Niño 1997–1998). A decline of protective measures due to the decentralization process and fragmentation of responsibilities probably contributed to the problem (Kroeger et al., 2002).

In line with Pérez (Pérez Gilberto, 2003), data on tuberculosis control can give some insight into the functioning of the whole Colombian health system, as suspicion of tuberculosis (and often diagnosis) occurs in the private sector while treatment and follow-up are the responsibility of MoH services. The steady and progressive decline in tuberculosis incidence

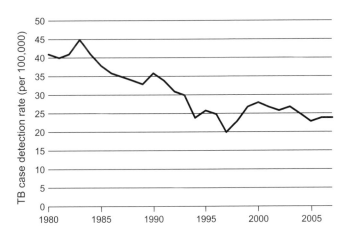

Figure 7.3. Tuberculosis (TB) notification rate, 1980–2007, as percentage. *Note:* TB case detection rate per 100,000 of population. Number shown is the notification rate of new and relapse cases. *Source:* WHO, Global Tuberculosis Control: Surveillance, Planning, Financing, Report. Geneva, 2009.

had a reversed trend in 1997 and rose steadily, from 8,042 reported cases in 1997 to 11,261 in 2002 (Pérez Gilberto, 2003). At the same time the already low notification rate further deteriorated with the introduction of the social security system, to reach an all-time low of 20–25% (see Figure 7.3). Other studies have shown a marked decrease in the number of tuberculosis patients under treatment (Kroeger et al., 2002).

It is difficult to disentangle the numerous determinants of tuberculosis incidence, among them Colombia's 5-year recession and the HIV epidemic. However, some control programmes' organizational features, related to the Colombian reform, have probably played a significant role:

- The reform caused fragmentation of responsibilities of the different aspects of diagnosis, treatment and follow-up of patients and contacts (Kroeger et al., 2002).
- Insurance companies and private health care providers are not prepared to spend time and resources on activities that are not rewarded financially (Lönnroth et al., 1999; Uplekar et al., 2001). Lack of health care–disease-control integration is known to reduce detection and cure rates while increasing delays for patients (Unger et al., 2003).

Financing

Health expenditure has skyrocketed since the introduction of managed competition in Colombia. On theoretical grounds, the trend could have been predicted as inherent to the system (Broomberg, 1994b). It has also been observed in other countries that have introduced a system based on a demand-oriented model (Labelle et al., 1994), from the US (Tabbush & Swanson, 1996) to Lebanon (Van Lerberghe et al., 1997) and Vietnam (Bloom, 1998).

The efforts of the Colombian government to increase its health care budget did not prevent private expenditures reaching 45% of total health expenditure in 1999 (more than 60% were out-of-pocket payments, the rest mainly employers' contributions). This is why, in a list of proportion of households with catastrophic health expenditure, Colombia ranked fourth out of 60 countries, after Vietnam, Brazil, and Azerbaijan (Xu et al., 2003). The cost escalation is probably due to the financing method. Rise in cost per capita for the contributory system (74% between 1997 and 2002) was comparable to the changes in the subsidized system (88% for the same period). By contrast the cost per capita for those who continued to be served by a system based on a supply-oriented model (the vinculados) remained under control between 1997 and 2002, increasing by 36% (Figure 7.4).

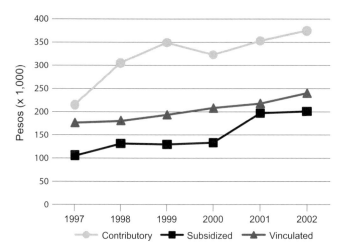

Figure 7.4. Evolution of cost per capita for the contributory and subsidized systems and the uninsured (vinculated), 1997–2002. *Source:* Departamento Nacional de Planeación et al. Proyecto: Cuentas nacionales en salud de Colombia. Síntesis general: aspectos conceptuales, metodológicos y principales resultados del periodo 1993–1999 Santafé de Bogotá D.C., 2001.

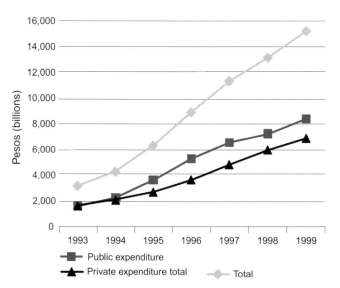

Figure 7.5. Public, private and total health expenditures, 1993–1999. *Source:* Ministerio de Salud de Colombia.Dirección general de Aseguramiento, Organización Mundial de la Salud, and Organización Panamericana de la Salud. Evaluación integral del equilibrio financiero del sistema general de seguridad social en salud. Bogotá, Colombia, 2001.

Although there was no strict regulation of contracts between providers and suppliers, there was a tendency to contract general practitioners on salary and to reimburse specialist and hospital services and procedures on a fee-for-service basis (Gutiérrez et al., 1996). Such a practice induced overconsumption of expensive care. Figure 7.5 shows that costs of health care delivery were out of control in the 1990s, probably because of this stimulation of high-cost care. Besides, the majority of the hospitals fulfilled both first- and second-line functions – despite evidence showing that the costs of handling first-line disorders increase with the institution's complexity (Van Lerberghe & Lafort, 1990).

Finally, the complex administrative structure has absorbed a substantial amount of funds (Figure 7.6). In 2001, 52% of the capitation fee was still spent on administrative costs (Organización Mundial de la Salud et al., 2001). In 1995 only 10% of the resources assigned to the subsidized system was spent appropriately, the rest was diverted into bureaucracy costs, frozen in bank accounts, or used in sectors other than the health sector (Jaramillo, 1997). This finding

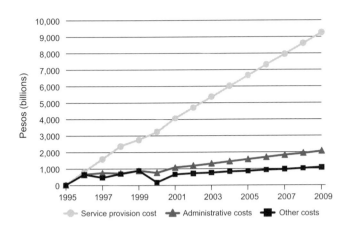

Figure 7.6. Health Promoting Enterprises – EPS: Expenditures 1996–2009. *Note:* Projection of trends from 2001 onwards. *Source:* Ministry of Health of Colombia (General Direction of Insurance) and Panamerican Health Organization. Integral Evaluation of the financial Equilibrium of the general System of social Security in Health. Bogotá, Colombia, 2001 p. 80.

echoes the comparison between Canada, which has a health system with a single purchaser and administrative costs representing 16.7% of health expenditure, and the United States, which has a health system with multiple purchasers and where this share of costs is 31% (Woolhandler et al., 2004).

Discussion

Can these disappointing outcomes be linked to the reform? Colombia's prolonged civil war has frequently been invoked to explain the poor results in the coverage, cost control and impact of the health insurance system. In 2001, 190,500 new refugees were registered in Colombia, bringing the total number of internally displaced persons (IDPs) to 720,000 (UNHCR, 2002). Although this number puts Colombia in the second rank of countries with IDPs, it represents only 1.7% of the total population, far from the target of 40% that must be included in the health insurance scheme to reach universal coverage.

Rather, we believe it is the inefficiency of the reform's approach, contracting out, that has undermined Colombia's health care reform. Total expenditure on health as a percentage of GDP stagnated at 3% during the period 1990–1995 (World Bank, 1999). In 1993 Law 100 was introduced at the behest of international development agencies (Bossert et al., 1998). This process attracted widespread support from sectors with significant influence on state decision making, such as senior health managers, pharmaceutical companies, medical manufacturers, and international health insurance corporations (Stocker et al., 1999). The Colombian government tried to accommodate their wishes (Restrepo & Valencia, 2002).

This conjunction of interests explains why health care expenditure almost doubled by 1997, to 5.5% (World Health Organization, 2000), while health care coverage remained below 55% and actual treatment rates decreased. The WB claims that countries with structural adjustment programmes spend more on health through public provision (van der Gaag & Barham, 1998). Hypothetically, in Colombia as in other countries, the bulk of this 'medical inflation' has been channelled to the private sector, the extent of which remains to be calculated.

The Colombian state has proved unfit to regulate and control the private sector. Is this a specific or a general feature of middle (and low) -income countries? Let us examine whether the public authorities in such countries possess the economic, technical and political capacity to face this challenge.

Firstly, European governments hold the purse strings; developing countries' administrations do not. Although the available data are not always reliable, the public share within total health care expenditure is obviously far greater in Western Europe than in developing countries. Public expenditure as a percentage of total expenditure on health amounts to 77.5% in Germany, 76.9% in France, 96.9% in the United Kingdom and 83.2% in Belgium (World Health Organization, 2000). By contrast public expenditure on health care represents 54.5% in Colombia, 48.7% in Brazil, 24.9% in China, 13% in India, 36.8% in Indonesia, and 28.2% in Nigeria. This paucity of funds also explains why so few developing countries have managed to apply the demand-side reforms recommended by the WB.

Secondly, as Figueras and Saltman (Figueras & Saltman, 1998) acknowledge, the success of reform strategies in Europe required 'the availability of public health skills to assess health needs, evaluate interventions and monitor outcome.' The management skills required for contracting out and regulating contractual arrangements seem well beyond the capacity of many developing countries, including MICs. One of the few published studies on contracting out to the private sector underlines the difficulties encountered in South Africa, a country with a mature public administration system (Mills, 1997). The author concluded that 'these problems are likely to occur to an even greater extent in countries with less well-developed systems of administration,' a conclusion shared by the authors of a case study from Zimbabwe (McPake & Hongoro, 1995).

Efforts by public authorities in the less developed countries to set care standards among private providers have remained inconclusive (Brugha & Zwi, 1998, Paredes et al., 1996) or failed (Kumaranayake, 1997). In Europe, as Figueras and Saltman (Figueras & Saltman, 1998) observe, in contrast to supply-side reforms, 'the existing evidence, taken together, appears to indicate that reforms have been decidedly more fraught – financially, politically, socially and even clinically – when undertaken on the demand side, specifically in the application of market-style incentives to individual patient-based demand. Measures such as choice of insurer, increased cost sharing at the point of use, or removing services from the publicly financed package of care have generated both equity and organisational problems.' These problems are even more acute in developing countries, where purchasing power is much lower.

Research suggests that contracting out is an acceptable alternative to public provision, if the following conditions are met: (a) real competition exists between competent and substantial private providers; (b) there is adequate government capacity to assess needs and to negotiate and monitor contract terms; (c) a legal and political environment exists that can enforce regulations and resist patronage and corruption (Mills, 1998). In industrialized countries it is clear that 'Managed market ... success will ultimately depend upon improvements in the underlying organisation, structure and functioning of the public sector' (Broomberg, 1994a). Based on these criteria, the only settings in developing countries where monitoring could be effective are urban centres in a few MICs with elaborate political and administrative structures and real competition between providers. Apparently, Colombia is not a member of this club.

Thirdly, the relative success of contracting out in France, Germany, and Belgium arose in a particular political and socio-economic context. Medical costs as a percentage of GDP are lower in Europe than in the United States, because of the supply-side cost-sharing. Although the 'poorest' still experience problems of access to health care, they represent only a minority in Western Europe. The main reason why these governments were able to secure access to (private) health care for the majority is that low-income groups managed to have their interests defended within the political system. In Western Europe workers' parties and mutual aid associations have been included in government health policy planning and administrations since 1945 and have acted as a counterweight to the vested interests (Criel & Van Dormael,

1999). In Europe social and health care policies were largely defined by 'the poor' and by their representatives, while in the United States and Colombia, policies for 'the poor' – in line with those favoured for developing countries by United Nations (UN) agencies – failed to improve social standards and to reduce medical costs. Health expenditure in the United States as a proportion of GDP is now the highest, by far, of all industrialized countries.

Unlike in Europe, the poor are rarely represented in the ruling circles of developing countries and so play little part in shaping health care policies or setting budgets. The Colombian reform aggravated this situation by undermining people's attempts to develop community health services (Restrepo & Valencia, 2002). This is a familiar feature of administrations in developing countries, when a ruling elite uses its monopoly power to weaken solidarity between rich and poor and so increase income inequality (Haubert et al., 1992).

In conclusion, the skyrocketing costs linked to the Colombian reform cast doubts on the efficiency of the new social security system, more so because the increase in spending is not related to an increase in real access to health services or to improvement in disease control. The impressive increase in public and private funds did not prove to be value for money. The Colombian case seriously undermines claims that the neoliberal international aid policy is evidence-based.

References

Almeida C., Travassos C., Céspedes J., et al. (2000). Efectos de la reforma de la seguridad social en salud en Colombia sobre la equidad en el acceso y la utilización de servicios de salud. *Revista de Salud Pública, Universidad de Antioquia*, **20**, pp. 9–19.

Ayala C. & Kroeger A. (2002). La reforma del sector salud en Colombia y sus efectos en los programas de control de tuberculosis e inmunización. *Cadernos de Saúde Pública*, **18**(6), pp. 1771–81.

Berman P. & Bossert T. (2000). *A Decade of Health Sector Reform in Developing Countries: What Have We Learned?* DDM Report No. 81. Boston: Harvard School of Public Health. Available at http://www.hsph. harvard.edu/ihsg/ihsg.

Bloom G. (1998). Primary health care meets the market in China and Vietnam. *Health Policy*, **44**(3), pp. 233–52.

Bossert T. J., Hsiao W., Barrera M., Alarcon L., Leo M., & Casares C. (1998). Transformation of ministries of health in the era of health reform: The case of Colombia. *Health Policy and Planning*, **13**(1), pp. 59–77.

Broomberg J. (1994a). *Health Care Markets for Export? Lessons for Developing Countries From European and American Experience.* London: LSHTM.

Broomberg J. (1994b). Managing the health care market in developing countries: Prospects and problems. *Health Policy and Planning*, **9**(3), pp. 237–51.

Brugha R. & Zwi A. (1998). Improving the quality of private sector delivery of public health services: Challenges and strategies. *Health Policy and Planning*, **13**(2), pp. 107–20.

Colombia Country Management Unit & PREM Sector Management Unit. (2002). *Latin America and the Caribbean region.* Washington, DC: World Bank. Colombia Poverty Report, Volume I.

Criel B. & Van Dormael M. (1999). Mutual health organisations in Africa and social health insurance systems: Will European history repeat itself? [editorial]. *Tropical Medicine & International Health*, **4**(3), pp. 155–9.

Departamento Nacional de Planeación, Dirección de Desarrollo Social, Subdirección de Salud, & Barón Leguizamón G. (2001). Proyecto: Cuentas nacionales en salud de Colombia. *Síntesis general: aspectos conceptuales, metodológicos y principales resultados del periodo 1993–1999.* Santafé de Bogotá D.C.

El Congreso de Colombia. (1993). Ley 100 de 1993. 100/Art. 162. 1993.

European Commission. (2002). *Communication From the Commission to the Council and the*

European Parliament: Health and Poverty Reduction in Developing Countries. Brussels, Belgium: European Commission. COM/2002/0129.

Félix M., Robayo G., & Valencia O. (2002). Hygeia no es Panacea. Condiciones para dialogar sobre cobertura de la seguridad social en salud. *Revista de Salud Pública*, 4(2), pp. 103–9.

Figueras J. & Saltman R.B. (1998). Building upon comparative experience in health system reform. *European Journal of Public Health*, 8, pp. 99–101.

Gutiérrez C., Molina C., & Wüllner A. (1996). Las Formas De Contratación Entre Prestadores y Administradores De Salud. *Sus Perspectivas En El Nuevo Marco De La Seguridad Social.* Santafé de Bogotá: Editora Guadalupe Ltda.

Haubert M., Frelin C., & Leimdorfer F. (1992). *Etats Et Société Dans Le Tiers-Monde. De La Modernisation à La Démocratisation?* Paris: Publications de la Sorbonne.

Hernández M. (2002). Reforma sanitaria, equidad y derecho a la salud en Colombia. *Cadernos de Saúde Pública*, 18(4), pp. 991–1001.

Human Development Network. (1993). *Health, Nutrition and Population.* Washington, DC: World Bank.

Jaramillo I. (1997). El Futuro De La Salud En Colombia. *La Puesta En Marcha De La Ley 100.* 3rd edn. Bogotá, Colombia: Tercer Mundo Editores.

Jaramillo J. (2002). Evaluación de la descentralización de la salud y la reforma de la seguridad social en Colombia. *GAC Sanit*, 16(1), pp. 48–53.

Kroeger A., Ordonez-Gonzalez J., & Avina A. I. (2002). Malaria control reinvented: Health sector reform and strategy development in Colombia. *Tropical Medicine & International Health*, 7(5), pp. 450–8.

Kumaranayake L. (1997). The role of regulation: Influencing private sector activity within health sector reform. *Journal of International Development*, 9(4), pp. 641–9.

Labelle R., Stoddart G., & Rice T. (1994). A re-examination of the meaning and importance of supplier-induced demand.

Journal of Health Economics, 13(3), pp. 347–68.

Lönnroth K., Thuong L. M., Linh P. D., & Diwan V. K. (1999). Delay and discontinuity – A survey of TB patients' search of a diagnosis in a diversified health care system. *International Journal of Tuberculosis and Lung Disease*, 3(11), pp. 992–1000.

Málaga H., Latorre M. C., Cárdenas J., et al. (2001). Equidad y reforma en salud en Colombia. X Jornadas Colombianas de Epidemiología. *Boletín APS*, 6(10), pp. 80–98.

Manning W. G., Newhouse J. P., Duan N., Keeler E. B., Leibowitz A., & Marquis M. S. (1987). Health insurance and the demand for medical care: Evidence from a randomized experiment. *The American Economic Review*, 77(3), pp. 251–77.

McPake B. & Hongoro C. (1995). Contracting out of clinical services in Zimbabwe. *Social Science & Medicine*, 41(1), pp. 13–24.

Mills A. (1997). Improving the efficiency of public sector health services in developing countries: Bureaucratic versus market approaches. In: Colclough E., ed. *Marketizing Education and Health in Developing Countries: Miracle or Mirage?*, Oxford: Clarendon Press, pp. 245–71.

Mills A. (1998). To contract or not to contract? Issues for low and middle income countries. *Health Policy and Planning*, 13(1), pp. 32–40.

Organización Mundial de la Salud, Ministerio de Salud de ColombiaDirección general de Aseguramiento, & Organización Panamericana de la Salud. (2001). *Evaluación integral del equilibrio financiero del sistema general de seguridad social en salud.* Bogotá, Colombia.

Pan American Health Organization. (2002). *Profile of the Health Services System of Colombia.* Washington, DC: World Health Organization.

Paredes P., de la Peña M., Flores-Guerra E., Diaz J., & Trostle J. (1996). Factors influencing physicians' prescribing behaviour in the treatment of childhood diarrhoea: Knowledge may not be the clue. *Social Science & Medicine*, 42(8), pp. 1141–53.

Pérez Gilberto R. (2003). La tuberculosis en Colombia. A propósito del Día Mundial de la Tuberculosis 24 de marzo 1882–2003 [Editorial]. *Repertorio de Medicina y Cirugía*, **12**(2), 2003.

Plaza B., Barona A. B., & Hearst N. (2001). Managed competition for the poor or poorly managed competition? Lessons from the Colombian health reform experience. *Health Policy and Planning*, **16**, pp. 44–51.

Preker A. S., Harding A., & Girishankar N. (1999). *The economics of private participation in health care: New insights from institutional economics.* Washington, DC: World Bank.

Profamilia Colombia. (2000). *Encuesta nacional de demografía y salud (ENDS) – Salud sexual y reproductiva en Colombia 2000.* Bogotá.

Restrepo H. E. & Valencia H. (2002). Implementation of a new health system in Colombia: Is this favourable for health determinants? *Journal of Epidemiology and Community Health*, **56**(10), pp. 742–3.

Riveros G. (2004). Diez años de la reforma a la seguridad social de salud en Colombia (1993–2003). *Isapre*. 2004. Ministerio de Salud de Colombia, PAHO.

Rutstein D. D., Berenberg W., Chalmers T. C., Child C. G., III, Fishman A. P., & Perrin E. B. (1976). Measuring the quality of medical care. A clinical method. *New England Journal of Medicine*, **294**(11), pp. 582–8.

Sen K. & Koivusalo M. (1998). Health care reforms and developing countries: A critical overview. *International Journal of Health Planning and Management*, **13**(3), pp. 199–215.

Stocker K., Waitzkin H., & Iriart C. (1999). The exportation of managed care to Latin America. *New England Journal of Medicine*, **340**(14), pp. 1131–6.

Tabbush V. & Swanson G. (1996). Changing paradigms in medical payment. *Archives of Internal Medicine*, **156**(4), pp. 357–60.

Unger J.P., De Paepe P., & Green A. (2003). A code of best practice for disease control programmes to avoid damaging health care services in developing countries. *International Journal of Health Planning and Management*, **18**(Supplement 1), pp. 27–39.

UNHCR. (2002). *Refugees by Numbers.* Geneva: United Nations High Commissioner for Refugees; 2002.

Uplekar M., Pathania V., & Raviglione M. (2001). Private practitioners and public health: Weak links in tuberculosis control. *Lancet*, **358**(9285), pp. 912–6.

van der Gaag J. & Barham T. (1998). Health and health expenditures in adjusting and non-adjusting countries. *Social Science & Medicine*, **46**(8), pp. 995–1009.

Van Lerberghe W., Ammar W., El Rashidi R., Sales A., & Mechbal A. (1997). Reform follows failure: I. Unregulated private care in Lebanon. *Health Policy and Planning*, **12**(4), pp. 296–311.

Van Lerberghe W. & De Brouwere V. (1989). Assessment of appropriate child care at district level: How useful are mortality rates? *Transactions of the Royal Society of Tropical Medicine & Hygiene*, **83**(1), pp. 23–6.

Van Lerberghe W. & Lafort Y. (1990). *The Role of the Hospital in the District: Delivering or Supporting Primary Health Care?* WHO/SHS/CC/90.2. Geneva: World Health Organization.

Westerling R. (2001). Commentary: Evaluating avoidable mortality in developing countries – an important issue for public health. *International Journal of Epidemiology*, **30**(5), pp. 973–5.

Woolhandler S., Campbell T., & Himmelstein D. U. (2004). Health care administration in the United States and Canada: Micromanagement, macro costs. *International Journal of Health Services*, **34**(1), pp. 65–78.

World Bank. (1997). *Health, Nutrition, and Population Sector Strategy.* pp. 1–112. 1997. World Bank. Part of the Health, Nutrition, and Population Series (HNP).

World Bank. (1999). *World Development Report 1998/1999: Knowledge for Development.* Washington, DC: Oxford University Press.

World Health Organization. (1999). *World Health Report 1999: Making a difference.* Geneva: World Health Organization.

World Health Organization. (2000). *World Health Report 2000: Health systems.*

Improving performance. Geneva: World Health Organization.

Xu K., Evans D. B., Kawabata K., Zeramdini R., Klavus J., & Murray C. J. (2003). Household catastrophic health expenditure: A multicountry analysis. *Lancet*, **362**(9378), pp. 111–7.

Yepes A. (2003). The violation of social rights within market rationale. In: *Social Watch. Annual Report, 2003.* pp. 100–1.

Yepes F. & Sánchez L. (2000). La reforma del sector de salud en Colombia: ¿un modelo de competencia regulada? *Revista Panamericana de Salud Publica*, **8**(1/2), pp. 34–41.

Section 3
Chapter

8

Impact of international health policies on access to health in middle-income countries: some experiences from Latin America

Chile's neoliberal health reform: an assessment and a critique

Unger J.-P., De Paepe P., Arteaga Herrera O., Solimano Cantuarias G. Chile's Neoliberal Health Reform: An Assessment and a Critique. PLoS Medicine 2008; 5(4) e79: 0001–0006.

Introduction

The Chilean health system has been studied extensively (Jack, 2000). Its current form is the result of a major reform undertaken by the Pinochet government following the coup d'état in 1973. Pinochet's reform established competition between public and private health insurers and promoted private health services, following neoliberal principles. Neoliberalism is an economic and political movement that gained consensus in the 1980s among international organizations such as the IMF and the WB. This movement demands reforms such as free trade; privatization of previously public-owned enterprises, goods, and services; undistorted market prices; and limited government intervention. After the publication of the World Bank's 1993 report, 'Investing in Health' (World Bank, 1993), Chile became a model for neoliberal reforms to health services.

In this Policy Forum, we assess the effects of the Chilean reform from Pinochet until 2005, and including the transition to democracy in 1990. We suggest that the use of Chile as a model for other countries of the health benefits of neoliberalism is seriously misguided. We stress the dominant role of the public health system in Chile, while most other studies have assessed the introduction of a private insurance sector as part of the neoliberal reform. Revisiting the Chilean health reform after 25 years, we come to new conclusions that could be important for countries such as Ecuador and Bolivia, which are preparing health reforms, and even for the United States, with its current debate on universal health insurance.

Pinochet's reform and its context

Chile has been a social laboratory, having experienced democratic liberalism (1958–1964), Christian Democratic reformism (1964–1970), democratic socialism (1970–1973), neoliberal authoritarianism (1973–1989), and three democratic coalition governments from 1990 to the present (see the Glossary at the end of this chapter for definitions) (Silva, 2005). The neoliberal reforms were not limited to the health system, but were also made to the pension system, in education, and through the privatization of state industries. Many of the changes in the health system were later conceptualized in WB-supported documents (Titelman & Uthoff, 2000).

In 1979, after having brutally repressed opposition to the 1973 coup against socialist president Salvador Allende, the Pinochet regime embarked on a sweeping health sector reform, based on neoliberal doctrines (Arteaga et al., 2002; Borzutzky, 2003; Reichard, 1996). The private insurances (ISAPRES) were developed alongside the state system and were intended to be the dominant one. The two systems followed completely different rationales: the public system, a traditional 'Bismarckian' social security system (members contribute a proportion of their wages to receive health services according to their need), promoted solidarity via risk-sharing and the internal redistribution of health care resources, while the private system offered health insurance policies corresponding to each individual's contributions.

The National Health Fund (FONASA) was created in 1979 as a public agency to collect and manage the financial resources coming from the compulsory contributions of employees who chose to remain in the public system (or who could not afford an adequate plan with an ISAPRES company), and from the national government's health budget. There are four categories of insured within FONASA; A, indigent; B, very low income; C, lower-middle income; and D, higher-middle income. Categories B, C, and D are entitled to choose health care outside the public provider system, with varying levels of co-payment. Category A members are limited to public services, both for primary care and hospital services.

ISAPRES was created in 1981 to manage the payroll contributions allocated to health care for those opting out of the state system. The private companies purchased most care from the private sector (Barrientos, 2002), which received an intense boost. The ISAPRES market offered no fewer than 8,000 different individual plans, designed according to sex, age, health risk, supplementary premiums, and co-payments. The market concentrated on relatively affluent clients with lower health risks: the mean income of ISAPRES members in 2003 was more than four times higher than FONASA members (Cid et al., 2006). The profit margins of ISAPRES exceeded 20%.

The National Health Service was decentralized into 26 autonomous territorial health authorities. These entities took over responsibility for hospital care, while PHC facilities were transferred to municipalities. The funding of public health services was drastically reduced (Vergara-Iturriaga & Martínez-Gutiérrez, 2006). Consequently, the supply of health care in public facilities was restricted.

In March 1990, a coalition of centre and left-wing parties came to power, and has remained in power ever since. Its social policy has been broadly 'social democratic,' seeking to attach a Western-style welfare state to a dynamic emerging market economy (Hiscock & Hojman, 1997). In the same year (1990) a government regulatory agency, known as the ISAPRES Superintendency, was created to establish some sort of regulation of ISAPRES. As Figures 8.1 and 8.2 show, public expenditure on health increased dramatically from 1990 (Programa de Naciones Unidas para el Desarrollo, 2002), to almost three times more in constant pesos. While the proportion of public expenditure on health remained fairly stable at around 3%, from a low of 2% in 1976, economic growth explains the increase in absolute numbers. Private expenditure remained stable as a proportion of GDP, but increased sharply in absolute numbers. To finance this increased public expenditure a tax reform was approved that reversed the tax reductions of the Pinochet years (Ffrench-Davis, 2002; Reichard, 1996; Vergara, 1996).

As the graph shows, there was a sharp increase in public health expenditure (in 2000 Chilean pesos) in Chile after 1990, with social democratic governments. A short spike can be observed during the socialist Allende government. The lower darker line represents public expenditure, the upper lighter one public expenditure per person (Programa de Naciones Unidas para el Desarrollo, 2002).

As a percentage of GDP, public health expenditure rose under the Allende government, then decreased sharply under the Pinochet neoliberal experiment, and is now stable at around 3% (Programa de Naciones Unidas para el Desarrollo, 2002).

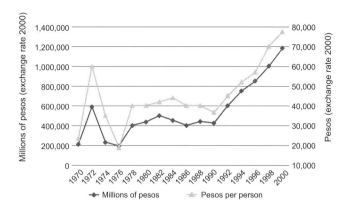

Figure 8.1. Public expenditure on health in Chile, 1970–2000 (in Pesos, 2000). *Source:* United Nations Development Programme (2002). Chile: 20 años de esquemas liberales en protección social. Taller Interregional.

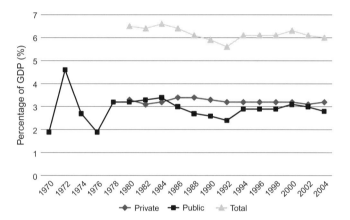

Figure 8.2. Health Expenditure in Chile, 1970–2004, as a percentage of GDP (Gross Domestic Product). *Source:* United Nations Development Programme (2002). Chile: 20 años de esquemas liberales en protección social. Taller Interregional.

However, none of the main features of the Pinochet reforms described above were substantially modified (Silva, 2005). More recently, President Lagos' government (2000–2006) initiated a new health reform plan (called Plan AUGE), aiming at better quality and shorter waiting times in the public sector and a minimum coverage plan in ISAPRES, but again, this policy remained broadly compatible with neoliberal reform.

The main features of Chile's neoliberal health reform

The partial privatization of social security

The compulsory contributions made by workers and employees go either to the public social insurer FONASA or to one of the private health insurers of ISAPRES. During Pinochet's regime, employers were relieved of the requirement to contribute on behalf of their employees. Table 8.1 presents the sources of health expenditure financing for the year 2003 (Vergara-Iturriaga & Martínez-Gutiérrez, 2006).

Out of Chile's population of some 16 million, 2.5 million of its more affluent citizens were members of private ISAPRES insurance companies in 1995 (this was the year in which membership in ISAPRES reached its peak, after which there was a decline). ISAPRES was legally entitled to set premiums based on individual risk factors. Although control over ISAPRES

Table 8.1. Sources of health expenditure in Chile, 2003 (millions of Chilean pesos)

	Payroll contributions	Tax-based	Out-of-pocket
ISAPRES	737.160	Unknown*	515.129
FONASA	477.142	706.518	202.530
Total	1.214.302	706.518	717.659

Note: *Subsidy for maternity licence, amount unknown.

Source: Programa de Naciones Unidas para el Desarrollo, 2002.

was strengthened by the creation of the Superintendency, problems remained with regard to catastrophic health expenditure for lower-income ISAPRES members. Under pressure from the Superintendency, ISAPRES decided in 2001 to cover some catastrophic conditions, but the level of the 'deductible' (the amount to be paid by the patient) remained very high.

ISAPRES membership reached 26% of the population in 1995 and declined to only 16% in 2006 – a small proportion of the population, and not the one most in need of health care. The decline was due to improved performance by the public sector, unemployment caused by the Asian crisis in the 1990s, the AUGE plan and the rising cost of private health plans. Some experts estimate that by 2010, ISAPRES may cover only 10% of the population (Araya, 2004).

Segmentation and lack of solidarity between two parallel health insurance systems

The ISAPRES system attracts the affluent, male, young, and urban. In the poorest quintile of the population only 1.6% are members of ISAPRES, compared with 50.5% in the richest (Vergara-Iturriaga & Martínez-Gutiérrez, 2006). Adult women pay up to four times more than men for their health plans, and the proportion of ISAPRES members over 60 drops dramatically since they face premiums of up to eight times as much as those of young adults. Adults over 60 are forced to enter FONASA. Some ISAPRES companies are in an oligopoly position: the main three firms share close to 80% of the market (Arteaga et al., 2002).

The state has subsidized ISAPRES in several ways. Firstly, until recently it subsidized ISAPRES to the tune of 2% of the salary of those who switched from FONASA to ISAPRES. Secondly, it pays for maternity leave for ISAPRES members. Thirdly, 25% of patients covered by ISAPRES receive services in public facilities because they cannot afford the co-payments (Larrañaga, 1997; Manuel, 2002). Almost half of all catastrophic events among children of ISAPRES members are treated in public hospitals (World Bank, 2000).

Moreover, FONASA finances the private health care sector (category B, C, and D patients can choose to be treated by private providers via a voucher system). The money transferred to the private sector in this way is substantial, greater than what is spent on municipal PHC (Rodríguez & Tokman, 2000).

The return of democracy: restoring an underfinanced public sector

The transition government inherited a series of problems with public health services from the Pinochet regime, including a major deterioration in the public infrastructure and inefficient management in the decentralized organizations (Manuel, 2002). Primary care services suffered from poor coordination between the regional health services and the municipal authorities. Working conditions and wages had deteriorated. Rural areas and poor urban districts were worst affected in the quantity and quality of the services provided, introducing regional differences unseen before.

From 1990 to 2002, however, tax revenues doubled and allowed for an increase in social expenditure of 240% over the same period. In 2000 expenditure on health care accounted for 7.3% of GDP: 3.1% on publicly provided care and 4.2% on private care. In 2004 out-of-pocket expenditures amounted to 27% of total health expenditure.

We turn now to an assessment of the impact of the reform, focusing on equity – in terms of finance, access and health status – and efficiency.

The impact of the reform: equity

Financial equity

Chile shares with Brazil the dubious distinction of having one of the most regressive patterns of income distribution in Latin America, and the distribution of spending on health is no exception. The private sector accounts for a disproportionate share of total health expenditure (38% of the total health expenditure was spent on 21% of the population in 2004) (Cid et al., 2006). This is a basic unfairness, and represents a lack of solidarity, since FONASA and ISAPRES have separate financing (Vergara, 1996).

Within the FONASA system, there is some internal redistribution between categories A-B and C-D, the latter helping to finance the health care of the former (Bitran et al., 2000). Between FONASA and ISAPRES there is some limited and indirect redistribution: ISAPRES members contribute directly to their individual health plans, but indirectly they make some contribution to the health care of the poor through the tax money received by FONASA (Savedoff, 2000), which accounts for half of its income.

Other dimensions of equity are also problematic. The ISAPRES system discriminates against women, whose participation in 2001 was only 34.4%, with lower-quality health plans than those of men (Arteaga et al., 2002). Access to ISAPRES health plans depends on income, and women generally have lower incomes or are outside the remunerated workforce. Insurance policies for women of childbearing age may cost four times more than men's policies (Pollack, 2002).

Equity of access to care

Considering the basic inequality of Chilean society and the unfairness of its health sector financing, one would expect access to care by the poor to be unequal as well. In fact the evidence is mixed: access to care is somewhat equitable, but quality of care is not.

Some data suggest relatively equitable access. In 1999 the utilization rate (consultations per person per year) for FONASA patients was 3.85% and for ISAPRES patients 4.12% (Rodríguez & Tokman, 2000). A 2003 national health survey (Ministerio de Planificación, 2003) showed that among those who reported having felt sick in the last month, 73.9% from the poorest quintile consulted with medical staff, compared with 79.7% from the richest.

But inequity may arise in the quality of health services. Frequency of surgeries and laboratory tests was positively correlated with income; more importantly, consultations with specialists were almost three times more frequent for patients in decile 10 than those in decile 1 (Ministerio de Planificación, 2003). Access to specialists appeared deficient in the public service: there were waiting lists of up to 4 years in some specialties, such as ophthalmology. Conversely, emergency visits were twice as frequent in the lowest income group.

Table 8.2. Percentage of total income per decile, 1969–2000

Deciles	1969	1989	2000
Poorest decile	1.3%	1.2%	1.2%
Richest decile	39%	41.6%	47%

Source: Programa de Naciones Unidas para el Desarrollo, 2002.

There are other reasons to believe that access is inequitable. Utilization rates differ greatly between poor and rich municipalities: for primary care, by a factor of 2.8, for emergencies by a factor of 3.9, and for inpatients, by a factor of 2.0 (Arteaga et al., 2002).

The 2003 CASEN survey (Ministerio de Planificación, 2003) indicated that only 57.5% of FONASA members described their health as good or very good, compared with 80.6% of ISAPRES members. This should be reflected in higher utilization rates for FONASA members, but as we have seen, the reverse is the case.

Equity of health status

The Chilean model of development has been associated with rapid economic growth: gross national product increased 7.9% per annum in the 1990s (Manuel, 2002). The country is ranked 22nd on the Global Competitiveness Index (GCI) (World Economic Forum, 2006), far ahead of any other Latin American country, and 37th in the 2003 Human Development Report, although its development model has created high social inequality. In fact inequality continued to increase even under the democratic post-Pinochet regime (Table 8.2).

Poverty (defined as being below the poverty line, determined annually for individuals and families) was sharply reduced under the democratic governments, declining from 45% in 1985 to 21.7% in 1998 (Raczynski & Serrano, 2002) and 13.7% in 2006 (Mideplan, 2009). But income inequality rose, making Chile 'the paladin [champion] of inequality' in the harsh words of Parada (Lezcano, 2005). Before 1970, Chile's Gini Index (a measure of income inequality on a scale of 0 to 100, where 0 is complete income equality and 100 is complete inequality) was under 45; in the 1980s, it jumped to 65. In 2003 it was 57.5, a very unfavourable figure compared with, for instance, Costa Rica's figure of 45.9. The richest 20% received 17 times more income than the poorest 20% (Raczynski & Serrano, 2002); for comparison, in the US this group received 8.9 times more and in Peru 10.5 times more than the poorest 20%.

In spite of this inequality, Chile's average health indicators are good, with high life expectancy and low infant and maternal mortality, even with 27.3% of children under 10 living in poverty in 2003 (Ministerio de Planificación, 2003). The relatively equitable access to health care probably played a significant role in this achievement, as did maternal and child protection programmes, carried out by the public sector. Still, the number of potential productive years of life lost is much higher in the poorest quintile of 20- to 79-year-olds in Santiago, 35% higher than in the richest quintile (Sánchez et al., 2005).

Another study suggests health inequities between municipalities: the tuberculosis incidence maximum/minimum ratio between municipalities was 5.53, and for child malnutrition it was 5.00 (Arteaga et al., 2002). The national department of epidemiology states that adjusted mortality for the poorest decile is 6.0 out of 1,000, versus 4.8 for the richest (Paz, 1998).

The impact of the reform: efficiency

Here the evidence is clearer. ISAPRES has hardly contained costs, and the ISAPRES companies never intended to do so: they have few incentives to be efficient buyers of health services

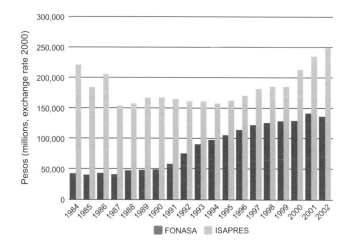

Figure 8.3. Expenditure per member, FONASA and ISAPRES, 1984–2002. *Source:* United Nations Development Programme (2002). Chile: 20 años de esquemas liberales en protección social. Taller Interregional.

for their clients. Instead they work hard to be efficient in the selection of their clients (they are allowed to refuse clients). Their focus is on low-risk, high-income patients, with the goal of making a profit. They spend 10 times as much on administration per member (Cid et al., 2006) and about 2 times as much on health care per member than FONASA (Figure 8.3), even though ISAPRES members are in better health and need less care (Titelman & Uthoff, 2000). To deliver care ISAPRES companies rely on a burgeoning private sector, reimbursed on a fee-for-service basis, which induces an increased supply of unnecessary but profitable services.

Discussion

Chile's health indicators are good, compared with countries with a similar GNP, such as Colombia and Argentina. These results are due in part to Chile's high economic growth rate and a spectacular reduction in poverty (Arellano, 2004; Hiscock & Hojman, 1997; Mideplan, 2009). Further significant factors are the high proportion of the population with access to drinking water and sanitation, and the high adult literacy rate and education level. But relatively equitable access to health care, mainly through public health insurance and public health services, which cover 80% of the population, played a major role in this achievement, as did maternity and child health protection programmes implemented through the public health network.

The democratic regime did not modify the essence of Pinochet's health reform. Key features such as social security privatization and the purchaser–provider split persisted. But public health expenditure was sharply increased to improve infrastructure, hire more personnel and provide better equipment and salaries. The ISAPRES companies were placed under the control of a government regulatory agency to avoid commercial excesses.

As for the role that health care has played in achieving Chile's favourable health indicators, a key conclusion from the foregoing analysis must be that results rested on the backbone of the public health system, which the neoliberal reforms were willing, but not able, to break. It is absolutely clear that the country's health indicators are not due to the superior access to health care enjoyed by the better-off minority, who in any case continued to rely significantly on the public system for many conditions and services. ISAPRES private health insurance never covered more than 25% of the population, and this proportion is now declining, thanks to a remarkable improvement in public health services. Even during the Pinochet regime the

Chilean system was basically a public system, accessible to the 75% of Chileans who could not afford private insurance with ISAPRES. The effects of the neoliberal health reform in Chile remain marginal.

The neoliberal health reform in Chile has created an unfair dual health system: FONASA and public services for the poor, ISAPRES and private services for the more affluent section of the population. ISAPRES now accounts for 40% of total health expenditure, on behalf of 16% of the population. The reform increased the incomes of private sector providers and decreased health system efficiency (through the incentive to overtreat inherent to fee-for-service payment, through much higher administration and marketing costs and through the fragmentation of service provision).

To present the Chilean reform as a model to be followed by other countries, as has been done by the WB and other international bodies, is to disregard the evidence, which tends to show that Chile's relatively successful health care provision has been achieved in spite of the reform, not because of it, or in fact because the intended neoliberal reform could not be implemented as foreseen. Another neoliberal reform, modified to avoid the segmentation that occurred in Chile, can be observed in Colombia, and the results are not encouraging.

A logical recommendation for a health system counter-reform in Chile would be to move from a multi-insurer scheme to a single public insurer scheme, as in Costa Rica. This single payer (and its members) would then still be able to choose between public and private providers, but with strengthened bargaining power. This would put an end to the unfairness of ISAPRES spending twice as much on their members than FONASA, although FONASA's members are a higher-risk population.

Glossary

Christian Democratic reformism: political parties based on Christian principles in a democratic regime; reformist as opposed to revolutionary. In many European countries Christian democrats have alternated in government with socialists. In Chile the Frei administration, from 1964 till 1970.

Democratic liberalism: in a democratic regime, a free or 'liberal' market with little state intervention (in fact, orthodox conservative economics). Not to be confused with 'liberal arts' or left-wing liberal democrats. In Chile the Alessandri government from 1958 till 1964.

Democratic socialism: regimes based on democracy and socialist principles like equity and solidarity; found in many European countries, such as Sweden. In Chile the Allende Popular Unity government from 1970 till 1973.

Neoliberal authoritarianism: orthodox neoliberalism combined with dictatorship. Neoliberalism demands reforms such as free trade, privatization of previously public-owned enterprises, goods, and services, undistorted market prices, and limited government intervention. In Chile the Pinochet regime from 1973 till 1989.

References

Araya E. (2004). En el 2010, sólo el 12% de la población estará en Isapres. 2004.

Arellano J. P. M. (2004). Políticas sociales para el crecimiento con equidad Chile 1990–2002. Santiago de Chile: Plataforma Universidad de Chile. report n°26. *Series Estudios Socio/Económicos.*

Arteaga Ó., Thollaug S., Nogueira A. C., & Darras C. (2002). Informacion para la equidad en salud en Chile. *Revista Panamericana de Salud Pública*, **11**, pp. 374–85.

Barrientos A. (2002). Health policy in Chile: The return of the public sector? *Bulletin of Latin American Research*, **21**, pp. 442–59.

Bitran R., Munoz J., Aguad P., Navarrete M., & Ubilla G. (2000). Equity in the financing of social security for health in Chile. *Health Policy*, **50**, pp. 171–96.

Borzutzky S. (2003). Social security privatisation: The lessons from the Chilean experience for other Latin American countries and the USA. *International Journal of Social Welfare*, **12**(2), pp. 86–96.

Cid C., Muñoz A., Riesco X., & Inostroza M. (2006). Equidad en el financiamiento de la salud y protección financiera en Chile: una descripción general. *Cuadernos Médico Sociales*, **46**(1), pp. 5–12.

Ffrench-Davis R. (2002). Distribución del ingreso y pobreza en Chile. In: Sáez J. C., ed. *Entre El Neoliberalismo y El Crecimiento Con Equidad: Tres Décadas De Política Económica En Chile*. Santiago De Chile.

Hiscock J. & Hojman D. (1997). Social policy in a fast growing economy: The case of Chile. *Social Policy and Administration*, **31**(4), pp. 354–70.

Jack W. (2000). *The Evolution of Health Insurance Institution: Theory and Four Examples From Latin America*. World Bank.

Larrañaga O. (1997). *Eficienia y equidad en el sistema de salud Chileno*. Santiago, Chile: United Nations.

Lezcano M. P. (2005). Solidaridad en el financiamiento de la salud. *Cuadernos Médico Sociales*, **45**(2), pp. 138–44.

Manuel A. (2002). The Chilean health system: 20 years of reforms. *Salud Publica de México*, **44**, pp. 60–8.

Mideplan G. d. C. (2009). *Resultados salud CASEN 2006*. Gobierno de Chile, Ministerio de Planificación.

Ministerio de Planificación. (2003). Encuesta de caracterización socioeconómico nacional 2004. Mideplan. *Encuesta de Caracterización Socioeconómica Nacional CASEN*. Ministerio de Planificación, Gobierno de Chile.

Paz X. (1998). Mortalidad y pobreza, análisis de comunas seleccionadas. *Boletín de Vigilancia Epidemiológica*, **1**(2), pp. 6–8.

Pollack M. E. (2002). *Equidad de género en el sistema de salud Chileno*. Centro Latinoamericano y Caribeño de Demografia (CELADE), División de Población de la CEPAL. Santiago, Chile.

Programa de Naciones Unidas para el Desarrollo Chile. (2002). 20 años de esquemas liberales en protección social. In: *Protección Social en una Era Insegura: Un Intercambio Sur-Sur sobre Políticas Sociales Alternativas en Respuesta a la Globalización*. Santiago, Chile. Mayo 14–16, 2002.

Raczynski D. & Serrano C. (2002). Nuevos y viejos problemas en la lucha contra la pobreza en Chile. Asesorias para el Desarrollo. Santiago, Chile.

Reichard S. (1996). Ideology drives health care reforms in Chile. *Journal of Public Health Policy*, **17**(1), pp. 80–98.

Rodríguez C. & Tokman M. R. (2000). *Resultados y rendimiento del gasto en el sector público de salud en Chile 1990–1999. Report n° 106. Serie Financiamiento del Desarrollo*. Santiago de Chile: Comisión Económica para América Latina y el Caribe (CEPAL).

Sánchez H. R., Albala C. B., & Lera L. M. (2005). Años de vida perdidos por muerte prematura (AVPP) en adultos del gran Santiago: hemos ganado con equidad? [Last years of life due to premature death in adults of greater Santiago: Did we win with equity?]. *Revista Médica Chile*, **133**(5), pp. 575–82 [in Spanish].

Savedoff W. D. (2000). *Is Anybody Listening? Ignoring Evidence in the Latin American Health Reform Debates*. Washington, DC: Inter-American Development Bank.

Silva P. (2005). Intellectuals, technocrats and social change in Chile: Past, present and future perspectives. In: Angell A. & Pollack B., eds. *The Legacy of Dictatorship: Political, Economic and Social Change in Pinochet's Chile*. Liverpool: University of Liverpool, pp. 198–223.

Titelman D. & Uthoff A. (2000). *Ensayos sobre el financiamiento de la seguridad social en salud. Los casos de Estados Unidos, Canadá, Argentina, Chile, Colombia*. Santiago: Cepal. Fondo de Cultura Económica. Comisión Económica para América Latina y el Caribe.

Vergara P. (1996). In pursuit of 'growth with equity': The limits of Chile's free-market social reforms. 264.0.

Vergara-Iturriaga M. & Martínez-Gutiérrez M. S. (2006). Financiamiento del sistema de salud Chileno. *Salud Publica Mexicano*, **2006**(48), pp. 512–21.

World Bank. (1993). *World Development Report 1993: Investing in Health*. Oxford: Oxford University Press.

World Bank. (2000). Chile Health Insurance Issues: *Old Age and Catastrophic Health Costs*. Washington, DC: World Bank.

World Economic Forum. (2006). *Global Competitiveness Report 2006*. Geneva: World Economic Forum.

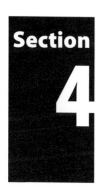

Section 4

Determinants and implications of new liberal health policies: the case of India, China and Lebanon

Introduction to Section 4

The three chapters in this section examine factors behind reforms of the health sector, most notably the financing of health services which, despite being undertaken over varying periods of time and in varied forms, retained the underlying common thread of rapid privatization and commercialization of health services. The approach to this section is an interdisciplinary one with historical, social, cultural and economic determinants of health reforms featuring in one or more of the chapters. In all three case studies the introduction of privatization whether of primary, secondary or tertiary care, has excluded large elements of the population from access to health care. In addition associated with this is a high risk of indebtedness and health related poverty, a phenomenon that is becoming increasingly widespread. All three countries also share regional variations in the experience of inequities with the urban employed having better access than the majority of the rural poor. Lebanon has the added burden of several decades of chronic conflict that has repeatedly affected its health infrastructure, in contrast to the rest of the Mashreq countries (generally speaking, the region of Arabic-speaking countries to the east of Egypt and north of the Arabian Peninsula) referred to in the chapter. In India the experience of financing will be varied by state, but the key-unifying factor is an almost complete absence of an evidence-base for donors and governments, from which policy decisions were made over the past two decades. The historical dimension of this section reinforces the often-missed perspective, that in order to plan for the future, we need to learn from the failures as well as the successes of the past.

**Section 4
Chapter**

Determinants and implications of new liberal health
policies: the case of India, China and Lebanon

9 Political and economic determinants of health care systems: the case of India

Qadeer Imrana (2009) Political and Economic Determinants of Health: the case of India in
Cook, H, Bhhatacharya, S and Hardy. A History of the Social Determinants of Health, Orient
Black Swan (eds), India pp. 228–248

Introduction

Politics, as the dynamics of managing stratified society, is linked to the control by different
social-strata resources and production systems. Indian society is differentiated along the lines
of class, caste, and gender among whom the rich peasantry and landlord-industrialists combine to control national politics. The former used their power to keep agriculture tax-free and
resisted land reforms, while the latter neglected the production of low cost basic consumer
goods in order to focus on an elite market. On the other hand, poor and marginal peasants,
agricultural labourers and a relatively small industrial working class constitute the majority
of the population – 93% of them are in the unorganized sector. In between come the middle
class whose growth, beginning in the 1970s, has expanded the market potential of India. Conflicts between these three broad groups, with different political interests, are often used by the
political forces for their own survival.

The development of the health sector in India reflects, to a large degree, the interest of
the dominant classes; this influence became more evident since the introduction of SAPs.
Notions such as CHC, the integration of disease control with medical care which were anti-
thetical to the spread of market forces, were replaced by essential primary care, and PPPs
under the aegis of SAPs.

Growth and reforms

Development in the 1970s

The slow growth rates in Indian industry and agriculture during the 1970s started a debate
on the nature of development itself. Officials blamed the failure of the rains, lack of resources
and high population growth for eating away at the fruits of development. But critics warned
against the misuse of protectionist policies by the powerful, the growth of industries for
luxury goods, reluctance to implement land reforms and agricultural taxes and the injudi-
cious use of international aid and grants (Chandrasekhar & Ghosh, 2000). They proposed
more stringent measures to hasten development for the majority instead of waiting for trickle-
down to take place.

The political configuration at the time did not permit this strategy and a general strike, in the context of the economic crisis, was dealt with by the declaration of a state of National Emergency in 1975. This resulted in the political defeat of the ruling party in the general elections of 1977. Nevertheless, this period catalyzed some sensitivity to basic needs and the government revived its Minimum Needs Programme (MNP) in the Sixth Plan covering employment, housing, health, education, sanitation, roads, electricity and water supply. The basic direction of development however remained the same with more loans and aid providing the basis for retaining the political status quo. Growing dependence on the WB and the IMF for loans at cheaper rates also paved the way for India to accept, first informally and then formally, the conditionalities of SAP in 1991.

The reforms in the 1990s

The growth rate over the 1990s declined from 7.8% (from 1980–1981 to 1990–1991) to 5.5% (from 1992–1993 to 2001–2002). Consequently, while growth in employment was 2.4% per annum in the late 1980s and early 1990s, from 1993–1994 until 2000 it fell to 1.0% per annum. This reduction was neither due to a higher population growth (that had actually declined from 2.1 to 1.93 over the same period), nor to increased educational opportunities for the young. In fact, compared to the 1980s when the labour force expanded at a rate of 80% of the population growth rate, during 1993–2000 it grew at half the rate of the population growth rate (Chaubey, 2002). During the period 1993–1994 to 1999–2000, the annual growth rate of rural employment was less than 0.6% per annum, far below the annual rate of growth of the rural population and the earlier rates of growth (Chandrasekhar & Ghosh, 2006). There was a similar position in urban employment. Unemployment level based on current daily status increased from 6.1% in 1993–94 to 7.3% in 1999–2000 to 8.3% in 2004–2005 (Himanshu, 2007).

Poverty estimates reveal that, though there had been a decline in the level of poverty during 1993–2005, the annual rate of reduction was lower than that in the 1980s (Table 9.1) (Himanshu, 2007). Income inequality estimates (measured by Gini coefficient) show an increase in the post-reform period as compared with earlier decades.

The promotion of Transnational Corporations (TNCs), the privatization of large elements of the public sector, the introduction of new technologies and the encouragement of Foreign Direct Investment (FDI) led to a further decline in employment, wage freeze, the erosion of worker's rights and the undermining of unions. The share of rent, interest and profits rose as the share of wages, in net value added, declined (Kumar, 2005b). Since 2001 the organized sector has shrunk to 7%, as the economic growth rate rose to 6.9% in 2004 (well below the expected 10%). However this did not change either the level of unemployment or the share of wages in net value added. Currently, the service sector

Table 9.1. Poverty and inequality estimates (URP, Official Poverty Lines)

	Headcount ratio			Gini		
	1983	1993–94	2004–05	1983	1993–94	2004–05
Rural	46.5	37.2	28.7	30.4	28.6	30.5
Urban	43.6	32.6	25.9	33.9	34.4	37.6

Source: Calculated from NSS Reports (various Rounds) cited in Himanshu, 2007.

contributes to more than two-thirds of the growth, whilst manufacturing has picked up marginally,[1] the primary sector has declined, and FDI has not gone beyond 0.5%! (Kumar, 2005a; Kumar, 2005b)

The cut back in public investments in rural development over the 1990s, from 14.5% to 6.0% of GDP, contributed to a reduction in the share of agriculture, led to huge indebtedness and sharp inequalities between rural and urban strata in particular, as well as large scale emigration from rural areas (Sen, 2003). In addition the shift to cash crops and the failure of new agricultural technologies increased the vulnerability of farmers. Between 2001 and 2006, some 8,900 farmer suicides were reported from the states of Andhra Pradesh, Karnataka, Kerala and Maharashtra (Suri, 2006). Food availability, as a 3-year cumulative average per head per year, came down from 177 kg in the early 1990s to 151.06 kg in 2000–2001 (Patnaik, 2004). Distorted development contributed to the social exclusion of the backward and scheduled castes from work and wages (Karan & Selvaray, 2008).

Assessment of the reforms

The SAP over the 1990s could, thus, not achieve much in terms either of growth rates (as compared to the past or to future projections) or of promised security nets. This dysfunctional growth de-linked local industry from agriculture, but integrated it into the global market as partners in production, producers of raw material, or as providers of markets. Since the rich peasantry also shifted its base to industry, business, service and construction, to align with the global elite, the remaining peasants were left politically unrepresented and unorganized to cope with new production patterns, pressures of the WTO, food product dumping, penetration of locally untested technologies (like BT cotton and GM food), paucity of loans and aid, and falling subsidies.

Cutbacks in welfare

Apart from the collapsed state of rural development, there were also sharp cutbacks in investments in other sectors directly linked to health. The implications of some of these are described below:

Food distribution

In 1997, the universal Public Distribution System (PDS) was replaced by Targeted PDS covering the population below the poverty line, and those just above the poverty line. Later, by 2003, the large buffer stocks of 45–58 million tonnes sharply increased the cost of maintenance. This cost was passed on to the beneficiaries by retaining the procurement price but raising the price of grain in the PDS. In 2006 private collectors were allowed to collect grain at prices higher than the official procurement price and export it. The official procurement prices were raised only towards the end of the collecting season. Thus, instead of protecting the poor, grain was sold to them at prices higher than those prevailing in the market (Raghavan, 2006).

---

[1] Services contributed as much as 68.6% of the overall average growth in GDP in the past 5 years between 2002–2003 and 2006–2007. Practically the entire residual contribution came from industry. As a result, in 2006–2007, while the share of agriculture in GDP declined to 18.5%, the share of industry and services improved to 26.4% and 55.1%, respectively. Economic Survey, 2006–2007, Government of India.

Curiously, duty-free imports of 800,000 tonnes of grain for the open market were initiated in the name of dwindling buffer stocks and low procurement. The government also sold the stock in the open market to private collectors in order to cut subsidies and economies but not to enhance food security (Raghavan, 2006). These are only some glaring examples of monetary efficiency at the cost of the populace at large.

Drinking water and housing

It is true that the resource requirements for providing safe drinking water are enormous. The Fifth Five Year Plan allocated a total of Rs. 8,100 million yet, by 1980, a population of 160 million remained without safe drinking water (Planning Commission Government of India, 1981). By 1991, 19% of the urban and 44% of the rural households remained without clean water. By the end of the 1990s the situation did not improve much (Mehta & Menon, 2001). In many states women had to walk between 100 to 400 meters to get 190 litres of water per day for a household, and yet the minimum norm of 40 lpcd (litres per capita per day) for humans and 30 lpcd for cattle could not be met for 590,724 habitations, especially when the quality and quantity were put together (World Bank, 2009).

Following the adoption of SAPs, however, the central government proposed 20% support to the States conditional upon accepting SAPs. The private sector and donor agencies such as DFID, Danish International Development Agency (DANIDA), the Swedish International Development Cooperation Agency (SIDA) and the WB played a crucial role in introducing demand-based, instead of need-based, projects with public participation and cost-sharing by beneficiaries (Mehta &, Menon, 2001). As a signatory to the International Drinking Water Supply and Sanitation Decade (IDWSSD) India accepted the emphasis on self-financing, demand-based response and the role of PPPs to promote viability, efficiency, sustenance and transparency. Over the 1990s a total of USD 260 million was received as aid but, by 1996, a country-wide crisis of declining ground water table and drying wells hit some 230 districts of 16 States and falsified these assumptions. It was then politically accepted that the task of supplying safe potable water was, 'beset with problems of sustainability, maintenance and water quality' (Planning Commission Government of India, 2006).

Like drinking water, housing too has been neglected and the neglect has increased over the past 15 years. In the urban metropolis housing schemes for workers were sacrificed and prime lands were provided to trade and commercial operations. The working class, a majority of whom were migrant labourers, was now declared as 'illegal encroachers' and stereotyped as dirty, criminals, thieves, worthy of eviction and clearance (Ramanathan, 2005). In the absence of proper and adequate housing this uprooted majority continues to live in slums, unauthorized, resettlement colonies that lack all basic facilities (Sunitha, 2005).

Health services

Before 1990, India had built a substantial infrastructure of different levels of institutions, a trained manpower, educational institutions and several disease-control programmes within its public sector. However, the process had been so heavily influenced by political decisions that it heightened, as in many other countries, an urban bias where manpower was top heavy with only a few paramedical workers who were poorly trained. The medical education system retained a framework created in the 1930s, and public health education remained limited and unresponsive to both current challenges and the needs of the public. Bureaucrats (often clinicians with poor knowledge of public health) dominated decision making, resulting in an inability to integrate levels of health care, with specific disease-control programmes, and generating a market perspective towards health systems. The Health Sector Reforms (HSR), were an integral part of SAP, and introduced major cuts in public expenditure and increased the distortions in several ways:

- The infrastructure was weakened to the extent that it failed to deal with epidemics particularly of plague and malaria. The closure of plague monitoring units in Gujarat, and the shortage of drugs for resistant malaria in the peripheral institutions of Rajasthan, are just two examples.

- A shrinking public health infrastructure, a shift away from even SPHC to primary level and essential care for the poor, forging partnerships with the private sector for secondary and tertiary care, forced majority of the population to depend on the emerging private sector.

- Nutrition, sanitation and safe drinking water, earlier a part of the peripheral health institution's functions, were now excluded and privatized, although the talk of inter-sectoral planning continued to prevail among policy making circles.

- Cost cutting and a techno-centric focus reduced public services to the so-called essential disease-control programmes (AIDS, malaria, tuberculosis), and Reproductive and Child Health care at the cost of priorities such as under-nutrition, diarrhoea, etc.

- Public sector doctors, with their class and training biases, often paid little attention to the social determinants of disease (Qadeer, 2006), and moved to the private sector thereby helping the process of aggressive privatization.

- In the name of increasing efficiency, public sector hospitals were also made to open up to private participation through casualization of the work force, contracting out ancillary services and providing space for installing hi-tech investigative services.

- A shrinking public sector was thus rapidly fragmented in the following manner:

  A. A division between medical care and public health (untenable theoretically) locked the state's capital investments in preventive programmes, while the private sector made quick and high profits from tertiary and secondary medical care.

  B. A de-professionalized peripheral service based on health workers, registered practitioners and paramedics, with inadequate institutional support for the rural poor was separated from the hi-tech specialized service for the rich in both rural and urban areas.

  C. Contrary to the earlier commitment to comprehensive integration, an integrated approach was adopted only in the Family Welfare Programme (FWP) at the cost of the programmes it integrated with (nutrition, anaemia control, and childcare among others). Malaria, tuberculosis, and AIDS control programmes were however verticalized with enhanced dependence upon donor aid.

  D. During this period, PDS, clean drinking water, sanitation and housing were domains also de-linked from the health sector.

Role of the state

The success of HSRs crucially depended on the withdrawal of the state from provisioning of medical care, wherever the private sector was ready to take over. The private sector negotiated to provide even primary level care, if it was ensured a social- or community-based insurance partnership with the public sector, its subsidies and support (Confederation of Indian Industry,

2008). This oversight function for the state has absolved the private sector from its responsibilities of self-regulation, maintaining quality, standardizing prices, and cooperating with the state. The state, in turn, provides tax exemptions, import subsidies, loans at low interest rates, land lease, partnerships, and a share in government insurance schemes. Legislative changes to accommodate Trade Related Intellectual Property Rights (TRIPS) and GATS regimes, shifting subsidies from the public sector, changing taxation systems, and opening up public institutions to private investments make 'governance' a key issue in HSR. Governance now distracts attention from the 'politics' of weakened institutions and the dictate of the donors.

The state has also been transformed into a client in order to purchase the technologies produced by TNCs and MNCs, and is advised to distribute these through primary level services and vertical programmes. India's Intensified Pulse Polio Immunization (IPPI) Programme is an example of an irrational programme that has no epidemiological basis but has opened a huge market for the sale of refrigerating equipment needed for vaccines. While the WB accepts the failure of the market, it still proposes PPPs on the assumption that the weakness in distribution would be compensated for by the public sector (World Bank, 2004) by merely putting the two together without any corrective interventions.

The evidence, though, is that institutions with contradictory objectives of providing services and maximizing profits, in the absence of accountable, self-regulatory mechanisms or a partner (not steward) with strong regulatory abilities, will tilt the balance in favour of the private sector. This is clear from the National Health Policy (NHP) of 2002 (Government of India, 2002) that bends backwards to allow the private sector to function as a purely industrial unit and to generate profits out of public subsidies into medical tourism, without being concerned about the consequences for the poor. The same Policy proposes that it is the public sector that should target the poor, while it also defends the right of professionals to engage in private practice (Government of India, 2002).

Who are the beneficiaries?

Politically, HSR was introduced in the name of improving equity. The impact on health and access to health, especially of the poor, are therefore worth examining.

Health status

The national health statistics record a slowing down of mortality declines after 1990. Death rates declined from 12.5 to 9.8 over the 1980s, and to 8.7 over the 1990s; in 2007 it got reduced to 7.4. IMR moved down from 110 to 80 and then to 70; by 2005–06 IMR was 57. Similarly, birth rates declined from 33 to 29.5 during the 1980s, to 26 by the end of the 1990s (Government of India, 2005) and then to 24.1 by 2006. The MMR, according to the two National Family Health Surveys (NFHS) published in 1992 and 2000, was 424 and 540 per 100,000 births (Government of India, 2000a). The slowdown in declines and stagnation in mortalities, and the continuing levels of poverty in India, match the global evidence of a link between death and disease and the standard of living. The stagnant IMR cannot be explained away biologically as the rates are still too high to be purely congenital or genetic, and therefore not amenable to change.

Many Asian countries have already achieved much lower levels of IMR (Bhutan, Sri Lanka, China and Iran); and in India itself, Kerala has an IMR of 40. As a current WHO study points out, poor-quality environment contributes to 25% of deaths each year and diarrhoea, malaria, lower respiratory tract infections and obstructive lung diseases are the prime causes, rooted in unsafe water and bad sanitation, housing and working conditions (Prüss-Üstün & Corvalán,

2006). In India the national morbidity statistic is of reported illness and is, therefore, often very loaded in favour of the rich, as the poor tend to under-report their illness. But both the National Council of Applied Economic Research (NCAER) and the National Sample Survey (NSS) data, which make trend analysis possible, show that the poor report higher morbidity due to diarrhoea and fevers and that, in the rural areas, reporting of acute disease is much higher in the households that fall in the lowest income deciles. For chronic illnesses, the difference is less, while in urban areas, the rich report much higher levels of chronic illness (Government of India, 2000b;National Council for Applied Economic Research [NCAER], 1992).

The declining sex ratio for the girl children is another indicator that reflects acute gender discrimination in India. While the national average is 993 girls for 1,000 boys, there are 45 districts in India where the levels are lower than 800 (10 of 17 districts of Punjab, 5 districts in Haryana) even though these are some of the economically better-off regions. Apart from these, the worsening food security situation compounds the crisis in the state of health and health care. The statistics on improving nutritional intakes, when disaggregated, show that almost 47% of the sampled population still gets less than 70% of the recommended calorific intake and 84% gets less than 90% (Qadeer, 2005). The latest round of the NFHS (III), published in 2006, reveals that there is an increase in the incidence of malnourishment and anaemia among women and children, compared to the previous round conducted during 1998–99. Thus, there is little evidence that HSR and SAPs have improved the lives of the poor or their access to health services.

The rural primary health centres provide not more than 10% of the total inpatient services. Hospital bed utilization for serious illnesses shows that the poorest 4 deciles constitute 60% of the users. They constitute 70–90% of the users of basic care (immunization, antenatal and delivery care) in public hospitals. The introduction of user fees, and other forms of privatization that increase the cost of care, has pushed them out of this public facility as well as the use of free beds (Mahal & Veerabhraiah, 2005). This is demonstrated by untreated cases of morbidity over the 1990s that stayed at 26% in rural and 19% in urban areas. The reason for this was primarily financial and physical inaccessibility of services (Government of India, 2000b). Even the private sector was expected to provide free treatment to the poor through 25% of its beds under the terms of the land lease (now 10%), but it rarely keeps its commitment, while the state ignores this omission (Qadeer & Reddy, 2006). What then, is the political agenda behind reforms?

The international politics of investing in health

Governments and corporations

With the decline of welfarism, intergovernmental cooperation between States has been replaced by the corporate sector (led by the WB) taking up health project financing in the third world. Corporate institutions such as the International Commission of Commerce (ICC) and Global Public–Private Partnerships (GPPPs) emerged in the 1990s to provide vaccines, drugs and equipment. These alliances were fully supported by the UN, private capital, multilateral organizations and the States – particularly of the First World (Buse & Gill, 2002), strengthened by trade agreements of the WTO. Local governments have been rendered ineffective by GAT provisions that deregulate FDI, services, technology and manpower transfer across international borders and lower national controls. TRIPS achieved the same by giving more control to the MNCs over drug, vaccine and equipment trade (Shaffer & Brenner, 2004).

Following 10–15 years of slowing down in the improvements of public health indicators and rising increased inequalities in south Asia with SAP and HSR, the more liberal elements among policy makers were compelled to accept the seriousness of these trends and take initiatives to contain them promising 1% of GDP (United Nations, 1998; United Nations General Assembly, 2005). Consequently, as GPPPs increased to protect MNCs from the high risk of investing in research into new drugs for the (Third World) markets, pressure also started building within the UN to keep alive its commitment to equality, tolerance, freedom and justice. It was argued that GPPPs must work with the WHO so that a compromise could be reached between profits and ethics. The hard liners among the international planners accepted the MDGs within the UN in 2000 and the creation of a Global Fund. However, as per the Global Monitoring Report (GMR) of 2005 (World Bank, 2005), they nevertheless linked the success of the MDGs to private sector-led economic growth, dismantling barriers to trade and increasing the level and effectiveness of aid, apart from scaling up services and poverty reduction strategies (PRSPs) that were primarily meant to promote technology transfers, irrespective of the local context of recipient nations (World Bank, 2009).

WB and WHO

Even after agreeing at the International Conference on Population and Development (ICPD) most rich countries failed to contribute even 1% of their GDP for population and development. To save the MDGs from a similar fate it was necessary to show the benefits of investing in health. For this, the WHO collaborated with the WB to set up a CMH that pronounced investing in health technologies as the cutting edge of health sector reforms, for promoting economic growth in poor nations (Commission on Macroeconomics and Health, 2001), not necessarily development. The CMH focuses on consolidating the link between investment in health and economic growth. The Commission sets its strategies on certain viewpoints:

1. Improvements in health translate into higher economic growth rates that, in turn, bring down the disease burden.
2. The real problem in poorer countries lies in bad governance with corruption, weak management, weaker public sectors and financial deficits.
3. The excessive disease burden is related to a number of identifiable conditions, for each of which a set of interventions are available to drastically reduce the burden.
4. Global and local partnerships mobilize both finances and implementers (NGOs) filling the gap created by a poorly developed public sector infrastructure.
5. Global initiatives in specific areas (vaccines and drugs) introduce rigorous methods of monitoring, evaluation, financial control and accountability.
6. Targeting the poor and a close-to-client approach are more efficient ways of reaching the poor.

Flawed assumptions

While health is important for individual earnings and family incomes, it is not that important for national economic growth rates unless the disease takes an epidemic form threatening to disrupt production systems. Poverty and disease in countries with large and young labouring populations, in fact, provide cheap labour by lowering wages and thereby enable capital to grow faster. The contemporary situation in India is an apt example of this. Despite falling food availability, stagnant or slow declines in mortality rates and high morbidity rates, its economic growth rates have been lauded worldwide. Historically too, it is evident that economic growth rates are determined by socio-economic structural and political transformations. The impact of health status on economic growth is a fall-out of this transformation but not a primary influence, in the absence of any radical structural or political shifts. The Indian strategy for planned development after 1947 (initial experiments with planning) and after 1991 (introduction of SAP) are two examples that show health may improve or decline depending upon the nature of structural shifts and not just the rate of economic growth.

The health problems of the Third World in general, and India in particular, are not as simple as they are often made out to be by technocrats. The relevant epidemiological triad of diarrhoea, pneumonia, and malnutrition is ignored.[2] The reason they are often left out by strategists is precisely because the known technological interventions are less efficacious and require addressing complex environmental issues, both social and economic. The strategy of mobilizing NGOs has evolved into another way of releasing the state from its political compulsions. The unquestioning acceptance by the majority of NGOs, of donor control, user fees and propagation of specific technologies eases the process of pursuing the corporate agenda of expanding medical markets. In fact the CMH makes a-priori assumption of the failure of the public sector without any hard evidence or comparison where appropriate with the private sector in terms of quality, reach and outcome of services.

The poor and the rich

The CMH strategy of close-to-client delivery and 'targeting' the poor for care is yet another recipe for weakening the concept of collective responsibility or solidarity necessary for cross-subsidizing large welfare systems with high levels of inequity (Maarse & Aggie, 2003). It fragments services into those for the poor run by the state, and those for which the market is responsible. It depends on expanding medical markets, transformation of the state into a client as well as a steward, shift of subsidies into the private sector and pushing the state to move out of the welfare sector to create space for the private sector. It accepts the international trade rules but protects the industry from lower prices in the name of, 'not undermine the stimulus to future innovation that derives from the system of intellectual property rights' (Commission on Macroeconomics and Health, 2001). The benevolence of the GPPPs and the corporate sector in drug production and donations and price discounts, which is lauded by the CMH, can be seen as a cover for capturing access and control over Third World markets (Buse & Gill, 2002). It also binds the states to donor-driven vertical national programmes, but often has little to do with improving the health of the poor.

The politics of knowledge

All political positions claim to be fighting poverty and disease but with very different understandings of the macro-processes and their implications for the socio-economic conditions that generate health or disease. In the sphere of health effort is focused to erase the memories of our past experiences with planning and classical public health and to push to centre-stage the biomedical model and its techno-centric approaches to disease control. The central issue

---

[2] India's inability to control high child mortality has been due to the futility of curative interventions without handling under-nutrition that itself causes diarrhoea and makes children more susceptible to infections. Estimates of causes of child deaths reported reveal that 70% of child deaths occur due to diarrhoea, pneumonia, malaria and malnutrition. *Lancet*, editorial, March 2005.

then is the ability to critically analyze the politics of policy and power balances within the country and the world outside.

New concepts and theories

Over the past 15 years a set of new concepts and theories from market economics have gripped public health and are continuously reshaping it. This new public health is anti-poor as it restricts their choices, controls priorities, and ignores the social determinants of disease and the need for genuine choices. It can easily be called a 'Malthusian public health' as it makes the poor responsible for their conditions and focuses on their numbers rather than on the causes of ill health. We have already pointed out the fallacy of the notion that ill health is a major cause of poverty. Now we will show how a set of international health experts have transformed the very notions of public health, health system, efficiency and definition of public good (Peters et al., 2002):

1. According to these experts, public health involves the programmes and institutions collectively organized by society to protect, promote, and restore people's health through the oversight of private and public actors. The function of public health is thus reduced to an oversight, while its overarching nature of linking primitive, preventive, curative and rehabilitative services is ignored.

2. The health system is confined to discrete institutions, ignoring the internal contradictions between the political notions of public and private. The social determinants of health are viewed as the external environment of the health system and excluded from all analysis for the sake of 'simplifying' things. The difference between health and health service system is thereby overlooked, the real notion of the porous boundaries of the health service system is rejected, and the crucial role of social determinants sidelined.

3. 'Efficiency and quality' of service are defined as good health status, financial protection (reduced direct and indirect costs), and patient satisfaction without making a distinction between effectiveness (power to cure), efficiency (cost of cure against coverage), and efficacy (relative efficiency compared to other interventions). Thus, patient satisfaction and technical and managerial cost remain central with no reference to full coverage of population, the need for cost optimization and of testing efficacy of the technology compared to other interventions. Unexpressed needs are not discussed at all in the discourse led by international experts and most donors.

4. The contestability of public goods is reinterpreted as 'the ability of entrepreneurs to penetrate the market' rather than goods for which there is no competition and that have high cost of exclusion. All services with low contestability and measurability are considered public goods and handed over to the public sector, while services with clear monetary returns and without long-term investment needs are allocated to the private sector! This transformation of a sector from service to private goods involves a change in definition that neither sees health services as an integrated entity nor a necessity for all. The services are fragmented and reorganized to suit the market, ignoring the issue of inability of buyers to make the right choices. Thus, the very reason for which health was considered ill suited for distribution through markets is obscured.

5. There is a move from equality to equity in this new frame. Inequality as we know it is defined as differentials in opportunities across groups. All differentials except for those arising out of biological factors and conscious choices are rooted in the structure of a given society. Equity is achieved by removing preventable inequality. Inherent in equity

then is the acceptance of the politically non-preventable inequality that varies with the politics that governs a system. Equity then not only is a move away from objective analysis of systemic structures but also a means of veiling political subjectivity. It has different standards of distribution for the unequals and when even those minimum standards are not rationally defined, it is a misnomer for an anti-poor bias. The transition from CPHC to SPHC, and then Primary Level Care, and now 'essential health care' is a vivid example of the shifting standards of equity of the political system.

Contemporary national health policies and their politics

Globalization challenges national health planning, by using international trade rules to bind it to economic growth rates, and tying national services to the global market by making national borders open to penetration by TNCs. Other than privatization, globalization has also pushed for deregulation and decentralization and often over-ruled national decisions regarding financing through its secret trade tribunal (Shaffer & Brenner, 2004; Smith, 2004). The influence of these on all the welfare sectors and the construction of new knowledge over the past two decades are reflected in the Five Year Plans of that period, the National Population Policy (NPP) 2000, and the Health Policy 2002. Apart from promoting crude privatization, pushing for the casualization of the work force in health, they have also brought investments in the health sector to the lowest ever level (0.83% of GDP in 2001–02) (Table 9.2), while establishing the two-child norm, targeting the poor, and linking services closely to small family norms.

Decentralization through local governments, that was to enhance people's participation, has been instrumental in shifting responsibility and financial burden on to the people. The Tenth Plan (2002–2007) carried over these policies until 2004 when the ruling party, proud of its economic growth rates, lost the elections due to rising disparities. The coalition government during 2004–2009 made the Common Minimum Programme (CMP) its focus. But it has continued to remain with the reform agenda, even though some progressive steps such as the Right to Information Act, the National Rural Employment Guarantee Act, and debt waiver scheme brought some relief to the rural population reeling under economic stress. It also promised a rise in public investment in health from 1% of GDP to 2–3%, and the introduction of the National Rural Health Mission (NRHM). Though this proportion is half of what other developing countries such as Sri Lanka, Brazil and South Africa spent on their health sectors, it was never achieved (United Nations Development Programme, 2008). Yet, within the SAP regime, these promises and the secular thrust generated hope among the poor and have helped the return of the leading political party in the name of inclusive development. The NRHM has in fact undermined the system by strengthening only village and block level institutions to promote reproductive health care while neglecting key intermediary PHC. The overemphasis on FWP and AIDS continues, as does the dependence on foreign aid. The NRHM has only emphasized a functional integration in the form of family planning through reproductive and child health, but integration of medical treatment and disease control has been grossly neglected.

Table 9.2. Trends in public investment on health in India (as % of GDP)

	1980–1981	1985–1986	1990–1991	1995–1996	2001–2002
Public Investment on Health	0.91	1.05	0.96	0.88	0.83

Source: Report of the National CMH in India, Ministry of Health and Family Welfare, Government of India, 2005.

Politics of support and resistance

There are three broad streams of approaches found among the ruling classes in India vis-à-vis economic reforms. Some work and support the reform process fully, some attempt to smooth the rough and painful edges of the reform process through the 'security net' approach, and there are people who argue that a security net is not possible within an existing macro frame that, at best, creates a market for poor quality goods for the poor.

Against, or with, these layers among the ruling classes, are the working people's class, caste, and gender-based organizations representing the urban poor, the dam oustees and other displaced persons, the marginalized peasantry, and industrial workers who define health as 'a roof over our heads,' work, 'two square meals' and 'schools and health services for our children' (the poorest slum dwellers in Hyderabad) (Kambhampati, 1994). They resist globalization by fighting against the process of economic adjustment and the intensification of their own exploitation by demanding the right to work, reservation in jobs, political participation, education and welfare for the poor; they also assert their entitlements for equality and improved health. In other words they ask for an analysis of the capitalist system itself and not just the containment of its crisis through improved equity and social capital. The consequential political tension between different constituencies at different levels is an important influence on health through shifting policies. The mirage of development with reforms is reviving this political tension and throwing up the question of whether HSR is indeed a fuel for capitalist growth or its nemesis, as distorted growth destroys labour, the very essence of capital? Enlightened planning demands that the lessons of the massive sterilization campaign in India during 1975–1977 under the National Emergency with the subsequent political mandate against the ruling party in the following elections, and the fall of the National Democratic Alliance in 2003 after its 'India shining' campaign, should not be underestimated. The health of the marginalized may not determine the economic growth of a democratic country, but it does affect its politics.

References

Buse K. & Gill W. (2002). Globalisation and multilateral public–private health partnerships: Issues for health policy. In: Lee K., ed. *Health Policy in a Globalising World*. London: Cambridge University Press, pp. 41–62.

Chandrasekhar C. & Ghosh J. (2000). *The Market That Failed. A Decade of Neoliberal Economic Reforms in India*. New Delhi: Left Word Books.

Chandrasekhar C. & Ghosh J. (2006). *Macroeconomic Policy, Inequality and Poverty Reduction in India and China*. IDEAs Working Paper Series. New Delhi: International Development Economics Associates.

Chaubey P. (2002). Unemployment. In: *Alternative Economic Survey 2001–2002: Economic `Reforms`: Development Denied*. Delhi: Rainbow, pp. 175–80.

Commission on Macroeconomics and Health. (2001). *Macroeconomics and Health: Investing in Health for Economic Development*. Geneva: World Health Organization.

Confederation of Indian Industry. (2008). *Health Insurance Inc.: Providing Health Insurance Access – The Road Ahead*. Mumbai: Confederation of Indian Industry.

Government of India. (2000a). *National Family Health Survey, India: 1993–1994 & 1998–1999*. Mumbai: International Institute of Population Sciences.

Government of India. (2000b). Morbidity and treatment of ailments: NSSO 52nd round (July 1995–June 1996). Sarvekshana, *Journal of National Sample Survey Organisation*, 23(3), pp. 43–78.

Government of India. (2002). *National Health Policy – 2002*. http://mohfw.nic.in/np2002.htm.

Government of India. (2005). *Health Information of India 2004*. New Delhi: Government of India, Ministry of Health and Family Welfare, Central Bureau of Health Intelligence.

Himanshu. (2007). *Recent Trend in Poverty and Inequality: Some Preliminary Results*. Mumbai: Economic and Political Weekly, February pp. 497–508.

Kambhampati A. (1994). *Health in the Priorities of Slum Dwellers: A Case Study of Habib Fatima Nagar*. Hyderabad: Jawaharlal Nehru University.

Karan A. & Selvaray S. (2008). Trends in Wages and Earning in India: Increasing Wage Differentials in a Segmented Labour Market. Geneva: International Labour Organization.

Kumar A. (2005a). Macroeconomic scenario. In: *Magnifying Mal-Development: Alternative Economic Survey*. London: Zed Books, pp. 22–7.

Kumar R. (2005b). Industry. In: *Magnifying Mal-Development: Alternative Economic Survey*. London: Zed Books, pp. 84–91.

Maarse H. & Aggie P. (2003). The impact of social health insurance reforms on social solidarity in four European countries. In: Sen K., ed. *Reconstructing Health Services: Changing Context and Comparative Perspectives*. London: Zed Books, pp. 117–32.

Mahal A. & Veerabhraiah N. (2005). User charges in India's health sector: An assessment. pp. 265–73. 2005. NCMH background papers: Financing and delivery of health care services in India. New Delhi: Government of India, Ministry of Health and Family Welfare, National Commission on Macroeconomics and Health (NCMH).

Mehta A. & Menon N. (2001). Drinking water. In: *Alternative Economic Survey, 2000–2001: Second Generation Reforms, Delusion of Development*. New Delhi: Rainbow Publishers, pp. 126–36.

National Council for Applied Economic Research (NCAER). (1992). *Household Survey of Medical Care*. New Delhi: NCAER.

Patnaik U. (2004). *The Republic of Hunger. And Other Essays*. Gurgaon, India: Three Essays Collective.

Peters D. H., Yazbeck A. S., Sharma R. R., Ramana G. N. V., Pritchett L. H., & Wagstaff A. (2002). *Better Health Systems for India's Poor: Findings, Analyses, and Options. 2002*. New Delhi: The World Bank.

Planning Commission Government of India. (1981). *Sixth Five Year Plan (1980–1985) Chapter 23. Housing, Urban Development and Water Supply*. 1981. New Delhi, India: Oxford University Press.

Planning Commission Government of India. (2006). *Towards Faster and More Inclusive Growth. An Approach to the Eleventh Five Year Plan (2007–2012)*. Working papers. New Delhi, India: Planning Commission Government of India.

Prüss-Üstün A. & Corvalán C. (2006). *Preventing Disease Through Healthy Environments. Towards an Estimate of the Environmental Burden of Disease*. Geneva: World Health Organization.

Qadeer I. (2005). Nutrition policy. *Economic and Political Weekly*, **40**(5), pp. 358–64.

Qadeer I. (2006). The real crisis in medical education. *Indian Journal of Medical Ethics*, 3(3), pp. 95–6.

Qadeer I. & Reddy S. (2006). Medical care in the shadow of public private partnership. *Socal Scientist*, **34**(3), pp. 4–20.

Raghavan M. (2006). Wheat imports: Food security or politics? *Economic and Political Weekly*, **41**(21), pp. 2057–9.

Ramanathan U. (2005). Demolition drive. *Economic and Political Weekly*, **40**(27), pp. 2908–11.

Sen A. (2003). Globalization, growth and inequality in South Asia: The evidence from rural India. In: Chandrasekhar C. & Ghosh J., eds. *Work and Well-Being in the Age of Finance*. New Delhi: Tulika Books.

Shaffer E. & Brenner J. (2004). International trade agreements: Hazard to health? *International Journal of Health Services*, 34(3), pp. 467–81.

Smith R. (2004). Foreign direct Investment and trade in health services: A review of the literature. *Social Science & Medicine*, 59, pp. 2313–23.

Sunitha D. (2005). *MPD-2021 and the Vision of a 'slum-free Delhi.' Draft Delhi Master Plan*

20121: Blueprint for an Apartheid City. New Delhi: Hazards Centre.

Suri K. (2006). Political economy of agrarian distress. *Economic and Political Weekly,* **41**(16), pp. 1523–9.

United Nations. (1998). *Master Plans for Development.* The Hague forum. Netherlands, The Hague.

United Nations Development Programme. (2008). *Human Development Report 2007/2008. Priorities in public spending.* New York: United Nations Development (UNDP).

United Nations General Assembly. (2005). *MDG Proposal.* New York: United Nations.

World Bank. (2004). *World Development Report 2004: Making Services Work for Poor People.* Washington, DC: Oxford University Press.

World Bank. (2005). Global Monitoring Report 2005-Millennium Development Goals: From Consensus to Momentum. Washington, DC: World Bank.

World Bank. (2009). *Poverty Reduction Strategies.* http://go.worldbank.org/FXXJK3 VEW0.

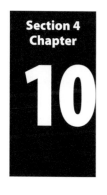

**Section 4
Chapter**

Determinants and implications of new liberal health policies: the case of India, China and Lebanon

10

An economic insight into health care provision in six Chinese counties: equity in crisis?

Lennart Bogg and Hengjin Dong

Background

China has, rightly, been noted for a health system which gives priority to the needs of the rural population, with an accessible network of basic health services, a preventative orientation and with innovative financial solutions. The Chinese health system has been reported to contribute to a better than expected population health status at a lower than expected cost (Halstead et al., 1985; World Bank, 1993). The acclaim for the Chinese health system influenced WHO to promote PHC and to launch the slogan 'Health for All by the year 2000' (Rohde, 1983).

Starting from the revolutionary decade of the 1960s, China developed a number of alternative and complementary health financing systems. Key characteristics of the different financing systems are laid out in Table 10.1. The delivery of basic health services for the rural population was closely linked to the rural health insurance, the Cooperative Medical System (CMS).

In the mid-1980s China, like many other countries, launched a health reform process. In many developing countries health reforms were not 'own' initiatives. Frequently they resulted from pressures for budget reductions in the context of structural adjustment programmes, often with severe implications for sectors such as health and education (Pinstrup-Andersen et al., 1987).

In China, health reforms may have been influenced by donor policy advice, although not necessarily driven by external pressures. The Chinese health reforms, for example, have been consistent with policy guidelines from the WB in the 1980s: decentralization of health management, introduction of user fees, privatization of financing and relaxation of government controls (Akin et al., 1987). These market oriented reforms led to problems with less access to health services for the poor in China (Taylor, 1992; World Bank, 2009). The impact of the Chinese reforms is reported to be among the most dramatic globally (Ma et al., 2008).

The Chinese government recently announced plans to redress setbacks and problems related to inequity, inadequate access for those in greatest need, quality problems, inappropriate provision of drugs, increasing antibiotic resistance and unreliable reporting due to perverse incentives (Hu et al., 2008; Liu et al., 2008; Wang et al., 2008).

The plans include a New Cooperative Medical System (NCMS), with, for the first time, budget contributions from the Central Government for rural health care. The funding will be strengthened with increased contributions from both local governments (counties and prefectures) and individual participants. The NCMS differs, however, in important aspects from the old CMS, something we will return to in the final discussion.

The privatization of farming from 1978 onwards removed the financial platform of CMS. In less than 15 years CMS participation dropped from around 90% of China's villages (1976) to less than 8% (Bogg et al., 1996).

As a consequence of the reforms, the public financial support for hospitals and village health stations was dramatically reduced, forcing doctors to increase fee revenue by expanding drug sales and seeking revenue from high-priced diagnostics and procedures (Chen, 1997;

Table 10.1. Characteristics of health insurance systems in China, 1965–2005

Health insurance systems	Enrolment	Premium	Service coverage	Claims refund system	Co-payments
Government health insurance (Gongfei)	Government employees and primary dependents (limited coverage)	Tax financed	Outpatient and inpatient services; drugs, tests, bed fees etc., except registration fee	Retrospective claims	Yes, flat rate contribution
Labour (enterprise) health insurance (Laobao)	Enterprise employees and primary dependents (limited coverage)	Varying; often covered by enterprise	Outpatient and inpatient services; drugs, tests, bed fees etc., except registration fee	Retrospective claims	Yes, flat rate contribution
Private health insurance	Voluntary or coverage purchased by employer	Varying	Outpatient and inpatient services; drugs, tests, bed fees etc., except registration fee	Retrospective claims	Yes, varying
Cooperative medical system (CMS)	Voluntary household, contingent on availability of CMS in the village	Varying, typically RMB 10–30 per year	Outpatient services at primary level (village health station); one day's issue of listed drugs, except registration fee	Prospective to primary providers, retrospective for hospital services	Prospective payment to providers
Prepayment systems; maternal immunization and child health	Women in fertile age, immunization aged children, school aged children	RMB 40–60, one-time premium	Yes, varying	Prospective payment to providers	Only registration fee, RMB 0.20 at primary level

Source: Adapted from Dong Hengjin; Health Financing Systems and Drug Use, doctoral thesis, Karolinska Institutet, 2000.

Dong et al., 1999; Wong & Chiu, 1998). Medical fees have become the dominant revenue source for the Chinese rural health system. The provision of medical services is influenced by the warped pricing and bonus systems. The most popular bonus system in the Chinese hospitals in the 1990s was the so-called Revenue-Related Bonus, linking the doctor's income directly to the revenue generated by the doctor's prescriptions and service provision (Liu et al., 2000).

According to a WB report, user fees provided 36% of the total health care resources in China in 1988 (Bumgarner, 1992). At the time it was considered a high level, but since then the proportion of revenue from user fees has reached even higher levels – 85% to 90% of the total rural health care financing less than a decade later (Bogg, 1995). Jun et al. report from a nation-wide household survey that, for the urban population also, the proportion of health care costs paid out-of-pocket increased in the 1990s, leading to a situation where not even all patients covered by government health insurance could afford advanced hospital care. The Chinese Ministry of Civil Affairs has warned that medical expenditures would be the leading cause of indebtedness among poor families in China (World Bank, 2009).

Yet Huang, in an early study of the impact of the Chinese health reform in Lin village, Fujian, based on data from 1984 to 1985, concluded that, although the privatization of health care initiated in June/July 1984 meant a shift towards more clinical care and out-of-pocket expenditure, it would not necessarily lead to a change in the national policy to control health expenditure. Neither did they accept that increased out-of-pocket expenditure would lead to a collapse of the entire health system or deterioration in the state of health within a short period (Huang, 1988). Gu and collaborators concluded that more research would be necessary to address the feasibility of funding the full range of rural health services out of community resources and to evaluate alternative financing models (Gu et al., 1993).

Equity – theory and evidence – Theoretical framework

Equity is defined as 'fairness', 'right judgment', 'principles of justice outside the common law or Statute law, used to correct laws when these would apply unfairly' (Hornby, 1980). Equity thus goes beyond equality, in that it has an ethical and moral aspect. Equity also differs from equality by being an impalpable concept, not easily measured. There are various definitions of equity (or inequity), more or less suited to varied operational perspectives.

Goddard and Smith observe that the concept of equity (in health care) remains somewhat elusive and that research evidence remains patchy and difficult to interpret (Goddard & Smith, 2001). Without a clear picture, even governments with a commitment to tackle inequities in access to health services face difficulties in making the right decisions. Goddard and Smith note that almost all empirical studies of equity in access to health care consider variations in treatment rather than variations in access, and that most exhibit little or no consideration of any theoretical framework.

Equity studies typically focus either on inequity in health status or inequity in access to health services, usually, in both cases, related to income. Studies of inequity in health examine the association between income differences and mortality rates. Health is usually measured by aggregate data; mortality rates, infant mortality or longevity. The relationship between health and income is termed gradient. Recent reports confirm a positive association between income inequality and higher mortality (Wolfson et al., 1999). As a policy response Deaton argued for income distribution or improving the income-earning abilities of the poor by education, rather than improving health through health sector interventions (Deaton, 2002). In Britain the government commissioned the Acheson Report, which led to measures aiming to improve the National Health Service (NHS), to provide income support for low-income groups, to improve education and employment opportunities, and to strengthen local communities and support vulnerable groups (Department of Health, 2001). Wilkinson found, by examining aggregate level data, that mortality is more related to relative income inequality than to absolute inequality and that national mortality rates tend to be lower in countries with smaller income differences, and that most of the long-term rise in life expectancy seems unrelated to economic growth (Wilkinson, 1997). Drever and Whitehead observed, however, a strong relationship between mortality and non-income socio-economic variables, expressed in a deprivation index, by analysis of data from English local authorities (Drever & Whitehead, 1995).

Inequities in the utilization of health care services are, reasonably, linked to indicators of socio-economic status. Health care services are generally expected to prevent or cure illness, to alleviate chronic illness and to avert premature death, although it has to be cautioned that evidence shows that health care only explains a modest part of health improvements (McKeown, 1980; Parkin, 1991).

China is, clearly, an example of a country of exceptional economic growth, with a five-fold increase of GDP per capita in the post-Mao period from 1978 to 2000. This growth has, however, been accompanied by growing disparities and a remarkable absence of improvements in the overall health of the population. The disparities in health between urban and rural areas and between West and East China are most stark and widening (Liu et al., 1999). The infant mortality rate (IMR) in 2006, was below 4/1,000 live births in the big cities Beijing, Tianjin and Shanghai, while the IMR in ethnic minority provinces Guizhou and Yunnan exceeded 50/1,000 (Gapminder Foundation, 2009).

Surveys have shown that 38% of peasants receive no medical treatment whatsoever when they fall ill, and 41% of those in need of hospitalization lack access (Gwatkin, 1999). These are facts which should suffice to point towards a collapse of the rural health system.

Yu and colleagues analyzed household survey data from three poor counties in Western and South China (Yu et al., 1997). They examined equity, with health care utilization as the criterion, in relation to per capita income, divided into three categories (low, middle and high). They reported evidence that user fees have a deterring effect on access for the low-income third of the population, particularly for inpatient care. Financial difficulties were the leading motive (55%) for not seeking care among the low-income group.

The European 'concerted action' research project (COMAC-HSR) in ten developed countries and the ECuity-projects, which compared inequality and inequity in health and health care across countries, produced a common research protocol and uniform methodologies for cross-country comparisons of inequity in the financing and delivery of health care (1987–1993). The COMAC-HSR studies examined vertical equity in financing of services – that is to say a regressive, proportional or progressive payment in relation to income for (same) health services, and horizontal equity in utilization. This would entail equal treatment for equal needs irrespective of one's income.

The studies were implicitly based on the assumption that income is the key predictor variable for inequity in financing and delivery of health care services. The variables sex and age were eliminated as confounding factors (Van Doorslaer et al., 1993).

Household income is, however, an aggregate measure for all the members of a household, although there are individual attributes such as age, health insurance coverage, educational or occupational status, and sex which are likely to influence care consumption.

Utilization is, in most equity studies, measured as an aggregate of all care expenditures, although different diagnoses have different socio-economic profiles and have different impact on the patient's well-being.

Most of the studies are descriptive with vague implications for health policy.

There are no previous reports examining the impact on equity (access/utilization) with respect to alternative health insurance systems.

Barnum and Kutzin defined inequity in health care as: 'involving interaction of the risks of illness across different social groups, the availability and use of services for the illnesses and the ability of different groups to pay' (Barnum & Kutzin, 1993). The definition involves both the needs aspect, that is to say the risk of illness, the utilization of services, and the financial ability across different socio-economic groups.

The following presentation is based on a conceptual framework, modified from a model by Whitehead (1997) reflecting the circular interrelationship between socio-economic status, health care utilization and health status (Whitehead, 1997). These include variables such as the following:

- Socio-economic factors influence morbidity;
- Different socio-economic groups may perceive illness differently in terms of need for care;
- Need is not only about people's perceptions of a need for care, but whether health care interventions can do anything useful towards satisfying their perceived need;
- How need translates into demand is influenced by alternative sources of care (e.g., in the family) but also by the health care system itself;
- People may have different knowledge and expectations of care and therefore differential demand;
- The actual translation of demand into utilization of care is dependent on supply, as well as different factors influencing access, for example economic, geographic, cultural, and organizational factors;
- The actual pattern of utilization of care will depend on the structure of the health system and its internal organization. Completing the first loop, utilization influences morbidity and 'need' related to this fact;
- The financial consequences of the utilization of care depends on the financing of the health system, the socio-economic characteristics of the particular society, and the household and the individuals contained within it;
- The financial impact will differ across disease categories and socio-economic groups. But completing the second loop, the financial impact will influence morbidity and may reinforce or counteract the health outcomes of care.

Objectives and assumptions

The aim of the study (1995–1997) was to assess how inequity in the financing and provision of health care in the six study counties was associated with socio-economic variables. The aim of this paper is to analyze what policy lessons can be learned from the first decade of health reform in China especially in relation to the design of the NCMS. It is important to study the reform process in China, not only from the perspective of the reforms affecting a large part of the world's population, but also for its potential policy relevance in other countries. Policy changes in China were probably driven by internal factors, and a strong desire to focus on economic development even at the cost of sacrificing investments in the social sectors, but they were also consistent with policy advice from the WB, as was the case for many countries (World Bank, 1992).

Equity studies usually examine utilization of health services in relation to income, which is a household level attribute. In the current study we examined both income and non-income variables, both at household and individual level. The variables, assumed to be relevant, at societal, household, and individual levels, respectively, are illustrated by Figure 10.1.

The specific aims were to assess:

- the degree of inequity in the financing of health services;
- the degree of inequity in the utilization of health services;
- the strength of association of key socio-economic determinants, with special interest in alternative health financing systems, with utilization of health care;
- the financial and health consequences of inequity in the utilization of health care.

Vertical equity in the financing of health services is examined from the criterion that equitable financing requires payment at least in proportion to income.

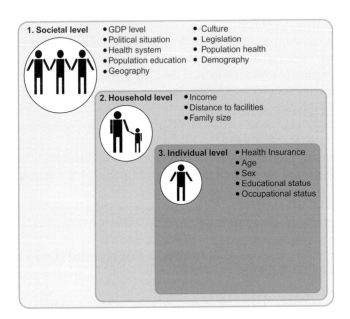

Figure 10.1. Model of attributes at societal, household and individual levels associated with utilization of health services. GDP, Gross Domestic Product.

Horizontal equity in utilization is examined from the criterion that the same needs should receive the same treatment irrespective of income, health insurance coverage, age, sex, educational or occupational status or geographical distance to health facilities.

It was assumed that inequity in access to health services is associated both with differences in household level attributes (income and geographical distance to health facilities) and individual level attributes (health insurance coverage, age, sex, and educational and occupational status).

The hypothesis was that alternative financing systems (out-of-pocket financing, the cooperative medical system, prepayment systems and other health insurance systems) differ with respect to inequity in utilization of health services.

Data and Methods

A household survey was conducted in 1995, in Central China. The survey covered 1,461 households, with a total of 5,756 respondents, selected through four-stage sampling in three provinces (Jiangsu, Anhui and Jiangxi).

The income data resulted from the question; 'What was your household's total income in RMB last year (1994)?' Health was measured by self-reported indicators: number of days within last month of illness, fever, cough, diarrhoea or blood in the stools.

Results

Indicator of health status

Figures 10.2 and 10.3 show the proxy indicator for health status, mean number of days with fever, by income quintiles (Figure 10.2) and non-income variables (Figure 10.3).

Figure 10.2 illustrates a near linear relationship between income and health. The differences in health status across the income categories are huge. The lowest income quintile had a 90% higher mean number of days with fever than the highest income quintile.

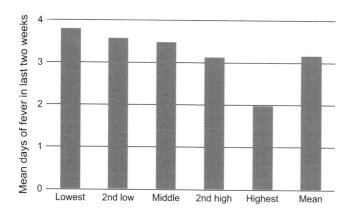

Figure 10.2. Indicator of health status by income quintiles.

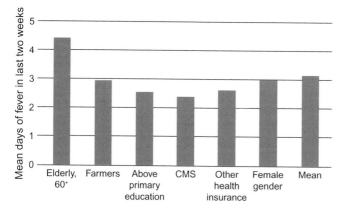

Figure 10.3. Indicator of health status by non-income variables. CMS, Cooperative Medical System.

Figure 10.3 shows that the non-income variables examined are also strongly linked to health status; the elderly suffered a higher than average number of days with fever, even higher than the mean for the lowest income quintile. Other categories examined – farmers, above primary educated; CMS participants; other health insurance participants and females – all had a lower than average number of days with fever. Those covered by CMS had a much lower number of days with fever, approximately 30% lower than the average, which could indicate that CMS participants went for treatment early, while non-participants waited until things got worse since they had no coverage.

The implications are that risk sharing within and across households had been reduced considerably with the demise of the CMS leaving the most vulnerable with the greatest exposure to poor access and ill health.

Co-variance between several of the variables can be expected. Multivariate analysis helps by reducing the risk of confounding. Table 10.2 is a summary matrix of multivariate analyses examining six alternative indicators for health status; severe (long duration) illness; number of days in bed due to illness; number of days with cough; number of days with fever, number of days with diarrhoea and number of days with blood in the stools.

Table 10.2. Financial impact, summary matrix of logistic and multiple regression analyses of socio-economic variables associated with health care utilization, self-reported difficulties in paying for medical expenditures (last visit), financial barriers to care and care-induced debt as dependent variables

Variables	Outpatient expenditures (excluding outliers)	Inpatient expenditures (excluding outliers)	Difficulties in paying for care (OR ML*)	Financial barriers to care (OR ML)	Care-induced debt (OR ML)
Household income		+0.243 (p=0.002)	0.7 (0.6–0.8)	0,8 (0.7–1.0)	0.9 (0.8–1.0)
Distance to county hospital	+0.094 (p=0.03)	+0.117 (p=0.12)			
Number of family members			1.1 (1.0–1.2)		
Co-operative health insurance			0.2 (0.1–0.5)		0.5 (0.2–1.1)
Other health insurance	+0,174 (p<0.0001)		1,4 (0.8–2.5)	3.2 (1.4–7.3)	0.7 (0.2–1.9)
Prepayment schemes			1,5 (1.1–2.0)	2.0 (1.2–3.5)	1.4 (0.9–2.1)
Aged 60 or more	+0.088 (p=0.04)	−0.194 (p=0.01)	2.2 (1.5–3.2)	2.0 (1.0–4.1)	1.2 (0.6–2.3)
Female gender		−0.142 (p=0.06)	1.0 (0.7–1.3)		0.9 (0.6–1.3)
Farmer by occupation		+0.233 (p=0.004)	1.8 (1.3–2.5)	1.5 (0.8–2.7)	1.9 (1.2–3.1)

Notes: *Odds ratio (OR with confidence interval) for logistic regression (ML) and beta (p value) for multiple regression (forward stepwise).

Severe illness was defined as being ill for at least 1 consecutive month. The definition yielded 90 positive cases (1.6% of the sample population). Logistic regression analysis identified two significant variables: age of 60 or more and CMS. Old age was, expectedly, associated with a much increased risk of severe illness, with an odds ratio of 5.2 (95% confidence interval [CI], 3.2–8.3). CMS was associated with much reduced risk of severe illness, with an odds ratio of 0.3 (95% CI, 0.1–0.8).

Other health insurance systems (than CMS) were associated with a non-significant increased risk of severe illness, OR=1.56 (p=0.12).

For the criterion 'number of days in bed due to illness,' three significant (p<0.05) predictors were identified; age of 60 years or more, occupation as farmer and other insurance coverage than CMS. All three had a positive correlation.

For the criterion 'number of days with cough,' CMS was associated with a lower number of days. Occupation as farmer was, again, identified with a positive correlation. Distance to nearest county hospital was negatively correlated. This may appear intuitively surprising. However, closeness to a county hospital indicates residence in a densely populated area, with possible higher risk of exposure to infection.

For the criterion 'number of days with fever,' two negative predictors were identified: household income and higher education; and one positive: old age.

Multiple regression analysis identified two negative predictors related to 'number of days with diarrhoea': household income and distance to county hospital.

Only 26 cases with 'days of blood in the stools' were reported. Multiple regression analysis confirmed only one predictor, occupation as farmer, with positive correlation. Since schistosomiasis is prevalent in the Yangtse Basin area it could be anticipated that farming would be correlated with the criterion.

Utilization of health services
Outpatient expenditures

Outpatient expenditures were analyzed by forward stepwise multiple regression.

The analysis was performed in two versions: with and without outliers. The alternative analyses yielded, as could be expected, quite different results. With all observations included, two significant explanatory variables – household income (positive correlation) and coverage by other health insurance systems (positive correlation) – were identified.

With outliers excluded (expenditure of at least RMB 500; 6 of total 535 observations), the low coefficient of multiple determination (R^2) increased from 0.012 to 0.046. Three significant explanatory variables, all positive, were identified: other health insurance systems than CMS, distance to nearest tertiary hospital, and age of 60 or more.

Inpatient expenditures

Inpatient expenditures were analyzed by forward stepwise multiple regression inclusive and exclusive of outliers.

The same explanatory variables were examined as for outpatient expenditure. Including outliers two explanatory variables were identified for the model, neither of which was significant. When outliers were excluded (expenditure of at least RMB 4000; seven of total 177 observations), the coefficient of multiple determination (R^2) increased considerably from 0.038 to 0.135.

Three significant explanatory variables were identified: age of 60 or more (negative correlation), household income (positive), and occupation as farmer (positive).

The elderly were predicted to have, on average, RMB 398 lower expenditure.

The age group of 60 years and more make up 8% of the population (actual numbers of elderly are among the highest in the world) yet consumed only 4% of the inpatient care.

The mean inpatient expenditure was predicted to increase by RMB 36 by each RMB 1,000 increment of household income. Farmers, on average, had RMB 314 higher inpatient expenditure.

The arbitrary and huge effect of the few high value observations was eliminated by the exclusion of outliers. The properties of the distribution of inpatient care expenditure came closer to normal distribution, skewness dropping from 5.4 to 1.3 and kurtosis from 36.4 to 1.2.

Indices of illness, utilization and financing

The Illness concentration index, the Le Grand index and the Kakwani index were calculated and compared with Denmark (1982), the UK (1985) and the USA (1980).

The Illness concentration index; inequity in health

The illness concentration index is a measure of inequity in morbidity. Individuals are ranked by order of their income, beginning with the lowest income. The illness concentration index represents the difference between the cumulated proportion of individuals and the cumulated proportion of illness for the ranked individuals. The illness concentration index can take a value from +1.0 (only the person with the highest income is ill) to −1.0 (only the person with the lowest income is ill).

Zero denotes morbidity which is not associated with income.

The illness concentration index for the six counties was negative both when using number of days with fever (−0.13) and days of cough (−0.12) as indicators, which confirms, expectedly, that the poorer suffer from a higher prevalence of morbidity. The levels fall within the range of the ten COMAC-HSR countries.

The Le Grand index: inequity in the utilization of health care

The Le Grand index is a measure of inequity in the access or utilization of health services. It relates utilization by income strata to need by income strata. If the Le Grand index is positive, there is inequity favouring the high-income groups, and if the index is negative, the inequity is favouring the low-income groups.

The analysis for the six counties yielded a Le Grand index of +0.32 for outpatient expenditures, when using days with cough as illness indicator, and +0.31 when using days of fever.

The Le Grand index was +0.21 for inpatient expenditures, when using days with cough and +0.20 for days of fever.

The results tell us that, in the six study counties, the poor do not have access to the same treatment for the same needs. The discrimination against the poor is higher than that observed in any of the ten COMAC-HSR countries.

The Kakwani index; inequity in the financing of health services

The Kakwani index was used to measure inequity in the financing of health services. The Kakwani index can take a value from +1.0 to −2.0. A positive value indicates progressive financing and a negative value regressive financing.

The Kakwani index for the six counties indicates an extremely high degree of regressivity in the financing of health services, even beyond what could be expected in a fee-for-service system, −0.73 for outpatient services and −0.94 for inpatient services. This represents a strong deviation from proportionality in the financing favouring the rich. The highest level of regressivity in the ten COMAC-HSR countries was recorded for the United States (1980) with −0.39 for out-of-pocket expenditures. The Kakwani index in the six Chinese counties, especially for inpatient services, was much more regressive than anything reported previously anywhere, reflecting the extreme level of inequity in the Chinese rural health system.

Financial hardships

Self-reported difficulties to pay for medical expenditures were analyzed by logistic regression analysis. Two questions related to financial difficulties were asked. One was a general question: 'Has your household experienced difficulties in paying?' This question yielded 1,807 positive responses of 5,414 valid observations (33.4%). The other was a more specific question: 'Last time you fell ill, did you have any difficulties in paying?' The second question received 232 positive responses out of 5,381 valid observations (4.3%). The analysis was based on the results of the second question.

The odds ratio for unit change indicated that coverage by CMS was negatively correlated with payment difficulties, OR=0.22, which implies that CMS does protect against financial difficulties. Coverage by prepayment system (PPS) was positively correlated, OR=1.49, which may seem surprising. However, prepayment systems primarily cover preventative low-cost interventions and do not cover costly curative care events. Other health insurance systems had non-significant correlation.

As could be expected, payment difficulties were negatively correlated with income, OR=0.71. Payment difficulties were positively correlated with age of 60 years and above, OR=2.22. The correlation for income and age were both highly significant (p<0.0001).

Being a farmer was correlated with an increased risk of payment difficulties, OR=1.84. Higher than primary education resulted in significant negative correlation, OR=0.63. Gender was not significantly correlated with payment difficulties.

Care-induced debt

Care-induced debt to providers, friends, relatives or money lenders was analyzed by logistic regression. There were 99 positive responses out of 5,433 observations (1.8%).

Two explanatory variables were identified with a significant correlation; higher education and farming. Higher education was related to a risk reduction by more than half. Being a farmer by occupation was related to a risk increase by nearly double.

Both household income and CMS had lower odds ratios: OR=0.87 and OR=0.48 (p=0.07 and p=0.09).

The most common way out of financial difficulties due to medical bills was to borrow from friends or relatives (73%). The average debt amount was RMB 1,640 (95% CI; RMB 1,019–2,262), substantial in relation to the annual household incomes. The lowest income decile had a mean annual household income of less than RMB 1,500. Of a total of 24 cases of care-induced debt of at least RMB 1,000, 7 cases occurred in the lowest income quintile and 6 in the second lowest. In other words more than half of the cases of severe debt afflicted the lowest two income quintiles. More than 1 in 4 inpatient visits (25.4%), but less than 1 in 12 outpatient visits (8.0%), resulted in care-induced debt. Inpatient costs more frequently caused care-induced debt, although, obviously, inpatient visits are less frequent than outpatient.

Financial barriers to care

Financial barriers to care were analyzed by logistic regression, based on the responses to the question: 'Did you resolve the difficulties by not seeking care?' as a dependent variable. There were 57 positive responses of a total of 5,434 observations (1%). Three significant explanatory variables were confirmed. For CMS, an odds ratio could not be calculated, since not even one CMS participant had to forego care due to financial difficulties. Surprisingly, other insurance systems were associated with a significantly higher risk of not seeking care due to financial hardship, OR=3.15. The reason could be that those covered by other health insurance systems tend to go directly to hospitals or specialized services, where they are offered more services and charged more. Prepayment systems were, similarly, correlated with a higher risk of not seeking care, OR=2.01.

Higher education was negatively correlated with not seeking care, OR=0.33. Old age and being a farmer were associated with a higher risk of not seeking care in the face of financial difficulties (p=0.05 and p=0.22, respectively). Household income was associated with less risk of not seeking care (p=0.08).

The analysis is summarized in a matrix (Table 10.2).

Discussion

We found important differences in the impact of alternative health insurance systems in the counties. The results indicate that the old cooperative medical system was powerful in reducing financial difficulties, while other health insurance systems were associated with an increased risk of not affording care. The population covered by CMS had, on average, a five times lower risk, after adjusting for other factors, of facing financial difficulties, a risk reduction by half of ending up in debt due to medical costs and, significantly, not one CMS participant had to forego care-seeking due to medical costs.

The population covered by the old CMS had a more than three times lower risk of illness for at least 1 month and a significantly reduced risk of suffering from a number of days of cough.

Other health insurance systems were associated with higher costs, without evidence of reducing barriers to care.

We believe that this is due to the prospective provider reimbursement system in combination with the gate-keeping functions directing CMS patients to local primary or secondary care facilities. The high degree of cost sharing for tertiary care and the administrative procedures limited the use of expensive curative services for CMS patients.

Patients covered by government or enterprise health insurance with retrospective reimbursement systems, had a higher proportion of curative services. The higher reimbursement rates increase the risks of moral hazard and supplier-induced demand.

The Central Government has supported policy initiatives towards the fast expansion of the NCMS in rural China (Gwatkin, 1999). It is clearly a good thing that the NCMS will bring in more funding and will have allocative function by bringing in Central Government funding. It is, however, a cause of concern that the NCMS is not a prospective system like the old CMS and it is not oriented to the basic care levels, which are geographically more accessible and less costly to users.

The rural population spent a considerable proportion of their income on health care. One inpatient visit in four resulted in care-induced debt, more frequently afflicting the poor. Thus, ill health completes the vicious circle by leading to poverty.

Inequity discriminating the poor in health financing and a strong bias against the poor and the elderly in illness prevalence and care utilization were observed in the study counties. High age was correlated with both higher needs and lower utilization. Only a very small proportion of the total inpatient services in the study counties were used by the elderly in contrast to the typical pattern in developed countries.

The multiple regression analysis confirmed that the low utilization by the elderly cannot be explained by confounding from income or health insurance coverage. This points to cultural or value factors within the families that restrict the medical access for the elderly.

The age distribution of inpatient costs in developed countries is typically U-shaped, high for the youngest, low for adolescent and active ages and highest for the elderly. Here, a rollercoaster distribution was observed with high expenditures for 0–5 years, low for 6–19 years, higher for 20–59 years and dropping dramatically for the 60+ category. This is an observation with serious potential implications, including control of infectious diseases.

The data reflects a significant negative correlation between household income and days of fever and days of diarrhoea, that is, the higher the income the lower the risk of illness, which is consistent with studies in other countries.

Individual non-income attributes (age, health insurance coverage, occupation, and education) were, however, also found to be associated with utilization of care, health status and financial consequences.

We did not find indications of geographical inequity (within the counties) in utilization. This is consistent with the analysis of Henderson and colleagues, concluding on the basis of an eight-province survey that China has achieved a very wide distribution of clinics and other services that are widely used by those who identify needs (Henderson et al., 1994). What we measured was intra-county geographic inequity, while Gustafsson and Zhong found that geographic inequity in China is more related to inter-regional differences (Gustafsson & Zhong, 2000). However, the fact that we did not find a significant inequity related to geographical access within the counties should not be interpreted as though there is no geographical inequity between counties.

On average, the lowest income quintile used more than 9% of their annual household income for inpatient care compared to less than 2% for the other income categories. One percent of the population did not seek care due to financial constraints. The poor appeared more prone to incur debt when faced with health problems, while the higher income groups more often stay away from the doctor, which could reflect less serious conditions. The results showed that the poor, the farmers and the elderly were more affected by illness and by more severe conditions.

More research, related both to the causes and the consequences of the lack of access to health care for the elderly, would no doubt be justified. It seems that families or the elderly themselves deem it not worth spending money on curing or alleviating their problems. This situation, obviously, impacts negatively on the quality of life of the elderly, but it is also likely to be counterproductive to the control of epidemic diseases. The tuberculosis control strategy is built on passive case finding (Bogg & Diwan, 1996). In rural China extended families are common. If the elder generation will not go to the clinic when they suffer fever and cough, it will not help no matter how effectively the younger generation is treated. The policy makers need to pay more attention to the low levels of care utilization for the rural elderly population and the non-financial barriers preventing their access.

The financing of health services needs to address two quite different sets of problems. First, and often most conspicuous, are the low-frequency high cost (LFHC) procedures, typically inpatient services. Inpatient care consumed 1.8% of the total self-reported household incomes in the six counties, but only in half of the cases the costs exceeded RMB 500. The aggregate cost of inpatient events above RMB 500 thus amounted to less than 1% of the aggregate household incomes. Yet they accounted for most of the financial difficulties for the affected families.

Second, there are high-frequency low cost (HFLC) procedures, often preventative by nature and typically performed as outpatient services. The HFLC events may not be so critical from the debt and poverty aspect, but should often be considered merit goods, specifically to have a value for the society over and above the value to the individual care consumer. The 'old' CMS was more geared towards the HFLC problems, while the NCMS is oriented towards catastrophic illnesses, that is to say the LFHC problems.

The small number of households faced with very high medical fees in the six counties suggests that policy measures, which support comprehensive health insurance that would cover the cost of LFHC events as well as incorporate a strong linkage to primary care and prospective provider reimbursements of the old CMS, are likely to reduce unhealthy provider incentives, and generate the most equitable option. This method should reduce the inequity both in access to health services and in the health and financial consequences as has been the case, following the for-profit commercial paradigm, illustrated throughout this book.

Acknowledgement: The financial support by Sida/SAREC, the Swedish International Development Cooperation Agency, the Department for Research Co-operation with Developing Countries, is gratefully acknowledged for support to Chapter 10 of Section 4.

References

Akin J. S., Birdsall N., & De Ferranti D. M. (1987). *Financing Health Services in Developing Countries – an Agenda for Reform*. Oxford, UK: World Bank Publications.

Barnum H. & Kutzin J. (1993). *Public Hospitals in Developing Countries: Resource Use, Cost, Financing*. Baltimore: Johns Hopkins University Press.

Bogg L. (1995). Health-insurance in rural Africa. *Lancet*, 345(8948), pp. 521–2.

Bogg L. & Diwan V. (1996). Tuberculosis control in China. *Lancet*, 347(9016), p. 1702.

Bogg L., Dong H., Wang K., Cai W., & Vinod D. (1996). The cost of coverage: Rural health insurance in China. *Health Policy and Planning*, 11(3), pp. 238–52.

Bumgarner J. R. (1992). *China: Long-Term Issues in Options for the Health Transition*. World Bank Country Study, Washington, DC: World Bank.

Chen J. (1997). The impact of health sector reform on county hospitals. *IDS Bulletin-Institute of Development Studies*, 28(1), pp. 48–52.

Deaton A. (2002). Policy implications of the gradient of health and wealth. *Health Affairs (Millwood)*, 21(2), pp. 13–30.

Department of Health. (2001). *Tackling Health Inequalities: Consultation on a Plan for Delivery*. http://www.dh.gov.uk/en/index.htm. London: Department of Health.

Dong H. J., Bogg L., Rehnberg C., & Diwan C. V. (1999). Health financing policies: Providers' opinions and prescribing behavior in rural China. *International Journal of Technology Assessment in Health Care*, 15(4), pp. 686–98.

Drever F. & Whitehead M. (1995). Mortality in regions and local authority districts in the 1990s: Exploring the relationship with deprivation. *Population Trends*, (82), pp. 19–26.

Gapminder Foundation. (2009). *Gaps Within China*. http://graphs.gapminder.org/world/china.php.

Goddard M. & Smith P. (2001). Equity of access to health care services: Theory and evidence from the UK. *Social Science & Medicine*, 53(9), pp. 1149–62.

Gu X. Y., Bloom G., Tang S. L., Zhu Y. Y., Zhou S. Q., & Chen X. B. (1993). Financing health care in rural China – Preliminary report of a nationwide study. *Social Science & Medicine*, 36(4), pp. 385–91.

Gustafsson B. & Zhong W. (2000). How and why has poverty in China changed? A study based on microdata for 1988 and 1995. *China Quarterly* (**164**), pp. 983–1006.

Gwatkin D. R. (1999). *Health care for China's rural poor; from research to policy in China's effort to reestablish effective rural health cooperatives*. International Health Policy Program (IHPP) Occasional Papers, pp. 1–57. Washington, DC: International Health Policy Program.

Halstead S., Walsh J. A., & Warren K. S. (1985). *Good Health at Low Cost*. New York: The Rockefeller Foundation.

Henderson G., Akin J., Li Z. M., Jin S. G., Ma H. J., & Ge K. Y. (1994). Equity and the utilisation of health-services: Report of an eight-province survey in China. *Social Science & Medicine*, 39(5), pp. 687–99.

Hornby A. S. (1980). *Oxford Advanced Learner's Dictionary*. Oxford: Oxford University Press.

Hu S. L., Tang S. L., Liu Y. L., Zhao Y. X., Escobar M. L., & de Ferranti D. (2008). Health System Reform in China. 6. Reform of how health care is paid for in China: Challenges and opportunities. *Lancet*, 372(9652), pp. 1846–53.

Huang S. M. (1988). Transforming China's collective health care system: A village study. *Social Science & Medicine*, 27(9), pp. 879–88.

Liu X. Z., Liu Y. L., & Chen N. S. (2000). The Chinese experience of hospital price regulation. *Health Policy and Planning*, 15(2), pp. 157–63.

Liu Y. L., Hsiao W. C., & Eggleston K. (1999). Equity in health and health care: The Chinese experience. *Social Science & Medicine*, **49**(10), pp. 1349–56.

Liu Y. L., Rao K. Q., Wu J., & Gakidou E. (2008). Health System Reform in China. 7. China's health system performance. *Lancet*, **372**(9653), pp. 1914–23.

Ma J., Lu M. S., & Quan H. (2008). From a national, centrally planned health system to a system based on the market: Lessons from China. *Health Affairs (Millwood)*, **27**(4), pp. 937–48.

McKeown T. (1980). *The Role of Medicine: Dream, Mirage, or Nemesis?* Princeton: Princeton University Press.

Parkin D. (1991). Comparing health services efficiency across countries. In: McGuire A., et al., eds. *Providing Health Care: The Economics of Alternative Systems of Finance and Delivery*. Oxford: Oxford University Press, pp. 172–91.

Pinstrup-Andersen P., Jaramillo M., & Stewart F. (1987). The impact on government expenditure. In: Cornia G., et al., eds. *Adjustment With a Human Face: Protecting the Vulnerable and Promoting Growth*. Oxford: Oxford University Press, pp. 73–89.

Rohde J. E. (1983). Health for all in China: Principles and relevance for other countries. In: Morley D., et al., eds. *Practising Health for All*. Oxford: Oxford University Press.

Taylor C. E. (1992). Surveillance for equity in primary health care – policy implications from international experience. *International Journal of Epidemiology*, **21**(6), pp. 1043–9.

Van Doorslaer E., Rutten F., & Wagstaff A. (1993). *Equity in the Finance and Delivery of Health Care: An International Perspective*. Oxford: Oxford University Press.

Wang L. D., Wang Y., Jin S. G., et al. (2008). Health System Reform in China. 2. Emergence and control of infectious diseases in China. *Lancet*, **372**(9649), pp. 1598–605.

Whitehead M.(1997). *Bridging the Gap: Working Toward Equity in Health and Health Care*. Karolinska Institutet, Department of Public Health Sciences.

Wilkinson R. G. (1997). Socioeconomic determinants of health – Health inequalities: Relative or absolute material standards? *British Medical Journal*, **314**(7080), pp. 591–5.

Wolfson M., Kaplan G., Lynch J., Ross N., & Backlund E. (1999). Relation between income inequality and mortality: Empirical demonstration. *British Medical Journal*, **319**(7215), pp. 953–5.

Wong V. C. & Chiu S. W. (1998). Health care reforms in the People's Republic of China: Strategies and social implications. *Journal of Management in Medicine*, **12**(45), pp. 270–86.

World Bank. (1992). *China: Long-Term Issues in Options for the Health Transition*. World Bank Country Study. Washington, DC: World Bank.

World Bank. (1993). World Development Report 1993: Investing in Health. Washington, DC: World Bank.

World Bank. (2009). *China: Strategies for Reducing Poverty in the 1990s*. Washington, DC: World Bank.

Yu H., Cao S. H., & Lucas H. (1997). Equity in the utilisation of medical services: A survey in poor rural China. *IDS Bulletin-Institute of Development Studies*, **28**(1), p. 16.

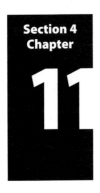

Determinants and implications of new liberal health
policies: the case of India, China and Lebanon

Health care financing and delivery in the context of conflict and crisis: the case of Lebanon

Adapted from: Sen, Kasturi and Sibai, Abla (2004). Transnational Capital and Confessional
Politics: the Paradox of the Health care system in Lebanon. International Journal of Health
Services, Volume 34, Nov. 3 2004. pp. 527–551.

Regional background – The Mashreq

Many countries in the Arab world promised education and health care free for all, as part of the
post independence revival of nationalism. However, a variety of factors prevented the development of universal access to health care. These include the high proportion of countries in
the region experiencing some sort of conflict: capital flight, a poor tax base and dependence
on donor assistance. There has also been a significant effect on the ability to deliver this promise due to the existence of oil-rich Gulf cooperation countries, whose high-tech, high-cost
medical priorities, have an impact on the nature of health services in other countries of the
region, through migratory flows and economic cooperation.

A focus on specialized rather than comprehensive care has also been encouraged by
donors, most notably the WB among others, through the doctrine of privatization and contracting out of health services, that has led to specialization often to the detriment of access
and equitable distribution of services (Kronfol, 2002).

Moreover, observers note that, in a majority of countries of the Mashreq region (the Arab-
speaking world stretching from east of Egypt to north of the Arabian peninsular), civil society
organization is weak and often unable to place pressure on their respective governments for
the basic rights of citizens (Jabbour et al., 2006).

In terms of health status, there are stark differences between individual countries with
non-communicable disease (NCDs) predominant in urban areas, whilst in rural areas
(with poor water and sanitation) infectious diseases predominate with higher levels of
maternal and infant mortality. Poor access to services and the high cost of medications has
an impact on the most vulnerable – women, children and elderly people. However, despite
the range of health problems reported, public health and prevention have a low priority
throughout the region, where the emphasis is on curative care. It is rare to locate variations in socio-economic status, age and gender in health status, reflecting the widespread
absence of citizens' rights.

The Arab Human Development Report (AHDR) highlighted several key dilemmas
facing the region as a whole. These include high levels of illiteracy, especially among
women; a lack of democratic government and civil society participation in politics;
high levels of military expenditure; and the effects of conflict and absence of freedom of
movement (related to occupations and wars among other factors) limiting the exchange
of information between citizens in the Arab region (United Nations Development
Programme, 2009).

The following chapter focuses on the Lebanon and examines issues of health financing and population access to the health sector in the aftermath of conflict. Lebanon straddles the traditional modern city versus rural divide, and one where policy is made within the context of complex donor pressures and confessional politics that reinforce division and inequality. This paper also explores some of the options for improving the state of health and health services for its citizens. The chapter is set in a historical context and considers the background to health services provision and the confessional political system that is predominant.

Background

Public health systems worldwide have experienced major structural changes during the past three decades. Among these included the rapid privatization of public provision and an increasing role for out-of-pocket expenditures for different elements of health care (Koivusalo, 2003). The ideological rationale of neoliberal strategy underpinning the changes has been to claim that market mechanisms are more efficient, provide better value for money and better quality of care, than public providers. Underpinning this case is an emphasis on the notion of 'consumer interest,' which its advocates claim may be better served through use of markets rather than the state in the provision of services (Newbrander, 1997; World Bank, 1993).

To a large extent this (neoliberal) paradigm has usurped and transformed the notion of 'the public' and of 'civil society' into a collection of individual consumers and individual providers. Nowhere is this paradigm better served than in Lebanon which witnessed a systematic erosion of centralized authority through prolonged wars and civil strife between 1975 and 1992 and again in 2006, and Israeli invasion and occupation. Set within a context of social and economic inequality, the war created a vacuum, which acted as a natural partner for the neoliberal agenda for commercialized and privatized health care. The Lebanese case provides an interesting example of the ability of transnational and globalized capital to combine its specific need for the accumulation of profit, with that of confessional groups at a local–national level particularly during prolonged crisis. However, the irony of the Lebanese context is that, unlike anywhere else in the world, reforms have been initiated to check the excesses of private provision in the health sector as indicated throughout the chapter.

It is evident that the fragmented nature of Lebanon's health system has also been reinforced and strengthened by geographical segregation and maintained through confessional stratification, unique to the country. However, within such a dynamic, private interests continue to be promoted though transnational capital, in partnership with local agencies. According to Harik it is this geographic concentration that has expanded or been restrained through war and conflict over the past 25 years that has served as the basis for 'local agencies' and which forms the pillars of a 'mosaic society' which involves a patchwork of localities that have been ruled by families for generations with the exception of Hizbollah where the leadership is elected (Harik, 1994).

Financing the health sector in Lebanon: historical measures

Historically the health and social sectors of Lebanon, unlike other countries of the Mashreq, have been largely managed through private and voluntary agencies. The direct role of the state as a provider has been limited to the provision of basic infra-structural support and the financing of the cost of care through various insurance schemes. However, despite the predominance of private providers, ironically their survival has been dependent upon extracting funds from the public purse.

In most countries the impetus for reforms arose out of a combination of laissez faire ideology coupled with weakened public provision (in terms of quantity and quality) and a growing external pressure for privatization. In Lebanon, however, the opposite has been the case. Here, the private sector (for-profit and not-for-profit) has been the mainstay of the health system throughout the past several decades. The reform programme for the health sector in Lebanon was accompanied by a number of feasibility studies of national accounts that have examined problems with the entire system, with focus on the excesses of private provision, increasingly dependent upon public subsidies as well as a large share of household expenditure. Despite its substantial public subsidy, private providers had, until recently, developed a reputation for providing services of high cost, uneven quality and a poor system of distribution, leading to gross inequality in terms of access to health care (Mechbel, 1997).

A review of the Lebanese health system and reforms highlights the fact that the state was forced to contract out health care to private providers as a result of the almost complete destruction of public health services during 17 years of war and invasion (1975–1992). While this has been changing, recently, it has been difficult to reverse this process in the aftermath of war because of vested interests embedded in the political and economic structure of the health sector, through powerful syndicates, professional associations (Order of Physicians and Pharmacists, for example), and the predominance of confessional political parties (Ammar, 2003).

The Lebanese health care system

Public health provision in the Lebanon has had a chequered and fragile history. At the turn of the twenty-first century the influence of the colonial power in evolving state paternalism was powerful. The role of the state in public health provision was defined to protect the poor from carrying 'contagious' diseases. The idea was to keep the poor apart from the rest of society in a manner not dissimilar to that of Victorian Britain. Thus laws were passed in relation to improving the supply of water and measures for sanitation were also developed by the state during the 1950s. However, beyond such measures little else of substance was achieved for public provision after independence (1943).

The experience of 'public provision', not unlike other countries of the Mashreq, was short lived. Between 1943 and 1958, the state built a network of district and rural hospitals operating within a referral system, but focused on servicing the under-privileged. But patients were required to prove hardship in order to be admitted for care, and thus the legacy and stigma associated with public provision remains. To add to this stigma the private sector has remained the most dominant and visible provider, despite its cost and exclusive nature of many of its elements. A large proportion of the population continues to rely upon health insurance, if they are in employment (more than 43% of the population are not covered by any insurance scheme) whilst the remainder, often only partially covered, resort to the Ministry of Public Health (MOPH), to trust-based and charitable institutions (faith-led), as well as individual loans when needing and unable to afford hospital care. There are also an increasing number of private providers, operating mainly as general practitioners (Mechbel, 1997) and a pool of highly specialized consultants. The culture of the health system influences health-seeking behaviour which is biased in favour of specialized care.

Protracted civil war coupled with several Israeli invasions and occupation damaged and weakened the institutional and financial capacity of the state and the public sector as a provider of health services. The historical trend towards political and social fragmentation was reinforced by war during which time one also witnessed the disintegration of MOPH and its associated services. Inevitably during this period there was no clear policy, no means to implement it, and no information database to work from (Mechbel, 1997). The few public health programmes such as vaccinations and mother and child health care were largely donor driven and pushed further into the hands of NGOs and international agencies.

One result was to encourage non-governmental groups and private sector providers to fill the gaps. These two sectors consequently witnessed a rapid and unprecedented increase in numbers and capacity to fill the vacuum. In part this expansion resulted in an escalation of costs as well as coverage through private health financing mechanisms. Fragmentation encouraged the expansion of a curative health care system with a focus on hospitals and centres for high technology services (Ammar et al., 2000). The overall effect of this was to create a health service which, led by private for-profit enterprises evolved into a supplier-induced service and in this way, shaped the current demand for health care (Ammar, 2003).

The greatest expansion in the health-sector during this period, and beyond, remained in the private for-profit sector with a concomitant proliferation in modern diagnostic techniques, equipment and services, such as MRIs (n=38), CT scans (n=104), and dialysis centres, all of which are disproportionate to the size of the population (Table 11.1). The availability of high-tech services in relation to population size is comparable and sometimes exceeds those of the OECD countries. There is hardly any emphasis on preventive or public health provision. It is evident that the past two decades of global restructuring of public health and welfare provision has meant that the private sector has rapidly risen to predominance, and much of this provision continues to be publicly subsidized. Oversupply in equipment led to a smaller market share per service, and thus to a higher cost per unit and inflated bills (Ammar, 2009). For advocates of neoliberal policies, this process has been beneficial, since in theory, it is supposed to provide more services than governments can afford and increase actual levels of investment in the health sector. However, the reality is often different and even among some advocates of the policies, there are doubts about whether such a rapid expansion of high-tech curative care can be

Table 11.1. Trends in 'high-tech' services and heavy equipment (1997–2007) and comparison with OECD

	Lebanon			Lebanon	OECD
	Number of units			Units per million	Units per million
	1997	1998	2007	2007	2007
Open heart surgery	12	16	22	5.7	3.3
Cardiac lab	19	24	32	8.3	5.2
Dialysis centres	39	45	55	14.2	
Lithotripsy	27	27	31	8.0	2.2
Kidney transplant	3	3	5	1.3	
Specialized centre for burned	2	2	1	0.3	
CT scan	54	60	104	26.9	20.6
MRI	12	16	38	9.8	9.8

Source: Ammar et al., 2000; Ministry of Public Health, 2007 and Syndicate of Private Hospitals, 2007; Organisation for Economic Co-operation and Development (OECD), Health data, 2007; Ammar, W. (2009).

beneficial to national health objectives. According to one such perspective, experience has shown that demand for curative health services from only those who are able to pay, and even if some of it is publicly subsidized, skews the health system away from promoting national welfare objectives and to meeting the needs of the population as a whole (Newbrander, 1997). It also contributes to a vertical health care system rather than one which is comprehensive.

Demographic transition and problems with data

In Lebanon, there are considerable gaps in demographic and epidemiological knowledge for most indicators. Data at the national level are scarce; the most recent census was conducted in 1932 when Lebanon was still a French mandate. There is a similar dearth of national-level socio-economic data, where the most recent studies conducted were in 1998 and 1999 and one in 2005, which are utilised for this chapter. Since independence in 1943 and for political reasons, efforts to collect demographic data and population statistics have not been welcome. Vital registration is unreliable while government statistical surveys and health statistics were, until very recently, non-existent (Sibai et al., 2002). Furthermore, there are considerable gaps in our current knowledge of the relative magnitude of major health problems and the proportion of these attributable to major risk factors. Epidemiological measures such as incidence, prevalence and mortality statistics for most diseases are mainly absent.

The limited data available suggest that the Lebanese population has witnessed a clear demographic transition in the past few decades. The decline in total fertility rates (from 2.5 in 1997 to 1.9 in 2004) has led to a lower proportion in the younger age groups and consequently to a narrowing down of the population pyramid's base. In contrast the proportion of the elderly Lebanese population, over 60 years, has increased from a value of 7.7% in 1970 (8.2% for females and 7.3% for males) to a value of 10.3% in 1996 (10.4% among females and 10.2% among males (Central Statistical Office, 1972; Sibai, 2001). Given the continuous decline in fertility rates and increase in life expectancy due to improved nutrition as well as medical interventions and technologies, this demographic transition is expected to continue positively in the coming decades (Sibai et al., 2004).

Despite the intrinsic problems with routine sources of data collection, several population-based and nation-wide surveys have been undertaken in Lebanon over the past decade. These include the Population and Housing Survey (PHS, 1995) which has been described as the most comprehensive nationally representative survey to be undertaken in Lebanon. This survey covered around 10% of the population and focused on basic socio-demographic characteristics of the population (Table 11.2). Following this survey, several others were conducted which included the National Household Health Expenditures and Utilisation Survey (NHHEUS) and the National Health Accounts (NHA) study (Ammar et al., 2000).

Table 11.2. Geographic distribution of population in the six Mohafazat: PHS 1995

	Beirut	Mount Lebanon	North	South	Bekaa	Nabatieh	Lebanon
Population (N)	407,403	1,145,458	670,609	283,057	399,891	205,411	3,111,828
Population (%)	13.1	36.8	21.6	9.1	12.9	6.6	100
Male/female sex ratio	94.6	99.2	98.9	97.3	101.7	94.2	98.8
Percent urban	100.0	92.5	64.9	72.4	65.6	70.4	80.8

Source: Adapted from Sibai, 2001 and Kronfol, 2002.

These two studies complement each other and cover roughly the same period (1998). These studies provided information for the first time on health financing agencies, insurance coverage, and health expenditures and suggest that throughout the country pockets of poverty are reflected by substantial variations in health status. More recent studies (2004) were also conducted by the Central Administration for Statistics, and the Ministry of Social Affairs in collaboration with the League of Arab States (the Arab Population and Family Household Health Survey-PAPFAM project), and the House-hold Living Conditions Survey (Administration Centrale de la Statistique, 1998; Central Administration for Statistics, 2009).

Socio-economic indicators and health expenditures

Geographically and administratively Lebanon is divided into six provinces or Mohafazats; these include the capital Beirut, Mount Lebanon, the North, the South, Bekaa, and Naba-tieh. The provinces are further sub-divided into 24 districts or Qadas. The districts follow geographic, political, social and historical divisions along the lines of confessional divisions. Tables 11.3 and 11.4 provide an indication of socio-economic conditions and household expenditures across the six Governorates in Lebanon. While it is important to note the enor-mous regional variation in these indicators, the tables hide the intra-regional variations, for example, of the pockets of poverty within Governorates. Moreover, the data do not include the Palestinian refugee population who continue to live in camps and mainly rely upon their own services that are largely funded by donor agencies such as The United Nations Relief and Works Agency (UNRWA). This population group experiences chronic poverty and high levels of deprivation. These refugees make up at least 10% of the total population and they live predominantly in the suburbs of Beirut and in southern Lebanon. In 2000 the total popula-tion of Lebanon was estimated at 3.5 million excluding refugees and the per capita income with substantial regional differences was USD 4500 ranking it as an MIC (United Nations Statistics Division, 2009).

Recent data from Lebanon suggest that up to 28% of the families are living below the abso-lute poverty line and around 8% live in extreme poverty, with wide disparities between governo-rates (Laithy et al., 2008). For example, while the North has 20.7% of the population, it includes 38% and 46% of the poor and extreme poor population, respectively. Between 1997 and 2000 and following the war of 2006, there has also been a worsening of the economic conditions with households gravitating towards lower income levels. Whilst these may fall in geographic con-centration, there is also evidence that declining economic conditions over the past 5 years have been paralleled by rising costs of health care that are borne largely out of pocket. Between 1994

Table 11.3. Selected socio-economic indicators and monthly income (2000)

	Beirut	Mount Lebanon	North	South	Bekaa	Nabatieh	Lebanon
Employed males (%)	74.8	74.4	78.7	79	74.5	75.6	77.3
Employed females (%)	35.1	23.7	17.4	18.7	12.1	15.0	21.7
Income (LL)/person/month (USD 1 = 1500 LL)	481	442	229	277	253	248	328

Source: Kronfol, 2002.

Table 11.4. Family expenditures at household level (%)

	Beirut	Mount Lebanon	North	South	Bekaa	Nabatieh	Lebanon
Food	31.9	33.6	33.8	37.0	37.7	37.7	33.9
Spends total income	53.1	51.3	42.8	51.9	62.4	62.4	51.5
Families in debt	36.4	25.4	42.7	31.8	17.8	17.8	30.6
Loans for living	9.8	10.7	22.8	15.3	7.8	7.8	14.9
Loans for schools	7.2	8.3	12.9	6.2	2.4	2.4	8.9
Loans for health care	5.1	3.5	6.6	5.2	1.5	1.5	5.1
Loans for dwelling	6.1	8.9	7.4	5.7	4.3	4.3	7.6

Source: Kronfol, 2002.

and 2000, for example, there was a 10% increase in out-of-pocket expenditures for health care (Ammar et al., 2000; Mechbel, 1997). More than 80% of health care costs were borne directly out of pocket, whereas approximately one-fifth was borne out of payment mechanisms created by the state (Ammar, 2009). There was little control over either the private or public dimensions of these expenditures since for the former, it is well nigh impossible to monitor private expenditure due to the reluctance of insurance companies to reveal details of charges for individual patients. In the case of public expenditure there are similar problems due to the multiplicity of state agencies dealing with health claims and the absence of monitoring of such mechanisms, resulting in a lack of information (Ammar, 2003).

What is especially significant are the high levels of the population (around 53%) who are not covered by any kind of health insurance schemes which affects their ability to afford health care. The MOPH argues, on the basis of recent surveys, that the patterns of utilization of health care show that health service usage is highest among low-income groups (Ammar et al., 2000). Nevertheless, this is also indicative of poorer perceived health status among low-income groups and a higher burden of out-of-pocket expenditure as the following details of household expenditure suggest.

The National Household Expenditure Survey (NHES, 2000) revealed that on average a Lebanese household would spend some 2,609,000 LL (USD 1,740), per annum on health care. Excluding major interventions, of this, 97% is spent on the private sector on the range of services available such as individual consultations and hospital care. A substantial part of this expenditure is on buying over-the-counter drugs. In this context it is likely that levels of self-medication are high coupled with iatrogenic complaints which potentially lead to additional expenditure. For the remainder, 2% is spent on the NGO sector and 1% only on the public sector (Ammar et al., 2000). On average households spend just under 15% of their income on health care as a share of total household expenditures. But households falling in the highest income group spent only 8% of their household expenditures on health services with the poorer ones spending more than twice as much – 20%. Within these figures there are regional variations with those households in Mount

Lebanon spending nearly twice as much as those in North Lebanon. On a per capita basis low-income households tend to make more visits but these are for outpatient services (Ammar et al., 2000).

Crisis of health finance and health care provision

It is evident that health financing in Lebanon is in crisis, with costs of health services showing linear increases over recent years (1992–2002), adding to the financial burden of the MOPH among others but especially so for households. For example, in 1992, the total amount spent on health services was USD 300 million or about USD 100 per capita (Mechbel, 1997). In 1998 this had increased to around USD 2,000 million and USD 500, respectively (Ammar et al., 2000). However, owing to cuts in government budget allocated for health in the past few years, to an important targeted reduction in out of pocket payments, an increase in spending from treasury source as well as a steady increase in the MOPH-subsidized admissions to public hospitals (Ammar, 2009), by the year 2005, the total amount decreased to USD 1,750 million and per capita health expenditure to around USD 460 (Table 11.5). Nevertheless, the share borne by the public sector has increased from around 18% to 29%, representing more than a 10 point increase through increasingly targeted support for inpatient and some outpatient services, although the bulk of payments is still derived mainly from households and direct payment at the purchasing point. While recent efforts made by the MOPH have been directed towards lowering out-of-pocket expenditures, the main challenge facing the Ministry today is the expenditure on pharmaceuticals. Recent data indicate that pharmaceuticals purchased through pharmacies, public bids and hospitals represent around 42% of

Table 11.5. Health expenditures (National Health Accounts, 1998 and 2005)

	1998	2005
Total population	4,000,000	3,870,000
Total health expenditures (mln USD)	1,996	1,750
Per capita health expenditures (USD)	499	452
Total GDP (mln USD)	16,200	21,607
Health expenditures as percent of GDP	12.32%	8.1%
Government budget allocated to health	6.6%	5.9%
Funding sources		
Public	17.98%	28.98%
Private		
Households	69.74%	59.82%
Employers	10.32%	11.17%
Donors/NGOs	1.96%	0.03%
Distribution of expenditures		
Public and private hospitals	24.5%	38.0%
Private non-institutional providers	41.0%	21.0%
Pharmaceuticals	25.4%	32.0%
Others	9.1%	9.0%

Source: Ammar et al, 2000; Ammar, 2009.

Table 11.6. Spending (in USD) on hospitals and pharmaceuticals by households and intermediaries in 2005

	Total hospitals (including pharmaceuticals)	Hospitals (excluding pharmaceuticals)	Pharmaceuticals (outside hospitals)	Total pharmaceuticals
Intermediaries	554,111	437,748	181,068	297,431
Households	116,927	92,372	432,507	457,061
Total	671,038	530,120	613,575	754,493
% of total health expenditures	37.55	29.66	34.34	42.22

Source: Ammar, 2009.

total health expenditures and almost half of household health expenditures go to purchasing drugs (Table 11.6).

Mechanisms of health finance

There are a number of health-financing mechanisms operative in the Lebanon. These include seven important public financing schemes – notably the National Social Security Fund (NSSF), the Civil Service Cooperative (CSC) fund, the Fund for Military Personnel (Army), and three others which are under the jurisdiction of the Ministry of Interior, and cover the Internal Security Forces (ISF), State Security Forces (SSF), and General Security Forces (GSF), and finally direct funding from the MOPH. These are the public funds, which (other than the MOPH funds) are all tied to employment with their levels of contribution dependent on both employer and employee resources. Although the NSSF is the most important source of public health insurance in Lebanon, the national Household Living Conditions Survey conducted in 2004 showed that only 23.4% of the population were covered by it (Ammar, 2009). According to the MOPH database, this may be an under-estimate of the true proportion of population enrolled in the NSSF.

There are numerous problems with such a system of duplication, covering for the same care by different ministries. This financing fragmentation is further challenged by the diversity in benefit package and of supervising authorities, making regulation and coordination more complex. The complexities of claiming and eligibility criteria mean that people often fall back upon MOPH funds, thereby creating additional financial burdens at the level of this Ministry (Ammar, 2003). For example, coverage through the NSSF ceases on retirement, which means that the elderly and poorer sections of the population have to rely on the MOPH welfare funds when in greatest need, unless they are able to pay themselves. Ongoing subsidies from the MOPH are a key factor contributing to periodic crises in health financing at the Ministry and serve the basis of health reforms proposed in early 2000.

Public versus private sector health coverage

There continues to be much debate over health coverage in Lebanon. According to recent household surveys in 2004–2005, only 47% of the population reported as having any kind of health coverage, whether public or private (Ammar, 2009). There is also considerable geographic variation in coverage, with the highest proportion living in the capital Beirut City (59.2%) and the lowest percentage of any coverage in more remote areas such as the Bekaa Valley (37.5%) and in Nabatieh in the south (39.4%). Among those with any coverage about

78% fall under various employment-based public-financing mechanisms. The largest source of financial coverage for this group is under the aegis of the NSSF consisting of around 51% of public coverage. The remainder (22%) were covered through an assortment of private for-profit and not for-profit schemes (Ammar, 2009). It is also important to clarify that coverage does not usually mean full coverage. In reality it can mean a significant sum of out-of-pocket expenditure as a top up, as it usually rises with age.

For the remaining 53% of the population who are not covered by any form of health insurance, the MOPH acts as the 'insurer of last resort.' It reimburses contracted hospitals for 85% of the bill, provides expensive drugs free of charge and finances the procurement of drugs for the chronically ill patients through selected NGO health centres. Theoretically this coverage is independent of the income or asset status of the individual. However, the nature and structure of health sector financing means that much of this type of funding is (a) for curative care with hardly any support for preventive or promotive health care, and (b) often requires a complex system for claiming, compounded by long waiting lists. This acts as a prohibitive factor for potential claimants, thus many are forced to pay for such services out of pocket. The complexities of claims from both public and private providers also means that people are discouraged not only from applying for but, most significantly, from using outpatient or any form of preventive care, where the onus for re-claiming costs lies with the patient rather than the provider. Inevitably this encourages greater hospital use over any other type of health service, since hospitals claim directly from the Ministries on behalf of patients. The Ministry subcontracts such services to many private hospitals where there is often little control or accountability. As a result MOPH expenditures on hospital care have sharply grown from 1994 to 2001.

The Ministry also covers total expenses for three main curative services: kidney dialysis, open-heart surgery and for cancer patients. Whilst this may be of great benefit to some, it remains an expense of growing concern to health planners due to the disproportionate share it takes out of the total budget for health care, financed by the MOPH. Increasingly this kind of subsidy, and the inability of the Ministry to influence the nature of intervention or the cost of it, has led to deficits in the health budget overall. Detailed information is rarely available but, in 1997, for example, the inability of the MOPH to curb hospital costs led to it paying out 60% of the budget of that year towards those specialists' interventions. This led the MOPH to be involved in a crisis in repayments to insurers that continues to have its repercussions (Ammar et al., 2000; TPA – MEDNET, personal communication, Beirut, December 2002).

Hospitals and public expenditure

A closer examination of the nature and structure of the hospital as provider would be instructive. Lebanon is a typical example of a laissez faire economy reflected particularly by the structure and functioning of its health sector and within this, most notably, the hospital sector. Over the past decade in particular, this sector has been characterized by unplanned expansion and high cost coverage, borne not out of health need but in order to maximize revenue. In this context the main difference between Lebanon and other countries of the region is that the public sector, through its contracting arrangements, foots the largest share of the health bill. Expenditure on hospital care through public finance mechanisms and other contractual arrangements is high. In the case of the MOPH 73% of its budget is utilized for hospital-based care (Ammar, 2009). As a result it is not surprising that expenditure on PHC services is very low and accounts for less than 5% of public expenditure. According to Ammar et al., the MOPH has often been unable even to disburse the amounts allotted to PHC and in some cases the allocation has been diverted to curative care services (Ammar et al., 2000). More recently, however, serious attempts have been made by the MOPH to regain leadership over community health services, including NGOs and PHC centres, contributing to preventive programmes carried out in collaboration with other agencies, such as the UN, WHO and Ministry of Social Affairs (Ammar, 2009).

During the past ten years (as in most other parts of the developing world), there has also been a shift towards large multi-specialty hospitals to emulate the 'teaching' hospitals in the West. The majority of hospitals are often linked to faith-led groups that have contractual arrangements with the state (usually the MOPH) for providing subsidized care. This structure originates from the period of the war (1975–1992) when most public hospitals were destroyed, either through internecine strife or Israeli bombing (Mechbel, 1997; Sen, 2002). This led to the state creating special financing arrangements with numerous private hospitals, where the public sector purchased their services. According to some observers the power of these hospitals was reinforced by the powerlessness and fragmentation of state structures (Ammar, 2003; Harik, 1994).

Hence, it was during this period of war that hospitals and hospital-based health care took on a momentum and became a powerful lobby with considerable influence on public expenditures on private health care as a whole. For example, the MOPH report showed that the hospitals, which receive the largest share of their costs through MOPH subsidies, tended to perform a large number of investigations and prescribe a number of drugs for each episode of hospitalization as a means of maximizing their revenues (Ammar et al., 2000). As a result MOPH expenditures on hospital care have grown sharply between 1994 and 2001, far exceeding the set budgets (Ammar, 2009).

During the past few years, however, and as new public hospitals (such as the Hariri Governmental University Hospital) are becoming operational, the MOPH made serious attempts to shift its hospitalization funding from contracting private hospitals to providing support to public ones. In addition during the same period, the MOPH introduced new contracting rules and took careful measures to control admissions, setting capitation levels for each private provider, automating admission authorizations and auditing of bills. All of this led to some control of budgets and a significant reduction in budget deficits, from around USD 2.6 million to almost nil in 2007 (Ammar, 2009).

Private sector coverage

While the proportion of people with a private insurance policy does not exceed 6.5% of the population (NHS, 2004–2005), the private insurance market has experienced rapid expansion in recent years in both the amount of coverage and type of insurance company. The market is highly fragmented providing both complimentary and comprehensive coverage. The fragmentation of this sector places citizens at a disadvantage when there is little knowledge of the best option to choose in terms of quality and cost of services. These insurance policies typically cover inpatient care, whilst outpatient services are covered with additional premiums and co-payments. According to one of the largest private insurance companies in the country, over one-third of the privately insured are also enrolled in the NSSF.

The private sector insurance market is taking full advantage of the system selecting the younger, healthier, and better-off clientele (Ammar, 2009). The burden of the severely ill, the older population, and those requiring expensive interventions is shifted to the MOPH. The process of duplicate cover and the cream-skimming of more expensive (and usually poorer) cases is iniquitous. It also encourages hospitals to undertake high cost interventions among the few with comprehensive coverage (through the public sector), since there are few mechanisms for recall and /or regulation.

Mutual funds

Part of the new reform agenda in Lebanon initiated during the late 1990s was to redress such imbalances and in particular the rising subsidies from state to private providers. In order to avoid the pitfalls of public and private insurance schemes and a growing crisis in the funding of health services, the past 12 years have witnessed a rapid increase in Mutual Funds which cover health expenses through a forum of syndicates which are occupationally based. The law governing mutual funds permits any group of 50 people or more to form a mutual fund. When the scheme began in 1991 under the aegis of the Ministry of Housing and Cooperatives, it covered only 66 individuals. However, by 1999, this coverage had increased to some 64,179 beneficiaries (Kronfol, 2002) and to over 150,000 by 2005 (Ammar, 2009), illustrating their popularity, owing to low risk and low premiums in comparison to many private insurance schemes. Under the Mutuality scheme, the linkage could be professional, faith-led or community based. Mutual funds are somewhat of a threat to the private insurance sector since they are allowed tax-free status and therefore viewed as at an 'unfair advantage' in a market which for private providers is otherwise a 'captive' one.

Non-governmental organizations

As with other non-public agencies, NGOs also grew in prominence during the period of war. Its constituents are mainly the poor and the uninsured, and it is likely that the skeleton services provided account for a large share in the patterns of ambulatory health care. The 1997 Household Living Conditions Survey indicated that 74% of outpatient visits took place in the private sector, and the remaining with the public sector NGOs dispensaries (Central Administration for Statistics, 2009). More recent evidence suggests that this percentage has been increasing of late, with enlargement of the MOPH PHC networks from less than 50 contracted centres before 2003 to 115 by 2007. The role played by these NGOs, supported by a strategic choice by the MOPH to invest minimally in basic equipment and essential drugs, has led to an upsurge in the number of individuals currently benefiting from their service (almost one-third), and consequently, in a significant decrease in out-of-pocket expenditures.

Overall, the NGOs play a limited role for inpatient care. The exception to this rule, however, is organizations such as Islamic Health Society whose network of health centres and hospitals have been increasing over the past 15 years. Between 1996 and 2001, for example, the period for which data are available, contributions to the social fund of the Islamic Society increased three-fold (Islamic Health Society, 2002). Much of this was invested in health services that are accessible to both the urban and rural poor. Whilst many of these facilities were systematically destroyed in the war of 2006, the group has worked hard to replace their losses and to be functional.

As is the case elsewhere in the world, the NGO sector concentrates on activities that are unprofitable for private sector providers. These include activities such as prevention and health promotion and community-based educational interventions (such as vaccination programmes and mother and child health care). Since NGOs are increasingly finding it difficult to raise funds for such services, many have been forced to operate on the same basis as 'semi-private' organizations and are having to charge for their services or renting out their facilities for the use of private doctors. The Islamic Health Society, which is one of the larger NGOs, charges a minimal fee of between 10 and 15 dollars per month, a practice that continues to provide extensive coverage to its own under-served populations.

Conclusion

In sum, Lebanon has a high cost health sector with a bill of around USD 1.75 billion (USD 450 per capita in 2005) and an overall share of the cost of health care constituting some 8.1% of GDP, a figure which is higher than most countries within the region. In spite of the achievements made in the past few years, in particular strengthening the role of contracted PHC and decreasing out-of-pocket expenditures, there is great concern about the ongoing malaise of the health sector in general and health services in particular that is applicable to the Mashreq as a whole. Moreover, despite guarantees of health insurance coverage from the state, among its endemic problems are the continued imposition of varied premiums for the same intervention or service; an oversupply of manpower and facilities (especially in the high-tech field), with an ongoing emphasis on technology-driven care; low occupancy of hospital beds; limited emphasis on preventive or promotive care; high cost and over-usage of pharmaceuticals, and limited, if any, controls on price increases. There is also concern that, given the high level of investment, there is little evidence of effectiveness in the delivery of health care (Ammar, 2003). Available evidence suggests that, with the exception of a small number of institutions, overall the system based on hospitalized care functions poorly with a very limited and highly specialized range of services. However, ,unlike in most other countries of the region, there have been some positive developments in Lebanon over the past 3 years. Despite its inherent weakness in state control, the MOPH has made a concerted effort to contain the excesses of the private sector, by establishing autonomous public hospitals, where care is subsidized, introducing careful controls over state supported private provision in hospitals, and, most significantly, making a conscious effort to divert from curative care by supporting primary care through the NGO sector (Ammar, 2009).

These measures could affect the dismal legacy of preventive and promotive care. For example, less than 2% of contacts with private practitioners are revisits with little continuity of care. Family health programmes were not well integrated and were fragmented between providers as well as being sparsely distributed. Moreover, despite the high levels of expenditure on health services (both public and private), child mortality in pockets of poverty in the country is high and many regions remain under-served for health services (Mechbel, 1997).

The reforms of the health sector in Lebanon, unlike in most countries of the world, entail changing the excesses of a market-led health system supported to date by the public subsidy of private providers. The degree to which this may be effective will depend upon class dynamics of Lebanese society led by confessional politics and, in particular, the pressure from civil society to rise above primordial ties and voice its support for a more rational and universal provision. Recent indications are that there is change in process; however, the degree to which the recent and substantial interventions will be effective in providing lower cost, comprehensive and balanced provision is yet to be seen, and dealing with the cost of medicines and high-tech medical equipment will be one of the major challenges.

References

Administration Centrale de la Statistique. (1998). *Conditions de vie des ménages en 1997 [Living conditions of households in Lebanon in 1997]*. Etudes Statistiques no. 9. Beirut: Administration Centrale de la Statistique.

Ammar W. (2003). *Health system and Reform in Lebanon*. Beirut: WHO Regional Office for the Eastern Mediterranean and Lebanese Ministry of Public Health.

Ammar W. (2009). *Health Beyond Politics*. Beirut: World Health Organization and Ministry of Public Health.

Ammar W., Azzam O., Khoury R., et al. (2000). *Lebanon National Health Accounts*. Beirut: World Health Organization, Ministry of Health, World Bank.

Central Administration for Statistics. (2009). *Living Conditions of Households. The National Survey of Household Living Conditions 2004*. Beirut: Lebanese Republic Ministry of Social Affairs, Central Administration for Statistics, United Nations Development Programme.

Central Statistical Office. (1972). *L'enquête par sondage sur la population active au Liban, 1970 [Survey of the economically active population in Lebanon, 1970]*. Beirut: CBO.

Harik J. (1994). *The Public and Social Services of the Lebanese Militias*. Oxford: The Centre for Lebanese Studies.

Islamic Health Society. (2002). *To Continue to be at Your Service: 1984–2002*. Beirut: Al Bana'a Society.

Jabbour S., El Zein A., Nuwayhid I., & Giacaman R. (2006). Can action on health achieve political and social reform? *British Medical Journal*, **333**(7573), pp. 837–9.

Koivusalo M. (2003). Health system solidarity and European Community policies. In: Sen K., ed. *Reconstructing Health Services: Changing Context and Comparative Perspectives*. London: Zeds Books, pp. 93–114.

Kronfol N. (2002). *The Lebanese Health Care System: Options for Reforms*. Cairo: World Health Organization.

Laithy H., Abu-Ismail K., & Hamdan K. (2008). *Country study: Poverty, growth and income distribution in Lebanon*. Brasilia: International Poverty Centre. Country Study no. 13.

Mechbel A. (1997). Health care reform in Lebanon: Research for reform. In: Nitayarumphong S., ed. *Health Care Reform at the Frontiers of Research and Policy Decisions*. Thailand: Ministry of Public Health, pp. 120–40.

Newbrander W. (1997). *Private Health Sector Growth in Asia: Issues and Implications*. Chichester: John Wiley and Sons.

Sen K. (2002). *Personal communication with Dar al Ajaza al Islamia-NGO*. Beirut, December, 2002.

Sibai A. M. (2001). The elderly in Lebanon. In: *The Status of Selected Social Groups in Lebanon*. Beirut: UNFPA and Ministry of Social Affairs, pp. 48–124.

Sibai A. M., Nuwayhid I., Beydoun M., & Chaaya M. (2002). Inadequacies of death certification in Beirut: Who is responsible? *Bulletin of the World Health Organization*, **80**(7), pp. 555–61.

Sibai A. M., Sen K., Baydoun M., & Saxena P. (2004). Population ageing in Lebanon: Current status, future prospects and implications for policy. *Bulletin of the World Health Organization*, **82**(3), pp. 219–25.

United Nations Development Programme. (2009). Arab Human Development Report 2004. *Freedom and Good Governance*. New York: United Nations Development Programme.

United Nations Statistics Division. (2009). Lebanon Country Profile. http://data.un.org/CountryProfile.aspx?crName=Lebanon.

World Bank. (1993). *World Development Report 1993: Investing in Health*. Oxford: Oxford University Press.

Principles for alternative, publicly oriented health care policies, planning, management and delivery

Introduction

Policy fundamentally determines both the delivery and management of health care. In theory policy makers should collect information on the performance of health services based on explicit criteria – which is what this section explores – in order to influence health care services and systems. In practice, however, this evaluation of field results and experiences has rarely taken place, leading to malfunctioning health systems in many regions of the world. We have argued that both alternative health care and models of service delivery should be promoted with appropriate resources while health professionals and citizens should have the opportunity to influence this process.

We have made a case throughout this book that neoliberal health policies have had a pernicious effect on health systems worldwide. However, challenging these policies also requires us to formulate alternative principles – not only for the sake of showing that another paradigm is feasible but also to offer different criteria for policy evaluation and to ground alternative initiatives in knowledge, experience, and history.

The first four sections of this book questioned the credibility of dominant health policies, for instance by contrasting them with success stories of heterodox health systems such as that of Costa Rica or the failures of others which, like Colombia, followed neoliberal policies. Whilst such evidence nested in practice is necessary, it is perhaps not sufficient to shake the conceptual model that has become so embedded in aid and trade circles. For instance, Costa Rica could be presented as an idiosyncratic accident of history. Since many other systems (from Spain to Sri Lanka) also made the political choice not to follow the dominant model, this section presents some principles which inspired these heterodox policies, together with other examples, derived from more limited, sometimes pilot, experiences in health services organization with a focus on public provision.

Whilst there has been an understandable worldwide preoccupation with the financing of health systems and health care, there has been little thought given in this process to the exclusive focus on cost-effectiveness: if efficiency is one criterion to assess health policies, it should be used together with others such as equity, access to, and quality of CHC.

Furthermore, there are reasons to believe that health systems structured along the 'cost-effective' definition of priority disease-control programmes end up being less efficient than others tailored to deliver CHC. The confusion between allocative and technical efficiency highlights a need to clarify public health methods since this is at the root of many of the problems, straining the conception of policies and systems that aim at delivering comprehensive care (Chapter 12, Part 2).

The paradigm shift proposed in this section relates to health systems' functions that have a social basis rather than a commercial motive. Such a basis assumes that health systems should secure universal access to CHC, but also that they should deliver them through publicly oriented services that are ideally co-managed by users and professionals under the guidance of the state. The rationale for these tenets lies in the concept of social justice, linked to an ethical framework. This includes values such as solidarity, democracy, and the universal right to health care premised on the satisfaction of essential human need. This section therefore offers those principles consistent with a very different set of values (and some evidence) for an alternative:

- health policy design (Chapter 13);
- health care delivery and management of services (Chapter 14);
- health planning (Chapter 15);
- disease-specific programmes management (Chapter 16).

Principles for alternative, publicly oriented health care policies, planning, management and delivery

Paradigm shifts in the health sector: mission and methods

Jean-Pierre. Unger and P. Van Dessel

Adapted from: J.-P. Unger. How could disease-specific programmes strengthen health systems delivering comprehensive health care? Strategic and technical guidelines. European Commission, 30 September 2008, Brussels.

Part 1: The need to alter health systems' missions to deliver comprehensive care

The strengthening of health systems appears to have become a motto for international health agencies since 2003, when the former director of the WHO, Jong-Wook Lee (2003–2006), called for a radical re-think of policy, if diseases are to be successfully controlled (Jong-Wook, 2003). This view has been echoed by his successor Margaret Chan. However, unlike the growing body of scientific papers that have begun to advocate the strengthening of health systems over the past several years, we would argue that health systems can only be strengthened if they are designed to deliver universally accessible comprehensive care. The remainder of this chapter outlines the rationale for this thinking.

Comprehensive health care: medical and managerial arguments

In a recent address to the 61st World Health Assembly, WHO Director, Dr Margaret Chan, acknowledged that the MDGs had stalled (see Section 1) (Chan, 2008). Besides the MDGs, the control of neglected diseases has also met with difficulties (see Section 1, Chapter 2).

The failure to make significant progress on health MDGs is surprising since they were limited to reducing maternal and child mortality and controlling a few diseases, which meant a considerable reduction of previous international commitments in health status as defined, for example, by the WHO in the 'Global Strategy for Health for All by the Year 2000' (World Health Organization, 1978; World Health Organization, 1981). However, it is our view that the abandonment of the principle of access to CHC in the MDGs as an explicit responsibility of a health system may precisely be the cause of this failure. This has been compounded by the segmentation and fragmentation of health systems worldwide (as illustrated throughout the chapters of this book). Discarding the idea of comprehensive care from the health MDGs has resulted in failure to progress in a number of areas of health care provision.

Whilst prevention is sometimes crucial to controlling diseases, comprehensive clinical activity that includes curative, discretionary individual care is a common denominator for the majority of disease-specific programmes: without Highly Active Anti Retroviral Therapy (HAART), tuberculostatics and anti-malarial drugs, for example, AIDS, tuberculosis and malaria control would be impossible. This also applies to the large majority of diseases, from chronic to those described as neglected diseases such as Guinea worm, schistosomiasis, and sleeping sickness. Moreover, case management is often the only practical control procedure, as in acute respiratory infections and adult tuberculosis. Even the disease-specific interventions that rely on environmental interventions, such as onchocerciasis and schistosomiasis, require individual pharmaceutical treatment.

The effectiveness of numerous treatments depends on early detection. The lethality and specific mortality of tuberculosis, severe malaria, and AIDS increase, for instance, with the delay in accessing clinical care as well as any delay in a doctors' ability to initiate appropriate treatment. This effectiveness also requires a working relationship between patients and health professionals, complemented by a tracing system for defaulters.

The best (and practically only) prevention for pulmonary tuberculosis is early detection and treatment – this entails detection as soon as possible following the onset of a cough. As early as 1963 it was already shown that 75% of tuberculosis patients detected by mass screening had consulted a physician previously (Banerji & Andersen, 1963). This reinforces the importance of access to CHC and the need also for the improvement of the quality of care.[1]

Thus one might argue that the number of diseases requiring clinical interventions, and the well-established need to reduce delay in seeking treatment through polyvalent services, makes it impossible to consider services geared to the delivery of vertical or indirect programmes (see Section 2, Chapter 4) as a gold standard for the organization of disease control. Finally, from a managerial viewpoint, health organizations need to be polyvalent, since disease epidemiology varies both geographically and chronologically. High-risk groups such as under-fives and pregnant women, chronic patients, and patients suffering from some tropical diseases would be served best within a polyvalent system which has the ability to cure acute patients, trace and secure follow-up of the chronic ones, distribute drugs as well as provide specific care to high-risk groups.

The financial case for CHC

The failure to progress on MDGs contrasts with official donor assistance (ODA) to the health sector which experienced a four-fold increase between 1992 and 2005 alone, and which has continued to increase largely due to the funding of disease-specific programmes (Shiffman, 2008). Taking advantage of an unprecedented exponential increase (see Figure 12.2), funding for HIV/AIDS has increased the most. In spite of this increase in funding, control efforts have had limited impact. Admittedly, a part of the reason for this lies in the environmental-, social-, and policy-related factors that may fuel the epidemic but this is not sufficient reason for this lack of progress (El Sadr & Hoos, 2008; Hanson & Hanson, 2008). We examine some of the underlying factors that in our view have contributed to the malfunctioning of international aid financing contributing to the intrinsic weakness of disease-specific and vertical programmes such as that of HIV/AIDS.

Already by 1986, the running costs of five disease programmes integrated with those of general practice were shown to be similar to those of five vertical programmes taken alone (USD 1–2 per capita yearly) (Unger & Killingsworth, 1986). How can this paradox be explained? Organizational structures that require independent staffing for each disease programme are expensive and difficult to sustain. Moreover, during the past two decades, the administrative

---

[1] Such access is necessary but not sufficient to enable detection. To permit MDs to screen effectively their patients, operational studies have to identify discriminatory signs and complaints which are sufficiently sensitive and specific (Baily et al., 1967).

and transaction costs related to disease-specific programmes have grown much faster than the operating costs of first-line health services.[2]

Different hypotheses on organization structures (integrated vs. vertical) inevitably lead to quite different cost estimates of health systems. In 2005, for example, the running costs of local health systems offering appropriate CHC were established at USD 10 in rural Zimbabwe (Vander Plaetse et al., 2005), three times less than the amount estimated by the Commission on Macroeconomics and Health 3 years earlier (e.g., as USD 32 in Uganda) (Preker et al., 2002).[3] Such a discrepancy can only be explained by the varied nature of health systems' functioning which in turn is confirmed by the huge variance in health systems efficiency, as shown by Figure 12.1.

A comparison between Vietnam and Cameroun (Table 12.1) also illustrates the heterogeneity of efficiency showing how different impacts on health status can be achieved at a comparable health expenditure rate, although it should be acknowledged that several factors outside of the health service system, such as the educational level of the population and its social organization, are likely also to contribute to reducing maternal mortality rates (MMR).

According to its 2007 report the joint United Nations Programme on HIV and AIDS (UNAIDS) is convinced that AIDS cannot be controlled without the strengthening of health

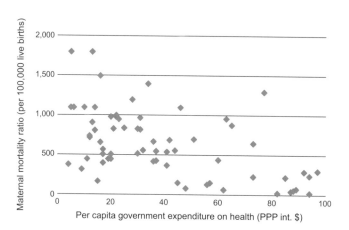

Figure 12.1. Maternal mortality rate (per 100,000 live births) as a function of public expenditure on health (PPP int. $) for 2005. *Source:* World Health Organization, 2009, WHO Statistical Information System (WHOSIS).

Table 12.1. 2000 public expenditure on health and MMR in Cameroon and Vietnam

	Public expenditure on health per capita	MMR (maternal deaths per 100,000)
Vietnam	13 USD PPP	130
Cameroon	17 USD PPP	730

Sources: World Health Chart, 2001, WHO/OMS, available at: http://www.whc.ki.se/index.php; WHO Maternal mortality reports, 1995–2005.

---

[2] In some central African states, a district medical officer earns 10 times less than poliomyelitis officers paid on international aid role.

[3] Besides methodological divergence, the difference in efficiency of health system organization is likely to explain the gap. While the authors of the Zimbabwean study had assessed the functioning costs of an organization delivering integrated health care and disease control, the Commission on Macroeconomics and Health rather elaborated upon those of several DSP put together (with heavy administrative costs).

systems (UNAIDS, 2007). On this point UNAIDS observes that: 'If the scale-up of HIV services continues at the same pace as in the recent past, the funding need is projected to reach USD 15.4 billion in 2010 (USD 13.4–17.6) and USD 22.5 billion in 2015 (USD 18.8–26.9). Yet even with such increases, the world will not reach universal access by 2010 or even by 2015. If current trends continue, only 4.6 million people would receive antiretrovirals in 2010, or roughly two-thirds of the number of people who needed antiretrovirals in 2006. By 2015 an estimated 8 million people would be on antiretrovirals.' The report continues: 'To meet the goal of global universal access by 2010, available financial resources for HIV must more than quadruple by 2010 compared to 2007 …' In spite of such a dramatic increase in aid to AIDS control (Figure 12.2), the funding gap is widening under the current strategy (Figure 12.3).

We view the reasons for the funding crisis of AIDS as three-fold:

- Progress on prevention is slow. In spite of the exponential increase in AIDS funding (Figure 12.2) the detection of new cases progresses three times faster than those put under ART (UNAIDS, 2008).
- Cases living close to health services were reached first and put on life long treatment. Due to staff shortages, often almost all staff time is devoted to those already on treatment. It is therefore increasingly difficult to recruit new patients in programmes (with equally low patient losses) unless staff numbers are increased and the strategy revisited.

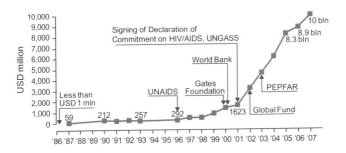

Figure 12.2. Total annual resources available for AIDS (1986–2007). The 1986–2000 figures are for international funds only; 2001–2007 domestic funds included; 1996–2005 data extracted from 2006 Report on Global AIDS Epidemic (UNAIDS, 2006); 1986–1993 data from Mann. & Tarantola, 1996. *Source:* UNAIDS & WHO unpublished estimates, 2007.

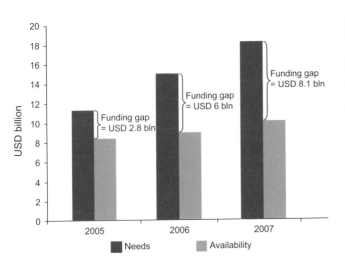

Figure 12.3. Funding gap between resource needs and resource availability 2005–2007. *Source:* UNAIDS report, 2007, Financial resources required to achieve universal acces to HIV prevention, treatment care and support.

- While the cost of ART has dropped, other treatment costs (e.g., of opportunistic infections) remain high due to the parallel, vertical organization pattern adopted by AIDS programmes in most countries.

In conclusion, integrated patterns delivering CHC are much cheaper than DSPs, with their parallel administrations. Boosted by unprecedented bureaucratic inflation, the administrative costs of current organizational patterns are not sustainable, even for the international donors. Instead CHC delivery encompassing polyvalent curative care and disease control will be affordable within integrated health systems only.

Social, economic and political reasons for CHC

Information on access to health care in LMICs is scarce. WHO statistical information systems do not provide indicators on health care accessibility or its utilization. Globally, this situation was known to be unacceptable as early as the year 2000. The limited evaluations that have been undertaken suggest that half of the countries of the world failed to provide their population with adequate access to health care (Department of Economic and Social Affairs, 2000). One in three in the poorest countries, for example, had little or no access to essential drugs (World Health Organization, 2000). Since 2000 access to and quality of health care is unlikely to have improved, and certainly not in Africa. Recent data provided by MPH theses from the region (Institute of Tropical Medicine, 2007) show utilization rates of first-line health services between 0.1 and 0.4 new cases per year per inhabitant[4] in West Africa and slightly more in Eastern and Southern Africa. For instance, chosen amongst tens of other such grey literature data, in the Bokande district Burkina Faso (population ± 260,000) in 2006, the utilization rate was 0.28 for those living less than 5 km from a facility, and 0.22 for the population living over 5 km.

Avoidable deaths, suffering, and anxiety linked to low access to health care have immeasurable, indirect consequences, one of these being expenditure on health care which is increasingly acknowledged as important if not a key factor of impoverishment in households in developing countries (McIntyre et al., 2006; Van Doorslaer et al., 2006; Xu et al., 2003).

In the industrialized world, even for-profit economic stakeholders have been advocating better access to health care in LMICs. For example, the European Federation of Pharmaceutical Industries suggests: 'Although patent protection has been blamed for problems with access to medicines, over 95% of all medicines on the WHO Essential Drugs list are off-patent, which means that they are freely available to all generic manufacturers, who can copy them at virtually no cost and market them anywhere in the world (European Federation of Pharmaceutical Industries and Associations, 2007). The website for the Pharmaceutical Research and Manufacturers of America also states that: 'Many developing countries are not adequately delivering basic health care services, including medicines, to their populations. Countries need functioning public health systems to get health care services and medicines to the sick' (The Pharmaceutical Research and Manufacturers of America, 2006). When the private sector calls for better public provision it is important to assess the possible underlying factors.

One of these is likely to be the need for political stability which is partly generated by improved access to health care and which can have far-reaching economic consequences outside of the health sector. It provides a stable base for investors engaged in long-term activities

---

[4] This amounts, on average, to one visit every ten years to one every two years to health services per inhabitant.

in a particular region. In Colombia for instance, many investors had become increasingly preoccupied by the inefficient, costly, and ineffective health policy in the country.

Conclusion

- More than disease control, access to good quality CHC is central to social and political stability because it answers to the demand for relief from suffering.
- Epidemics and pandemics will not be controlled unless health care is made comprehensive and acceptable in those health facilities where disease programme interventions are delivered – that is, in general, public services.
- To the extent that AIDS and multi-resistant tuberculosis pandemics threaten the security of industrialized countries, these countries need to acknowledge that a strategic change is needed for the benefit of their own citizens.

Part 2: The need for a methodological shift to determine priorities in health policies

Why are public health methods an issue? The methods often used to define specific programmes have a political dimension that has been largely neglected. This political aspect appears when such methods have led decision makers to adhere to an ideologically motivated policy that is often at the core of specific programmes. This can be illustrated with the use of disability-adjusted life years (DALYs) and quality-adjusted life years (QALYs), two indicators of cost-effectiveness which were devised to prioritize disease-control programmes and were the mainstay of health policy making throughout the 1990s.

> **DALYs and QALYs**
>
> The disability-adjusted life year (DALY) extends the concept of potential years of life lost due to premature death to include equivalent years of 'healthy' life lost by virtue of being in states of poor health or disability (World Health Organization, 2008). One DALY can be thought of as 1 lost year of 'healthy' life, and the burden of disease can be thought of as a measurement of the gap between current health status and an ideal situation where everyone lives into old age, free of disease and disability. The quality-adjusted life year (QALY), is a year of life adjusted for its quality or its value. A year in perfect health is considered equal to 1.0 QALY (World Health Organization, 2008). The value of a year in ill health would be discounted.

The concepts of DALY and QALY were disseminated by the 1993 WB report 'Investing in Health.' However, aid programmes established to reduce the 'disease burden' managed in this view to largely evade the need for a real evidence base (for the definition of priorities, see examples in Section 1). Many observers have argued that the concept and practice of 'burden of disease' in health programming has operated as a ploy to sell a policy – which is the policy to restrict health care delivery in public services to disease- and risk-specific programmes.

Furthermore, it is not only the application of the prioritization of disease but also its (utilitarian) rationale which is discriminatory. According to M. Segall: 'For allocative efficiency … people are to be prioritised for care, not in terms of the seriousness of their state of health, but according to their ability to contribute to aggregate societal health gain.' (Segall, 2003). The notion of societal gain implicit in the concepts of QALYs and DALYs is steeped in neoclassical economics, and remains highly subjective; in the case of who is a burden, for example, will be defined by hand-selected economists, rather than by the public health scholars and professionals in any particular region. This approach inevitably discriminates against treatment of the old, the chronically ill, and the disabled, while failing 'to make a qualitative distinction between treatment to save life ('the rule of rescue') and treatment to reduce morbidity' (Hadorn, 1991).

Under an egalitarian framework, an alternative way of priority setting would be based on the quest for maximum state of health (of which someone is capable). This quest leads to formulate health objectives in terms of appropriate access to care of good quality – which is not incompatible with economic development, which is premised on equity and the incorporation of social–cultural perspectives.

Accordingly, in order to meet access requirements, LICs should be covered with sufficient public health centres and general hospitals while their package of activities should be defined on the basis of the full use of both their infrastructure and staff skills, as defined by managerial experience in different environments. Then health centres should provide care covering the intersection between the community's demand for accessing polyvalent care and need defined by health professionals. Therefore, this package – the problem-solving capacity of health facilities – should be improved through continuing medical education and local knowledge transfer techniques. These would include in-service training, technical/psychological coaching, and practical rotations in a referral hospital.

The shift in the methodology of priority setting will have consequences for the 'right to health care' promoted by the WHO. Instead of describing its content on the grounds of programmatic outputs (MDGs plus a few other DSPs), this shift will enable us to consider, as a right, access to health centres and a referral hospital delivering comprehensive care. As in Western Europe people have a right of access to a family doctor and referral hospitals. Since World War II this approach has guaranteed one of the best means of access to health care in the world. Unlike in managed care settings, this positive dimension of access and reasonably sound efficiency did not require France, Belgium and Germany to provide a precise definition of the care delivered by family doctors, for instance. Notice that, with accurate task shifting, family doctors can be replaced by nurses and medical assistants. This would still represent major progress because health centres and district hospitals together can offer a solution for up to 95% of health problems provided that:

- DSPs are not permitted to strain access to polyvalent curative consultations during, say, half a day every day, 6 days a week (Section 2, Chapter 4);
- Managed care techniques are not permitted to strain the needed balance between the doctors' therapeutic freedom and his/her quest for rationalization of clinical decision making (see Section 6, Chapter 19, Part 1).

Finally, besides health services outputs, priorities in health policy need to encompass steps in services and systems development, possibly at the expense of disease-control ambitions. Conditional priorities – priorities defined on local conditions – are to be introduced in health planning, which requires de-concentration within the government administration. Such decentralization pattern has not been deemed to be compatible with the central administration of disease-control programmes by international aid agencies (Brinkerhoff & Leighton, 2002). To take advantage of de-concentration, professionals in charge of health services need to have a strategic know-how about health services development (see Section 6, Chapter 20) which public health academic units should follow up and place within a conceptual framework.

References

Baily G. V., Savic D., Gothi G. D., Naidu V. B., & Nair S. S. (1967). Potential yield of pulmonary tuberculosis cases by direct microscopy of sputum in a district of South India. *Bulletin of the World Health Organization*, 37(6), pp. 875–92.

Banerji D. & Andersen R. (1963). A Sociological study of awareness of symptoms among persons with pulmonary tuberculosis. *Bulletin of the World Health Organization*, 29, pp. 665–83.

Brinkerhoff D. & Leighton C. (2002). *Decentralization and Health System Reform. Insights for Implementers.* Bethesda, MD: Partners for Health Reformplus (PHRplus).

Chan M. (2008). Address to the 61st World Health Assembly. http://www.who.int/dg/spe eches/2008/20080519/en/index.html.

Department of Economic and Social Affairs. (2000). *Charting the Progress of Populations.* New York: United Nations Population Division. ST/ESA/SER.R/151.

El Sadr W. M. & Hoos D. (2008). The president's emergency plan for AIDS relief – Is the emergency over? *New England Journal of Medicine*, 359(6), pp. 553–5.

European Federation of Pharmaceutical Industries and Associations. (2007). *Building Healthier Societies for Better Global Public Health.* http://www.efpia.eu/Content/Default .asp?PageID=395.

Hadorn D. C. (1991). Setting health care priorities in Oregon – Cost-effectiveness meets the rule of rescue. *Journal of the American Medical Association*, 265(17), pp. 2218–25.

Hanson S. & Hanson C. (2008). HIV control in low-income countries in sub-Saharan Africa: Are the right things done? *Global Health Action*, 1, doi: 10.3402/gha.v1i0.1837.

Institute of Tropical Medicine Antwerp. (2007). *MPH Programme – Health Sector Management and Policy, 2005–2007 data.* Antwerp: Institute of Tropical Medicine.

Jong-Wook L. (2003). Global health improvement and WHO: Shaping the future. *Lancet*, 362(9401), pp. 2083–8.

McIntyre D., Thiede M., Dahlgren G., & Whitehead M. (2006). What are the economic consequences for households of illness and of paying for health care in low- and middle-income country contexts? *Social Science & Medicine*, 62(4), pp. 858–65.

Preker A. S., Langenbrunner J., & Suzuki E. (2002). *THE GLOBAL EXPENDITURE GAP, Securing Financial Protection and Access to Health Care for the Poor.* Washington, DC: Commission on Macro Economics and Health, The World Bank.

Segall M. (2003). District health systems in a neoliberal world: A review of five key policy areas. *International Journal of Health Planning and Management*, 18 p. S5–S26.

Shiffman J. (2008). Has donor prioritization of HIV/AIDS displaced aid for other health issues. *Health Policy and Planning*, 23(2), pp. 95–100.

The Pharmaceutical Research and Manufacturers of America. (2006). *Health Care in the Developing World.* http://world.phrma.org/.

UNAIDS (2007). *Financial Resources Required to Achieve Universal Access to HIV Prevention, Treatment, Care and Support.* Geneva: UNAIDS.

UNAIDS(2008). 2008 *Report on the Global AIDS Epidemic.* Geneva: UNAIDS. UNAIDS/08.25E / JC1510E.

Unger J. P. & Killingsworth J. R. (1986). Selective primary health care: A critical review of methods and results. *Social Science & Medicine*, 22(10), pp. 1001–13.

Van Doorslaer E., O'Donnell O., Rannan-Eliya R. P., Somanathan A., Adhikari S. R., Garg C. C., Harbianto D., Herrin A. N., Huq M. N., Ibragimova S., Karan A., Ng C. W., Pande B. R., Racelis R., Tao S., Tin K., Tisayaticom K., Trisnantoro L., Vasavid C., & Zhao Y. X. (2006). Effect of payments for health care on poverty estimates in 11 countries in Asia: An analysis of household survey data. *Lancet*, 368(9544), pp. 1357–64.

Vander Plaetse B., Hlatiwayo G., Van Eygen L., Meessen B., & Criel B. (2005). Costs and revenue of health care in a rural Zimbabwean district. *Health Policy and Planning*, 20(4), pp. 243–51.

World Health Organization. (1978). Declaration of Alma-Ata. In: *Report of the International Conference on Primary Health Care, Alma*

Ata, USSR, 6–12 September 1978. Geneva: World Health Organization, pp. 2–6.

World Health Organization. (1981). *Global Strategy for Health for All by the Year 2000.* Geneva: World Health Organization. WHA34.36.

World Health Organization. (2000). *Medicines Strategy: Framework for Action in Essential Drugs and Medicines Policy 2002–2003.* Geneva: World Health Organization.

World Health Organization. (2008). *The Global Burden of Disease: 2004 update.* Geneva: WHO Press, pp. 1–160.

Xu K., Evans D. B., Kawabata K., Zeramdini R., Klavus J., & Murray C. J. L. (2003). Household catastrophic health expenditure: A multi-country analysis. *Lancet,* **362**(9378), pp. 111–7.

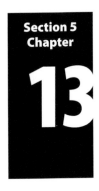

Principles for alternative, publicly oriented health care
policies, planning, management and delivery

Principles for an alternative, social and democratic health policy

Adapted from: Unger J.-P., De Paepe J.-P., Ghilbert P., Soors W., Green A. Integrated care: a fresh perspective for international health policies in low and middle-income countries. International Journal of Integrated Care 2006; 6. ISSN 1568–4156.

Introduction

In Section 1, we reviewed the role that international aid and health policies have played in the disappointing health sector results in LMICs. Both policies are neoliberal in their promotion of commodification of health care. We argued that the combination of government-operated DSPs together with privatized health care services constrained both programme performance and people's access to care. Whilst we also recognized other factors that contributed to this failure (including, for example, state crisis, debt, corruption and patronage), we concluded that the only way forward was to support an alternative aid policy towards health services.

In this chapter we call for the promotion of a publicly oriented integrated health sector as a cornerstone of such a health policy, conceived to overcome the fragmentation and segmentation of LMIC health systems as it currently exists. We define 'publicly oriented' as opposed to 'private for-profit' in terms of objectives and commitment, not of (government vs. private) ownership. The combination of public aims and co-management with users and health professionals gives the name 'social-and-democratic' to such a policy.

We outline health system-specific strategies consistent with this policy, with the potential to improve both health care and disease control in LMICs.

A social-and-democratic health policy and a publicly oriented health sector

The core of this proposed policy is a publicly oriented health sector. We believe that the classical division of health facilities by ownership has lost its relevance. In many countries not all government structures are 'publicly oriented' (with a social mission), nor do all private services always seek profits first. Not all NGOs are publicly oriented with some NGOs, including faith-based organizations, following a for-profit or a proselytizing rationale. As such a classification based on aims and commitment is proposed, using the framework developed by Giusti and colleagues (Giusti et al., 1997). According to Giusti, publicly oriented, as opposed to private for-profit, health care organizations are facilities and systems whose *raison d'être* is the response to the health demand and needs of the population. Publicly oriented services aim to balance the concerns of the patient, the community, the state, and professionals in care delivery and management. In contrast private for-profit services focus

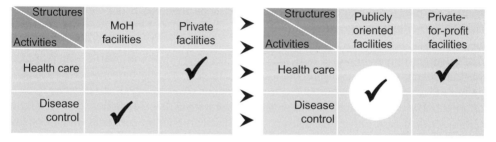

Figure 13.1. A proposal for a more integrated policy. MoH, Ministry of Health.

primarily on financial profitability and treat corporate and health professionals' income as an end in itself. This classification enables the formulation of quality standards for publicly oriented health care delivery (Section 5, Chapter 14), which can inform teaching, research, partner identification, contracting, management, evaluation and health policy design. Providers from non-governmental organizations, including denominational as well as from community-owned or other social security organizations, could belong to this publicly oriented health sector alongside government facilities belonging to the MoH and city councils.[1] Their social mission and management would be to balance the interests of individuals and society. Such a broadened publicly oriented sector allows wide geographical coverage, integration of disease control in services in a manner that attracts patients, together with equitable access to quality health care. Management contracts can be designed to secure a co-management structure that involves the participation of key stakeholders – including the community in all publicly oriented facilities – and the delivery of health care responding to specific quality criteria to a defined population. Such contracts could help to distinguish those with a social motive from the others. In other words we acknowledge that there is a gradient of grey between health organizations and facilities with a commercial versus a social mission, both in government and private services (Peters, 2009). However, we wish to promote a not-for-profit sector (delivering individual curative care and integrated disease-specific interventions) which would abide by clear quality standards thanks to appropriate contracts, resources and control. The grey area would then disappear and the two sectors would progressively become clearly dichotomic (Figure 13.1).

We will classify development strategies for publicly oriented health services according to an organization-based typology of health systems as defined by Mintzberg (Unger et al., 2000). This categorizes organizations into five clusters depending on their prime coordinating mechanism, key level, and type of decentralization. As such we start by examining strategies adapted to three types of health systems: machine bureaucracies, professional bureaucracies and divisionalized forms.

Machine bureaucracies

Machine bureaucracies are found in West and Central African countries, in the Andes, in Central America and in many Asian public services. They are based on clinical standards (set by technical committees) and thus standardization of work processes. Peripheral units are highly

---

[1] Such an approach is meant to overcome the fragmentation and segmentation of services with a social mission as in the vast majority of LMICs, not in the rare countries such as Costa Rica not subject to this disorder.

specialized, have limited autonomy, and a reduced scope of output. In our view this managerial configuration is inappropriate for highly diversified types of health care that dispensaries and hospitals need to deliver. To the contrary, disease-control programmes can, to a large degree, successfully standardize work processes. This is why health ministries with powerful vertical programmes tend to display many of the features of machine bureaucracies. Each programme focuses on a narrow output (such as vaccination coverage rates), and develops its own information system and parallel management control systems. It focuses its research agenda on the burden of disease, rather than delivery of care. Each programme competes with the others for scarce funding. Such systems have a powerful techno structure but a weak apex, which tries to achieve coordination mainly through formal planning and control mechanisms.

Machine bureaucracies face four interlinked challenges (health care, economic, political and managerial) to achieve adequate publicly oriented health systems.

The health care challenge: pursuing a health ideal compatible with Hippocratic principles

Confining public services to disease-control units leads to under-utilization of the skills of professionals as they are obliged to concentrate on a few, defined, pathologies. This is dubious not only from an efficiency viewpoint, but also from a medical ethics perspective. LMIC patients are similar to service users elsewhere in the world in their need to be considered as people rather than as cases and to access health care irrespective of the form of suffering (Haddad et al., 1998; Tarrant et al., 2003). There is, therefore, a need for a broad application of the Hippocratic ideal, putting family and community health care at the core of services. To implement such an agenda, first-line health professionals need both the will and the skills to interact with patients and communities to solve health problems, in environments where poor communication has been widespread and where pre-graduate education of health professionals has often not included psychosocial care. Until teaching programmes go beyond the biomedical paradigm, additional in-service training and coaching will be necessary to develop bio-psychosocial, patient-centred care (see Section 6, Chapter 19) and to increase the problem-solving capacity of first-line services. Rotations in district hospitals can teach primary care practitioners relevant know-how. Computerised self-teaching programmes based on complaints instead of diseases (Van den Ende et al., 2000) can also improve clinical decision making. Strategies to improve general practice in first-line health services are discussed in Section 6, Chapter 18.

District hospitals are expected to offer the four major specialties (internal medicine, surgery, OB-GYN and paediatrics). They should be included as part of the rationale of developing a publicly oriented health care system as the indispensable complement of the primary care practitioners' frontline provision. The key distinguishing feature of peripheral hospitals, in contrast with first-line facilities, is their capacity to handle medical and surgical emergencies. Together health centres and district hospitals are capable of solving 95% of health problems (Shaw & Elmendorf, 1994), when under a management that integrates resources and structures and with a sustainable operating budget (see Section 5, Chapter 15).

The economic challenge: sustainable, viable finances

Free health care at the point of delivery is clearly desirable from the perspective of accessibility, especially in LMICs. Free health care includes free drugs, tests, exams, X-rays, referral, hospital admission and more. If, as in Uganda, health consultation is made free but some of these items are not provided and must be individually purchased by the patient, 'free' health care becomes instead an obstacle to access to care as it prevents community co-managed health centres from competing with private pharmacies in drug delivery. A number of Latin American countries (Costa Rica and Cuba, and more recently Chile, Brazil, Uruguay and Venezuela) who did not follow the market-based rationale of international aid agencies set up instead public systems delivering free health care and competing with a non-subsidized private for-profit sector. Costa Rica, Chile and Cuba are now among the best examples of health status in the continent (Pan American Health Organization, 2004). At one stage Zimbabwe, Lesotho, and Kerala (India) (Rosenfield, 1985) also achieved outstanding results under a government/state health care delivery system. It took them, for example, only a few decades to achieve mortality reductions where European countries had needed more than a century for the same (Okuonzi, 2004). None of these health systems were machine bureaucracies.

Based on a sample of 18 LICs, the IMF estimated in 1995 that between 1983 and 1990, central government expenditures for health accounted for only 0.4% of GDP, compared to 2.8% for defence (Chu et al., 1995). The IMF authors contrasted this with the need for health expenditure which LICs face. Paradoxically, affordability could be within reach: there are reasons to doubt whether the cost of comprehensive care necessarily exceeds that of a few vertical programmes put together (see Section 5, Chapter 12). Basic health services' requirements appear moderate enough to understand that political will – in both poor and donor countries – is at least as important as the country's GDP and that some LICs and all MICs have the economic potential to finance adequately their health sector.

The problem is to finance publicly oriented services in a sustained manner beyond projects' deadlines in countries where the government's social commitment is weak. Theoretically the Bretton Woods institutions (IMF and WB) could lend a hand by imposing increased social health expenditure in debt and loan negotiations. But over the last decade this has not happened. It is of paramount importance, therefore, that national pressure groups campaign to get LMIC government health budgets increased. Groups representing health professionals (such as the Thai Association of Rural Doctors) and mutual aid associations representing users need to lobby governments and political parties to commit funds. In Egypt, Mali and other countries, communities involved in pilot projects managed to influence national health policies temporarily. These experiences give credit to externally funded pilot projects aimed at the development of community health centres.

Hospital care and drugs represent the main financial constraint for the sick, and communities are too poor to take over health care expenditures. User fees may improve financial accessibility if, and when, they succeed in reducing the total cost of a sickness episode (spanning from illness onset to cure) faced by the patient. To achieve such results mechanisms to pool risk for items such as drugs, laboratory tests, and medical images are needed. Pre-paid schemes can increase solidarity between the sick and the non-sick, fee per sickness episode improves continuity of care and solidarity between the moderately and the severely ill, whilst established health committees may help to define exemptions.

The Bamako Initiative, a large-scale experiment launched in 1987 by UNICEF and WHO, proved capable of improving government health services in some countries where it had been implemented. Revolving funds used to purchase essential generic drugs were negotiated against social control of government and NGO health facilities. Communities were drawn into the management of these funds in order to counter-balance the power of civil servants. Mali, where health sector reform – best known for its community-owned health centres – was introduced in 1990, saw service utilization rates more than double (Maiga et al., 1999). In Benin and Guinea, where the Bamako Initiative was most successful, service utilization rates increased even more significantly (Levy-Bruhl et al., 1997). Admittedly, in many of the 35 other countries where it was implemented, the Initiative failed to improve utilization rates. Specifically, it failed when cost recovery could not reduce the total sickness episode's costs for the user. We also now know that, to increase the success rate of the Bamako Initiative, specific initiatives are needed to improve care acceptability and bio-psychosocial care.

At the global level, international aid can be urged to reorient disease-control budget lines towards the financing of publicly oriented health systems and services. To spend such funds governments and aid agencies could deploy a contracting-in approach. This implies that aid should promote supply-side financing, which is not synonymous with mere support for the MoH as it can encompass all the institutions making up the publicly oriented health sector.

The political challenge: democratizing the health sector

In the past, health systems such as those of Botswana, Zimbabwe, Costa Rica and Kerala State in India have also managed to achieve decent access to good health care because they were monopolistic publicly oriented health care providers. They were also built on a strong social commitment, which is not easily replicable. How then can publicly oriented services be promoted in LMICs where governments badly lack this and incorporate the support of communities?

Indeed, there is one LMIC social feature which favours such a plan. In many shantytowns and rural areas it has been observed that different forms of solidarity or communal self-help are often extensively practiced. This often takes care of elementary schools, waste dumping, water supplies, legal advice, access to telecommunications, and even roads. To some extent such community organization substitutes for the limits of family solidarity and of ailing state health services. The social-and-democrat policy that we propose builds on this potential. In a true political sense our strategy thrives on community development leading to democratization of health services. Community development could inject a degree of pluralism into health services' management under certain conditions. Firstly, the political nature of such participation is critical if it is not to be hijacked by dominant community groups. Secondly, basic quality of health care in publicly oriented facilities is an important pre-condition for community interest in services co-management.

Because of the undemocratic nature of a number of LMIC states, emerging social-and-democrat health policies will initially have to forego any influence on policy design and limit their ambitions to increase the accountability and responsiveness of operational public services through community participation and social control. In hospitals and dispensaries such strategies contribute to bringing together the professional, cultural, and political identities of health professionals, as they root medical practice in a social project and open up avenues to traditional cultures in modern societies, by involving communities in the management of a social sector.

Unfortunately, community participation has often led to demagogic decisions based on unrealistic expectations and insufficient information on technical issues. Mutual control of stakeholders with opposed interests (e.g., professionals and users) can to a certain extent limit them. In practice, health facilities' management boards should consist of patients' and professionals' representatives, MoH district managers, and possibly representatives of any cooperation agencies involved in the region.

Such an approach aims at establishing a constructive dialogue between community associations, health professionals, and government through co-management. It does not aim to replicate the history of the European mutual insurance, with the approach of purchasing care in the private sector and, in theory, improving its quality (Bennett et al., 1998). That would be an illusory task (Criel & Van Dormael, 1999). Neoliberal policies follow this approach by promoting mutual health organizations (MHOs) independently from health care management. All too often, in Africa, MHO coverage remained stuck at disappointing low levels (Waelkens & Criel, 2004). One way of rescuing the concept of mutual health associations in LMICs is to offer them the opportunity to co-manage publicly oriented facilities. This is in line with our strategy.

The managerial challenge: successful and appropriate decentralization

Decentralization of power from central to district government levels can be an important opportunity for community participation, sustainable development and efficient use of resources through adaptation to local needs (see Section 5, Chapter 15).

Decentralization was implemented by colonial authorities in many LMICs in the late 1950s and re-emerged in the 1970s for various reasons. These included objectives of overcoming constraints on development and improving community participation. By the end of the 1980s WHO was promoting districts as baseline administrative units for decentralized health systems (World Health Organization, 1987). Since then many developing countries have adopted a district policy, to improve management and to make top-down (designed at central level of MOH) and bottom-up (conceived by peripheral health professionals together with users and communities) planning meet. Districts can be viewed as integrated local health systems requiring:

- First-line and hospital facilities as operational tiers interconnected under a single administrative umbrella;
- A capable executive team enjoying a degree of autonomy and authority over the health services, able and willing to coach health professionals (Segall, 2003) (Section 6, Chapter 18). International aid could help recruit experienced staff for district management with a responsibility to improve health care and disease control (possibly in pilot projects designed to expand) instead of deploying them only in disease-control programmes (Kelly, 1999). The district executive teams (the middle line managerial level) could be multi-institutional and work alongside MoH health officers; they could include the best health professionals from any of the organizations locally involved in health care activities – although still remaining under MoH leadership.

The managerial potential of district executive teams is linked to their responsibility, which encompasses a two-tiered system, a large population (from 150,000 to 300,000 people) and many professionals. This potential can be enhanced with technical assistance. In the 1980s several African national initiatives targeted district teams with ad hoc in-service training, coaching, and technical support (in Senegal, Burkina Faso, Mali, Congo, for instance) (Unger et al., 1989).

Motivation of staff is a key issue for care delivery and system development. An appropriate practitioners' income, often an unfulfilled need in LMICs, is necessary but not sufficient for these purposes. The UK approach to professionals' remuneration that mixes salaries, registration-based bonuses and partial fee-for-service, could be tested in LMICs.

Other factors such as living and working conditions and job satisfaction are critical. Some health professionals find additional motivation in the Hippocratic ideal of subordinating personal interest to that of the patient. Others may be inspired by faith, politics or a quest for social recognition. They can gain strength by a health service organization able to appeal to their complex professional, political, religious, and philosophical identities. The enlargement of health service responsibilities from disease control to health care delivery provides the opportunity for the use of wider skills and thus motivation from professional identity. It also provides better opportunities for long-term career progression.

Many health professionals have tested original, effective solutions to problems specific to their health systems. As a general recommendation all central level staff of MoH should aim at collecting these experiments and feed with them the design of national health policies. In practice this is rarely done.

Professional bureaucracies

Western European Bismarckian health systems[2] and private for-profit sectors in developing countries generally share the features of professional bureaucracies. They are characterized by standardization of professional skills rather than output, a high degree of autonomy for working units, and weak vertical and horizontal integration. The key component of these organizations is the operating core. In professional bureaucracies health professionals defend their autonomy against the influence of the central apex and techno structure is weak. Medical doctors work without technical supervision, on-the-spot training or evaluation. Their outputs remain almost totally unstandardized, thereby increasing the cost of care. Self-employed professionals may invest in training to increase their technical skills, because increased prestige gives them even more freedom in decision making and revenues. The major drawback is that their mission, as they perceive it, is almost exclusively professional, that is to say medical, to the neglect of organizational aspects, resulting in poor integration and inefficient practices.

In such settings, there are various challenges. Firstly, there is a need to develop systemic links between first-line services and hospitals (including referral systems, technical support by specialists, and communication between primary care practitioners and specialists). Secondly, teams are necessary to bring together doctors and other practitioners such as medical assistants, nurses and physiotherapists. There is also a need to introduce reflexive methods to continuously improve quality of care (such as medical audit, technical supervision, coaching, self-learning methods). Lastly, the regulation capacity of LMIC administrations needs to be strengthened.

Experiences in Belgium have helped address the first three challenges in developing countries, and although it may not always be feasible to export this experience, it is worthwhile describing its process. Firstly, the 'Study Group for a Medical Reform' demonstrated the potential for an independent research and training unit disseminating specific quality criteria for health care delivery (Mercenier, 1971). It managed to promote integrated health centres that nowadays represent between 5% and 10% of the country's first-line care. Secondly, the federation of these health centres acquired influence at national policy level. Finally, the

---

[2] Bismarckian health systems are mainly financed by social contributions. In Beveridge health models health care is financed by the government through tax payments. In practice there is a continuum between the two models. Particular health systems can then partly be defined by the proportion of the two mechanisms used to base health care financing.

15 years experience of the Local Health Systems project suggests that motivated profession-als from first-line services and referral hospitals can take over some district team tasks even in the absence of a formal management structure and with only modest funding. With the technical assistance of an academic unit, voluntary networks of health professionals from functional units used their influence to improve coordination between hospitals and first-line health services, hospital management, clinical decision making, service organization, and quality of care.

In terms of control and regulation, European features should be treated even more cau-tiously in LMICs. So far, there is no single experience that suggests that the French, Belgian and German health systems can be exported. The creation of a welfare state in Western and Northern Europe arose from unique socio-political circumstances in a particular histori-cal context (Baldwin, 1990; Flora & Alber, 1981). European governments provided access to health care for the vast majority of their population only when low-income groups suc-ceeded in defending their interests within the political system. In the aftermath of World War II workers' parties and civic associations were able to incorporate their social agenda into government policy, planning and administration. Since 1945 they have acted as a coun-terweight to the vested interests of health care professionals and private providers. As a consequence social and health care policies in Europe were largely defined by 'the poor' and their representatives. Social protection developed in tandem with democratic rights. Insti-tutional welfare for the population as a whole, based on solidarity through taxes, became the norm (Spicker, 2004). A similar evolution took place outside Europe in countries such as Canada and New Zealand.

By contrast, in the USA social and health care policies were created for 'the poor.' Residual welfare, not solidarity, has been the norm. This narrow concept of welfare as a safety net, confined to those who are unable to manage otherwise, can be traced back to the English Poor Law (1598–1948). In the second half of the twentieth century it has been reinforced by neoliberal ideology and has subsequently received worldwide promotion by policy makers and aid agencies.

In the USA this evolution triggered a series of consequences for health care. In 1970 total expenditure on health was below 7% of GDP in all High-Income Countries (HICs). By 2003 it was around 9% of GDP in countries as far apart as Canada, the United Kingdom (UK), New Zealand and Sweden. However, in the USA, health expenditure reached over 15.2% in 2005 (World Health Organization, 2008) and is still rising. It would be hard to interpret these figures as the price to pay for higher quality. By the turn of the century the USA continued to lag behind the health systems of equivalent countries in terms of solidar-ity, equity and financial access. A predominant share of private expenditure in total health expenditure illustrates low solidarity: private expenditure totalled 56% of total health expenditure in the USA in 2000, compared to 30% in Canada, 21% in New Zealand and 15% in Sweden. Low public insurance coverage affects access and efficiency, and reflects inequity: public health insurance coverage reached no more than 27.8% in the USA in 2007 (DeNavas-Walt et al., 2008), against 100% in Canada, the UK, New Zealand and Sweden. Maternal mortality is an indicator sensitive to care accessibility: while in 2000 US maternal mortality was still 17/100,000, Canada was 6, New Zealand 7, and Sweden only 2/100,000 (World Health Organization, 2003). It is difficult to escape the conclusion that the US health policy is inefficient (Organisation for Economic Co-operation and Development, 2002) and ineffective.

Such policy-induced inefficiency is likely to pose bigger problems in LMICs, where access to health care is even more constrained by the prevailing poverty. Moreover, in LMICs, the poor rarely take part in shaping policies or setting budgets. A common sight in developing countries is a lack of social pluralism in government decision making, which tends to increase inequality (Haubert et al., 1992). The elite that concentrate power in many LMICs have little interest in redistributive policies. Indeed more than a few LMIC governments willingly adapted their policies to neoliberal aid conditions (Navarro, 2004). As a result of this concentration of power and the influence of private doctors, improvements in the regulatory capacity of LMIC governments remain a challenge.

Divisionalized forms

According to Mintzberg, divisionalized systems provide interregional coordination whilst allowing regional difference based on geographically defined health districts and regions. Until some years ago, the UK, Costa Rica, Chile, Sweden, and Jordan had such health services that tackled disease-control and health care challenges simultaneously and allowed a degree of autonomy and decision making capacity at the periphery. These systems favour both accessibility to health care and user participation. While they have proved to be amongst the best, they share two specific drawbacks. Firstly, bureaucratization resulting from managed care (introduced during the last 15 years) that is symptomized by a plethora of guidelines, mechanistic evaluations and administrative tasks which affect the motivation of professionals, as well as their problem-solving capacity. Secondly, some countries lack reflexive methods. Both professional associations and political groups have proved essential to defend the public mission of divisionalized national health systems and improve their operations. We concentrate here on their technical challenges.

Technical and psychological support to health professionals

While some degree of clinical decision making standardization is needed, improvements in health care quality cannot rely solely on managed care techniques (Section 6, Chapter 19, Part 1) that, in many systems, have grown unduly. Alternative techniques are available. Coaching, also known as individual, dynamic guidance to professionals is available to support motivation and quality of care. It is broader than traditional continuous professional development as it offers psychological support to professionals and teams as well as assessment of individual and group learning needs based on observation and discussion. Coaching builds upon numerous methodologies (Section 6, Chapter 19). Experience with coaching in LMIC pilot projects suggests that it helps to bridge the gap between health care delivery and management. It certainly is an innovative tool to identify learning needs, which traditional continuous professional development is unable to fulfil (Norman et al., 2004). Furthermore it can strengthen common culture and practice (Glouberman & Mintzberg, 1998). In addition to coaching, action and operational research, and specific forms of audit led by the professionals themselves, instead of external evaluators, can be valuable devices to improve reflexivity in divisionalized health systems.

An ideal organizational model?

Which organizational configuration is likely to support such managerial techniques? It needs to foster a high degree of professional staff initiative, community participation, action and operational research, continuous evaluation and managerial autonomy. An organizational form worth consideration at least is adhocracy, defined by Mintzberg as a configuration coordinated chiefly by mutual adjustment and characterized by horizontal job specialization based on formal training (Mintzberg, 1993). An adhocracy performs ideally in complex environments. Its managers become functioning members of the team. It is called operating adhocracy if its main purpose is to produce creative solutions to unique problems on behalf of its clients, as in health care. In an operating adhocracy the administrative and operating work tends to blend into one single effort. However, though appealing at the level of the service providers, a health organization as a whole cannot be a pure adhocracy. As a system encompassing both health care and disease control, it also tends to give middle managers the authority to control their own units, resulting in a configuration that Mintzberg describes as the divisionalized form (Figure 1-2, p. 10). When in balance, the resulting structural hybrid (Figure 1-2, p. 10) becomes a divisionalized operating adhocracy.

Conclusions

Solidarity through publicly oriented services is needed to avoid a problem in many LMICs. This has entailed full health care services for the rich and ineffective disease control for the poor (delivered in public services, starved of patients despite the fact that many of them are supposed to be candidates of disease-control programmes) (Section 2, Chapter 3). A publicly oriented health sector defined by motive, and able to balance individual and collective interest, allows the successful integration of disease control with health care and equitable access to health care.

We favour a pluralistic social representation within, and an increased accountability of, health institutions. If communities are to support public services, health professionals and policy makers must aim at improving care quality. Our proposed social-and-democrat policy thus relies on consistent medical, managerial, socio-political and economic features: family and community health care delivered by decentralized units, local health systems, and community development of public services in machine bureaucracies. Under such an approach professional and political identities may echo each other and become an active motivational force. A political and technical terminology common to those who endorse the principles presented here would further strengthen this strategy.

Stakeholders outside the health sector may have an interest in supporting such a proposal on different grounds. If Western politicians ignore the avoidable suffering, mortality and anxiety in LMICs, they cannot ignore the global political instability when 60% of the world's population lives with less than USD 2 per day and is lacking not only access to work and shelter, but also access to health care, compounding matters. Throughout the industrialized world conservative politicians should understand that it is difficult to restrain economic migration without first improving conditions in emigrants' countries. They also ought to be aware that family-planning initiatives and AIDS control programmes fail when they are not integrated into health services offering acceptable health care. Social democrat politicians would find support with voters by exporting mechanisms that favour solidarity and that form the foundations of democracy. Green politicians could be inspired by the opportunity to put social control of the state apparatus into practice in contexts where communities still exist.

As committed and progressive health professionals we should tirelessly explain to all people, parties, and policy makers the importance, choices, and stakes of international health policy. Together we can bring disease control and health care back in step with ethical principles and desired outcomes, and contribute to a fairer and safer world.

References

Baldwin P. (1990). *The Politics of Social Solidarity. Class Bases of the European Welfare States 1875–1975*. Cambridge, UK: Cambridge University Press.

Bennett S., Creese A., & Monasch R. (1998). *Health Insurance Schemes for People Outside Formal Sector Employment*. Geneva: Division of Analysis, Research and Assessment, World Health Organization. ARA Paper number 16, WHO/ARA/CC/98.1.

Chu K., Gupta S., Clements B., et al. (1995). *Unproductive Public Expenditures: A Pragmatic Approach to Policy Analysis*. Washington, DC: International Monetary Fund.

Criel B. & Van Dormael M. (1999). Mutuelles de santé en Afrique et systèmes nationaux d'assurance-maladie obligatoire: l'histoire Européenne se répétera t'elle? *Tropical Medicine & International Health*, 4(3), pp. 155–9.

DeNavas-Walt C., Proctor B. D., & Smith J. C. (2008). *Income, Poverty, and Health Insurance Coverage in the United States: 2007*. Washington, DC: U.S. Census Bureau. pp. 60–235.

Flora B. & Alber J. (1981). Modernisation, democratisation and the development of welfare states in Western Europe. In: Flora P. & Heidenheimer A. J., eds. *The Development of Welfare State in Europe and America*. London: Transaction Publishing, pp. 37–80.

Giusti D., Criel B., & de Béthune X. (1997). Viewpoint: Public versus private health care delivery: Beyond the slogans. *Health Policy and Planning*, 12(3), pp. 192–8.

Glouberman S. & Mintzberg H. (1998). Managing the care of health and the cure of disease. *Health Care Management Review*, 26(1), pp. 56–69

Haddad S., Fournier P., Machouf N., & Yatara F. (1998). What does quality mean to lay people? Community perceptions of primary health care services in Guinea. *Social Science & Medicine*, 47(3), pp. 381–94.

Haubert M., Frelin C., & Leimdorfer F. (1992). Etats et société dans le Tiers-monde. De la modernisation à la démocratisation? Paris: Publications de la Sorbonne.

Kelly M. (1999). A donor's perspective on tuberculosis in international health. *Lancet*, 353(9157), p. 1006.

Levy-Bruhl D., Soucat A., Osseni R., et al. (1997). The Bamako initiative in Benin and Guinea: Improving the effectiveness of primary health care. *International Journal of Health Planning and Management*, 12(Supplement 1), pp. S49–S79.

Maiga Z., Traore F. N., & El Abassi A. (1999). La réforme du secteur santé au Mali, 1989–1996. In: Kegels G., et al., eds. *Studies in Health Services Organization*. Antwerpen: ITG Press, pp. 1–132.

Mercenier P. (1971). Pour une politique de santé publique. *Intermédiaire*, pp. 1–9.

Mintzberg H.(1993). *Structure in Fives. Designing Effective Organisations*. New Jersey: Prentice-Hall Inc.

Navarro V. (2004). The world health situation. *International Journal of Health Services*, 34(1), pp. 1–10.

Norman G. R., Shannon S. I., & Marrin M. L. (2004). The need for needs assessment in continuing medical education. *British Medical Journal*, 328(7446), pp. 999–1001.

Okuonzi S. A.(2004). Dying for economic growth? Evidence of a flawed economic policy in Uganda. *Lancet*, 364(9445), pp. 1632–7.

Organisation for Economic Co-operation and Development. (2002). Assessment and recomendations. In: *Economic Survey – United States 2002*. Paris, France: Organisation for Economic Co-operation and Development, pp. 7–18.

Pan American Health Organization. (2004). *Core Health Data System. Special Programme for Health Analysis (SHA)*. Washington, DC: Pan American Health Organization (PAHO).

Peters D. H.(2009). Increase access to health services by the poor, but don't blame 'privatisation' or export British prescriptions to developing countries. *Lancet Rapid Responses*, 339(b2337). 2009.

Rosenfield P. L.(1985). The contribution of social and political factors to good health. In: Halstead S. B., et al., eds. *Good Health at Low*

Cost. Proceedings of a conference held at the Bellagio Conference Centre, Bellagio, Italy, April 29-May 3, 1985. New York: Rockefeller Foundation, pp. 1–248.

Segall M.(2003). District health systems in a neoliberal world: A review of five key policy areas. *International Journal of Health Planning and Management,* **18,** pp. S5–S26.

Shaw R. P. & Elmendorf A. E.(1994). *Better Health in Africa. Experience and Lessons Learned.* Washington, DC: World Bank.

Spicker P.(2004). *An Introduction to Social Policy.* Aberdeen, Scotland: The Robert Gordon University.

Tarrant C., Windridge K., Boulton M., Baker R., & Freeman G.(2003). How important is personal care in general practice? *British Medical Journal,* **326**(7402), p. 1310.

Unger J. P., Daveloose P., Ba A., Toure-Sene N. N., & Mercenier P.(1989). Senegal moves nearer the goals of Alma-Ata. *World Health Forum,* **10**(3–4), pp. 456–63.

Unger J. P., Macq J., Bredo F., & Boelaert M.(2000). Through Mintzberg's glasses: A fresh look at the organisation of ministries of health. *Bulletin of the World Health Organization,* 78(8), pp. 1005–14.

Van den Ende J., Van den Enden E., Bisoffi Z., & Lagana S.(2000). Kabisa 2000(CDROM). *2000.* Antwerp: Prins Leopold Institute of Tropical Medicine.

Waelkens M. P. & Criel B.(2004). *Les mutuelles de santé en Afrique sub-saharienne. Etat des lieux et réflexions sur un agenda de recherche.* Washington, DC: The World Bank. Health, Nutrition and Population (HNP) Discussion Paper.

World Health Organization. (1987). *Report of the Interregional Meeting on Strengthening District Health Systems Based on Primary Health Care, Harare, Zimbabwe, 3 to 7 August 1987.* Geneva: World Health Organization. WHO/SHS/DHS/87.13, Rev.1.

World Health Organization. (2003). *Maternal Mortality in 2000: Estimates Developed by WHO, Unicef and UNFPA.* Geneva: World Health Organization.

World Health Organization. (2008). *World Health Statistics 2008.* Geneva: Word Health Organization.

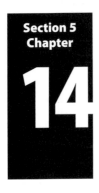

14 Quality standards for health care delivery and management in publicly oriented health services

Adapted from: Unger J.-P., Marchal B., Green A. Quality standards for health care delivery and management in publicly-oriented health services. Int J Health Planning and Management 2003; 18: S79-S88.

Throughout this book, we have advocated the delivery of CHC. But the expected output of publicly oriented services also needs to be defined. This chapter therefore aims at specifying quality standards for health care delivery and management when the goal is not-for-profit. It argues that there is not one medicine, nor one science for the management of health but two, according to whether their purpose is social or commercial. The proposed criteria may be viewed as a complement to medical ethics (deontology).

Introduction

As early as 1997, an editorial in the *British Medical Journal* (BMJ) stated a case for a shared code of ethics that might bond all health care stakeholders into a consistent moral framework (Berwick et al., 1997). To elicit comments and discussion the multidisciplinary 'Tavistock group' issued five ethical principles that should govern all health care systems (Smith et al., 1999), in essence:

- Health care is a human right.
- The care of individuals is at the centre of health care delivery, within an overall preoccupation for generating the greatest possible health gains for groups and populations.
- The responsibilities of a health care delivery system include the prevention of illness and the alleviation of disability.
- Cooperation between providers and with those served is imperative.
- All individuals and groups providing access or services have a continuing responsibility to help improve its quality.

This paper elaborates these principles further in two directions. Firstly, it develops a set of quality standards based on ethical principles intended to regulate health care delivery and service management. In doing so we aim to clarify in tangible terms the meaning of 'quality' of health care – a fashionable, but rather ill-defined policy issue. The paper focuses on primary care services, although the principles apply to other levels of care as well.

Secondly, it applies these principles to 'publicly oriented' health services. Indeed health systems are generally pluralistic, incorporating organizations ranging from private for-profit, NGO, governmental, municipal, denominational, mutual aid and social security. According to the framework of Giusti et al. (1997) we classify these organizations as 'publicly oriented' health care organizations and refer to facilities and systems whose *raison d'être* is to respond to the health needs and demands of the population. They aim to provide a service to patients that is equitable, sensitive to community requirements, and sets priorities according to need. In other words they are defined in terms of their mission, rather than their ownership. State-operated health facilities are not automatically 'publicly oriented' as degrees of internal privatization might exist and may give rise to management for-profit and the sharing of benefits amongst professionals. On the other hand, many NGO facilities are often 'publicly oriented' in their calling, although private in terms of ownership. In this paper our view is that 'publicly oriented' refers to a definition based on public interest and not on government ownership.

Our proposed principles are designed to influence health care delivery and management in all services operating in the public interest, by serving as a basis for:

- management contracts between health authorities and 'publicly oriented' services;
- audits of health services, as regards the content and aspects of service to be assessed;
- statutes, objectives, and benchmarks for 'publicly oriented' organizations (NGOs, municipality, government and mutual aid association);
- formulation of hypotheses in research and evaluation;
- design and teaching of health services managerial strategies;
- dissemination in and by health professional networks;
- health policy proposals for and by political bodies.

The definition and assessment of quality standards in health care is a political as well as a technical issue. In this paper we explore how the adoption of what might be termed 'humanistic' criteria for quality health care could have a positive influence on the development of the health sector. Indeed health professionals, health care managers, policy makers, consumers, and professional associations seeking to encourage social accountability in health care within government, municipal, and NGO health organizations could use them as guidelines. The likely impact of a new service compact based on these principles, between patients, health professionals, and the government on health care delivery and management is contrasted with care provided by market-based, for-profit organizations. The reasons why this sector is reluctant to adopt the proposed standards in many developing countries are explored in this document.

Ten principles as a basis for health care delivery in the public interest

We propose ten axioms to be the basis of quality in 'publicly oriented' health care systems and services. In doing so we were initially inspired by the Groupe d'Etude pour une Réforme de la Médecine (G.E.R.M.), which defined axioms 3, 4, 8, 9, and 10 (Groupe d'Etude pour une Réforme de la Médecine [G.E.R.M.], 1971; Mercenier, 1971) and which were further developed through extensive experiences in the field over the past decades. A first set defines the individual's interest in health care:

1. Each individual has the right to access quality health care at a cost within their reach without jeopardizing the economic security of the individual and his or her family.
2. Quality care is patient-centred (Brown et al., 1986; Engel, 1977) and continuous, and reduces suffering, disability, anxiety, and risk of premature death.
3. Clinical practice must be effective and, therefore, rooted in evidence-based medicine. Decisions that are not based on scientific criteria should be acknowledged as such by the provider in an explanation to the patient.

4. Quality care enhances the patient's autonomy (Beauchamp & Childress, 1994), makes him/her less of a hostage to the disease and its treatment, and respects the decision-making capacity of patients.
5. There is a need for a balance in care between effectiveness and efficiency,[1] between the medical handling of the psychosocial dimension of care and the quest for patient's autonomy, and between rationalization of treatment and response to a patient's demand. The practitioner should strive to maintain this balance through dialogue with the patient.
6. Health professionals should use their knowledge for the benefit of their patients, before their own advancement or that of an employing organization.
7. Health professionals should recognize the multiple causes of ill health and actively engage in wider activities to promote good health and prevent disease.

A second set of axioms balances these individual interests with the population's collective interest:

1. Well-being, defined as the satisfaction of basic needs (food, housing, education and health), is a pivotal human right. Health professionals have a duty to respond to such needs in a way that entails solidarity between the rich and the poor, between the healthy and the sick, and between the moderately and the seriously ill.
2. 'Publicly oriented' health care delivery decisions should be driven by equity. In the presence of scarce health care resources, equity may demand that a limit be placed on personal health care consumption in the wider interests of universal access according to need.[2] Conflicting health objectives should be resolved in the joint interest of the patient, and the community and the nation concerns (since the last two actors often co-finance individual health care). 'Publicly oriented' decision making in an account-able and transparent manner is needed to prioritize health care activities.
3. 'Publicly oriented' health care delivery should be holistic, culturally and gender sensitive (Brody, 1999) and should strengthen the health care capacity of individuals and their community. Collective reflection and community action are essential contri-butions to the development of 'publicly oriented' health systems and services, and should be fostered throughout such services (World Health Organization, 1978). In practice publicly oriented services should be co-managed with representatives of the communities, users and professionals under state stewardship.

Principles in practice

These principles are unlikely to be applied in the private for-profit sector of developing coun-tries. Some independent doctors may pursue these criteria and, in the industrialized world, some indeed (partly) do. However, in LICs profit is necessarily more an end in itself because of the fragile economic situation of the vast majority of health professionals. These conditions are likely to deter private for-profit providers from adopting these principles. These argu-ments can be further elaborated by comparing the application of the principles in five main aspects of health care delivery, respectively, in 'publicly oriented' and market-based systems:

---

[1] This contrasts with the Hippocratic Oath, which favours effectiveness above any other consideration.
[2] Public management should aim at health sector productive efficiency, which refers to the entire health care public system and not just to one isolated institution.

care delivery (clinical practice, family medicine, community medicine and disease control), and service management.

Care delivery

The axioms set out above that define the individual's interest in health care are stated as principles. In this sense readers are free to accept or reject them. However, continuity of care, patient-centred care, the quest for patient autonomy, and evidence-based medicine can be argued as pre-conditions for effective care. They are both an end and a means. For example, when decisions about treatment are made on a shared basis, adherence is likely to increase. In other words health care that promotes the patient's autonomy is likely to be more effective.

Clinical practice

In 'publicly oriented' health care systems, both the individual patient and the community become stakeholders in clinical decisions. At this point, owing to the scarcity of resources, the requirement that is placed on health professionals to deliver optimum quality of care needs to be matched with a concern to contain costs. Similarly, health professionals need to balance rationalization imperatives imposed by protocols of disease-control programmes with the flexibility needed in patient-centred care (with regard to use of drugs, for instance). They must strive to optimize the balance between health care provision in the community and the rights of the individual. In practice epidemiology should play a pivotal role in clinical decision making. An essential drug policy, epidemiological knowledge, evidence-based medicine, and appropriate diagnostic and therapeutic technology are other key elements in effective and efficient health care provision. In the for-profit sector clinical decisions are taken on a case-by-case basis with the objective of maximizing patient benefit. Effectiveness usually outweighs efficiency, especially because of inherent incentives to over-consumption. In particular the health professional's income and a facility's revenue are usually dependent on the volume and the complexity of diagnostic and therapeutic interventions. This explains why for-profit hospitals in the USA lead to increased spending on health care, while being less efficient than public institutions (Woolhandler & Himmelstein, 1999). For the same reason publicly financed, but privately delivered, care in industrialized countries is likely to be inherently less efficient than publicly financed and delivered care (Havighurst, 1977; Silverman et al., 1999) – although not all public systems achieve their potential for efficiency. Health maintenance organizations that combine the functions of both financing and provision will consider maximizing efficiency as a prime objective and therefore may be an exception. However, the improvements may be largely absorbed by the profits taken.

Family medicine

In our view, patient-centred care, the pivotal feature of family practice, is the best mechanism for health care delivery in 'publicly oriented' first-line services. Such practice is characterized by an assessment of social, family, psychological, and somatic factors that may influence the health problem and its solution. It implies a provider-patient negotiation of a therapeutic and/or preventive strategy appropriate to the specific needs ('patient-centred care'). Several managerial strategies are available to progressively apply the principles of patient-centred care in developing countries (see Section 6, Chapter 19).

Family practice was never a characteristic of colonial health policies. Indeed its features were conceptualized after the colonial period. However, it did not emerge after independence in the majority of developing countries (Van Dormael, 1995), and holistic care is somehow at odds with government services preoccupied with disease-control activities.

Some crucial aspects of family practice are also at odds with the profit motive. In making clinical decisions the family practitioner faces dilemmas that lie at the very heart of patient-centred care. Does the problem need to be medicalized? Should it be treated biomedically or psychosocially? Should the patient be treated as an individual to the exclusion of all else or with reference to his or her environment (Kunneman, 1995)? Even in industrialized countries, only a minority of health professionals, usually socially and/or politically motivated doctors, address these issues with respect of their patient's autonomy. In developing countries promoting patient autonomy may not prove feasible if health care financing is inadequate and practitioners are forced to depend on health care over-consumption for survival. Other barriers include perceived class differences between providers and patients, the varying degree of professionalism, and the role of personal relationships that can all affect the feasibility of family medicine.

Consequently, shared decision making about case management, an essential element of patient-centred care, is very difficult to achieve in private for-profit practice and 'internally privatized' government facilities in developing countries. In these situations any attempt to increase efficiency and patient autonomy will be at the expense of profitability.

Community medicine

'Publicly oriented' and for-profit health care organizations are very different in the way they treat the interaction of professionals with the local communities. 'Publicly oriented' delivery adhering to the quality standards enters into a dialogue with local groups and other services in order to solve individual and community health problems. Resolving some patient problems (such as drug abuse, violence, and disease due to poor sanitation) requires the participation of providers in community forums. More basically, health care services cannot be 'publicly oriented' and accountable to their clients where the government is the sole authority and if no weight is given to the voice of the community. These considerations have given rise to the discipline of 'community medicine', which is in fact family medicine revisited. Individual and family health problems are addressed whilst giving due consideration to the collective needs of the community. It is of limited interest to most private doctors because it involves a number of unpaid activities, mostly amongst poor patients, rather than amongst the better off – the core of their clientele in developing countries – and the delivery of 'public goods' cannot be charged to the patients. Moreover, community medicine's aim of empowering the community cuts across the grain of market-based health care delivery. In practice private doctors tend to interact with communities primarily to recruit clients. When private doctors are paid by mutual aid associations, the 'public' or 'private' character of their practice depends to a large extent on whether they are supervised by a health professional concerned with the public interest.

Disease control

See Section 2 and Section 5, Chapter 16.

Service management

'Publicly oriented' management should ensure access to quality health care for a defined population. This implies acting upon the quality of, and access to, care in all accessibility forms: financial, pharmaceutical, geographical, intra-institutional, cultural, and psychological. By contrast market-based management aims at securing access to quality health care only for those who can pay.

Managers of 'publicly oriented' facilities should also adopt a systems management approach, treating health facilities, resources and processes as complementary parts of the same system, in order to ensure flexible resource utilization, achieve economies of scale, and improve access to care (Berman & Rose, 1996). Systems management as applied to the health sector is generally not relevant to market-based management because, in the latter, profitability primarily determines the decisions made and the investment required. Furthermore, in developing countries where the private sector has not achieved the degree of complexity necessary to allow it to share resources across health units, a systems management approach is particularly unsuitable.

These managers should also supervise both health care and disease control; if these activities are separated into distinct service structures, the disease-control objectives tend to overwhelm wider health care goals (see Section 1, Chapter 2).

The objectives of community participation in the provision of health care differ also according to the management rationale. Four different (though not mutually exclusive) objectives could be:

- community participation is considered an appropriate method of resolving health problems identified by governments and aid agencies;
- these problems are defined in dialogue with communities;
- co-management of 'collective' health facilities;
- community organization as a goal per se.

The last three objectives are typical of 'publicly oriented' management. By contrast social control upon private for-profit health facilities may reduce profits made by investors and the income of health professionals, and thus conflicts with the objectives of market-driven management. Under these circumstances, transparency and the democratization of health facilities are simply not relevant.

They are also not relevant or even unwanted for health services charged with delivering disease-control programmes and managed by objectives, ignoring the broader demand for health care.

Health systems

In developing countries, health care delivery is broadly classified into one of three categories with some overlap (Green, 1987). One category is market-based and driven mainly by profitability. The other two share a mission to work in the public interest. 'Official' health services comprise primary facilities and hospitals under the control of the government or municipalities. In contrast community-based health care organizations such as local pre-payment associations, mutual solidarity networks, village and neighbourhood committees, run their own facilities. NGOs are active in both the first and third categories.

Our proposed compact requires that, if any of these sectors receive public funds (including international aid), they should abide by the ethical principles laid out above.

Conclusion

We have proposed ten axioms for the organization of medical practice in 'publicly oriented' health services in developing countries. These could form the basis of a new contract between the public, health professions, health care providers, and the government. Since ancient times medical deontology has set out to inform doctors' freedom of decision making in the interests of the patient. In 'publicly oriented' health care delivery medical practice should also take into account the collective interests of the community alongside the interests of individual patients.

We are aware that only strong motivation – and reasonable income – can drive health professionals to adopt these standards. Improving this motivation by strengthening the social and moral status of health professionals is one of the greatest challenges facing current health policies (Marchal & Kegels, 2003). In our opinion the advantage of employing such criteria for teaching, research, contracting, evaluation, management, and policy design lies precisely in their ability to bridge the gap between the professional and the social-political identity of health professionals. In so doing they make use of the professed ethical motivation of health professionals and politicians which has to date been little explored and therefore, probably, under-estimated.

References

Beauchamp T. L. & Childress J. L. (1994). *Principles of Bio-Ethics*, 4th edn. Oxford: Oxford University Press.

Berman P. & Rose L. (1996). The role of private providers in maternal and child health and family planning services in developing countries. *Health Policy and Planning*, **11**(2), pp. 142–55.

Berwick D., Hiatt H., Janeway P., & Smith R. (1997). An ethical code for everybody in health care. *British Medical Journal*, **315**, pp. 1633–4.

Brody H. (1999). The biopsychosocial model, patient-centered care, and culturally sensitive practice [editorial; comment]. *Journal of Family Practice*, **48**(8), pp. 585–7.

Brown J., Stewart M., McCracken E., McWhinney I. R., & Levenstein J. (1986). The patient-centred clinical method. 2. Definition and application. *Family Practice*, **3**(2), pp. 75–9.

Engel G. L. (1977). The need for a new medical model: A challenge for biomedicine. *Science*, **196**(4286), pp. 129–36.

Giusti D., Criel B., & de Béthune X. (1997). Viewpoint: Public versus private health care delivery: Beyond the slogans. *Health Policy and Planning*, **12**(3), pp. 192–8.

Green A. (1987). The role of non-governmental organisations and the private sector in the provision of health care in developing countries. *International Journal of Health Planning and Management*, **2**, pp. 37–58.

Groupe d'Etude pour une Réforme de la Médecine (G.E.R.M.). (1971). *Les lignes de force d'une politique de santé*. In: *Pour Une Politique De La Santé*. Bruxelles: La Revue Nouvelle, pp. 9–17.

Havighurst C. C. (1977). Controlling health care costs: Strengthening the private sector's hand. Journal of Health Politics, *Policy and Law*, **1**(4), pp. 471–98.

Kunneman H. (1995). De huisarts als normatieve professional. Dilemma's in een postmoderne wereld. In: Bakker R., et al., eds. *De Huisarts in 2010: Perspectieven Voor Medische Zorg*. Utrecht, The Netherlands: De Tijdstroom, pp. 147–61.

Marchal B. & Kegels G.(2003). Health workforce imbalances in times of globalisation: From brain drain to professional mobility. *International Journal of Health Planning and Management*, **18**, pp. S89–S101.

Mercenier P.(1971). Les objectifs de l'organisation médico-sanitaire. In: *Groupe d'Etude pour une Réforme de la Médecine (G.E.R.M.): Pour Une Politique De La Santé*. Bruxelles: La Revue Nouvelle, pp. 67–72.

Silverman E. M., Skinner J. S., & Fisher E. S. (1999). The association between for-profit hospital ownership and increased Medicare spending [see comments]. *New England Journal of Medicine*, **341**(6), pp. 420–6.

Smith R., Hiatt H., & Berwick D.(1999). A shared statement of ethical principles for those who shape and give health care. A working draft from The Tavistock Group. *Journal of Nursing Administration*, **29**(6), pp. 5–8.

Van Dormael M.(1995). Médecine générale et modernité. Regards croisés sur l'occident et le tiers monde. Thèse de doctorat en sciences sociales, Université Libre de Bruxelles.

Woolhandler S. & Himmelstein D. U.(1999). When money is the mission: The high costs of investor-owned care. *New England Journal of Medicine*, **341**(6), pp. 444–6.

World Health Organization. (1978). Declaration of Alma-Ata. In: *Report of the International Conference on Primary Health Care, Alma Ata, USSR, 6–12 September 1978.* Geneva: World Health Organization, pp. 2–6.

Principles of publicly oriented health planning

Adapted from: Unger J.-P., Criel B. Principles of health infrastructure planning in less developed countries. Int J Health Plan Manag 1995; 10: 113–128.

The following planning principles are designed for decision makers at central level but also for those responsible for local health systems and health districts. These principles organize the functions and relationships of health systems components (first-line health services, hospitals, and programmes). This relatively old paper has been inserted in this book because we feel the principles it offers are still relevant for strengthening health systems. The principles were formulated to make the most efficient and effective use of health care facilities and resources. They contribute to updating the concept of PHC, which re-emerged in the international policy agenda in 2006 (when the Director of the Pan American Health Organization [PAHO] took the initiative to revive this strategy) (Macinko et al., 2007).

Introduction

The highly varied efficiency in health systems and the international financial crisis may oblige MoHs to rationalize their structures of health care provision and to focus on the allocation of scarce resources to the most efficient types of facilities in their respective health systems. The aim of this chapter is to assess some of the principles for the identification of these entities, the definition of their functions and their relationships to the other elements (such as disease-specific organizations, social services and academic institutions) in the health system. We also hope to support the identification of the resources needed and the means of interaction of the health structures with the communities they serve.

Key principles

An integrated health system

Several health systems (public as in Spain and non-profit private as in the Kaiser Permanente) are featured with some or all of the following characteristics of an integrated health system. They are amongst the best performers in their category in delivering CHC even though their public and private status would have an impact on access. The reader will judge the extent to which one explains the other while getting acquainted with the rationale of integrated systems, a concept derived from managerial experience with polyvalent health care delivery.

This principle of an integrated health system argues the need for a specificity of, and a complementarity between, the various tiers in the health system.

Not all facilities are equally fit to provide a given service. This is a quite straightforward statement that seems obvious at first glance. Yet, notwithstanding its common sense, it often lacks operationalization in health planning terms. The arguments underlying this statement are two-fold: there is an economic rationale on the one hand, and a functional or technical one on the other. Nobody questions the relevance of having hospitals host and centralize technology and expertise. There is far less consensus, however, when the question arises whether hospitals are to deliver first-line health care, that is to say the care tradition-ally delivered by polyvalent health workers (such as a general practitioner). The assumption that hospitals should do so is often an implicit one. Indeed many authors describe 'primary programmes' delivered by hospitals (Chiphangwi, 1987; De Boer & McNiel, 1989). In the case of Zimbabwe, for instance, it is illustrative that the facilities in the vast majority of the districts are either 'rural health centres' or 'district hospitals.' For the urban or semi-urban population living around the location of the hospital, it is taken for granted that the hospital is the place to provide primary care to its surrounding communities. The implicit assumption is that a health centre is a valid option for the delivery of primary care to rural communities; but not so for urban communities where the district hospitals' outpatients departments will take up that role. Furthermore neoliberal health policies often granted financial and managerial autonomy to hospitals (the 'management-property split') without securing any regulatory and control environment. The importance of the professionals' and health workers' income was linked to the hospital benefits (for instance, bonuses in China). Autonomously managed government hospitals in low-income settings thus tend to admit a middle-class child with diarrhoea rather than a township woman in need of a caesarean section, in order to keep costs down.

We challenge these beliefs and practices on the grounds of the following arguments.

Identical health care becomes increasingly expensive when it is delivered by 'higher' levels in the health care system (Van Lerberghe & Lafort, 1990). There must, therefore, be one type of facility that is more efficient and more effective than others when it comes to solve a given health problem. We think that a hospital is not fit to provide first-line health care. Indeed:

- it is too big a structure for staff and community members to know each other and as a result comprehensive and continuous care are jeopardized from the start – for instance, the population served by hospitals is so large that home visits meant to ensure continu-ity of care are impracticable;
- integrated care (in particular family medicine) is hampered by the division of labour inherent to large entities;
- the technical and organizational complexity of hospital operations is hardly compatible with a process of participatory management;
- a high number of primary cases presenting at hospital level results in under-utilization of the qualifications of its staff. Furthermore, involvement of the hospital into primary care fosters the perception in the community that a health centre really is only the 'second best' solution.

The role of first-line health services is to deliver care that is comprehensive, holistic, con-tinuous and integrated (Groupe d'Etude pour une Réforme de la Médecine [G.E.R.M.], 1971), a principle that was implemented in the Kasongo project (Kasongo Project Team, 1981). Many of the factors conditioning comprehensiveness, continuity, and integration of care can only be met by a health facility responding to the following characteristics: a mod-estly sized building with not too big a staff, a relatively small population to care for, and a close relationship between staff and people.

A sick person is more than a sick deficient liver or a weak heart; he or she is also anxious about what the future may bring. A child with measles is more than merely the victim of a virus; he or she may also become malnourished. A woman with a tenth child may be very eager not to have future pregnancies, but she does not dare to express it, under her circumstances. The process of decreasing the suffering (present or potential) is greatly enhanced when the intervention proposed by the health worker takes into consideration the multiple dimensions of the health problem (that is to say by including elements apart from the purely biological one). Because of this complexity, the management of a patient must be a holistic one (Armstrong, 1979) if it is to be effective.

Care leading to a useful end is called continuous. It should not be limited to the issuing of a prescription. For instance, if a patient has no money, then he will not purchase the drugs. Similarly, a patient with tuberculosis, in the absence of conditions that would motivate him to complete his treatment, is likely to stop his treatment as soon as he feels better. If care is to be continuous, then it should be holistic. A holistic approach also implies that the health worker can offer the most appropriate type of care for the problem the patient presents at a given time and in a given context; curative or preventive or promotional care, or a combination of them. It is, other things remaining equal, easier to offer such integrated care if curative and preventive cares are being coordinated within one single, small unit.

Much has been written about the value of community care in improving the quality of care. It is likely to succeed only if a number of structural and organizational changes are met: for instance, the existence of real dialogue between health service and community; the organization of defaulter tracing with the possibility of carrying out home visits, and the implementation of a continuity 'friendly' fee system (Criel & Van Balen, 1993). Integration of care, in itself a condition for having holistic care, implies a good knowledge of the patient and of his social environment and an appropriate individual information system The point is that holistic, integrated, and continuous care can only be delivered under certain structural and organizational conditions; factories such as hospitals do not fit these conditions and are therefore the wrong structures to deliver that kind of care.

These arguments, together with the trade-off between the need to centralize technology on the one hand, and the need for health facilities to be readily accessible, strengthen the idea that each level within the health pyramid should provide a given type of care. Each level should provide those services for which it is most fit, without at the same time offering services for which another level is most appropriate. Therefore, an overlap of activities should be avoided. An occasional diversity of functions can be accepted if, for instance, a multiplication of urban hospital facilities is to be avoided.

While nobody denies the usefulness of a consistent health care pyramid, the principle of the specificity of each level of care is described only exceptionally.

Since the levels of health care services must be specific and since it is desirable that people are treated as close as possible to their domicile, the links between the different health care levels must be defined unequivocally, corresponding to the definition of an integrated system. In practice a health system should meet the following five criteria:

- The system should contain no functional gaps: most of the situations must be covered in such a way that the vast majority of the health problems encountered can find an appropriate solution somewhere within the existing health pyramid. The overall effectiveness of the system can thus be ensured. The definition of health system functions should be based, as a priority, on the intersection of community population demand (curative care being the most common one) and needs (as defined by professionals).

- The system should avoid any functional overlapping among its different levels (principle of specificity), with a few exceptions, such as the function of a district hospital being fulfilled by higher level hospitals (for example, provincial or regional hospital).
- The patients should be taken care of at the level that is best able to manage their problems. An organizational consequence is that barriers (financial, intra-institutional, psychological, geographical and other obstacles) hindering the flow of referred patients within the system should be avoided as much as possible. The first level of care should be the entry gate into the system. Indeed the likelihood that health problems will be solved under level 1 infrastructures' jurisdiction is very high (90–95%). The problem will not only be solved in a more efficient way, but also in a more effective way. A WB study, carried out 23 years ago, expressed the importance of health posts as follows: 'But even in their present, imperfect state, health post programmes are quite possibly competitive with the other available modes of service delivery when compared with them in cost-effectiveness terms' (Gwatkin et al., 1986). Other studies have yielded similar conclusions (Adekolu-John, 1979; Van Lerberghe & Pangu, 1988). Because of the principle of specificity, barriers to a direct access to second-line professionals (such as through higher fees, system of appointments) should be used as incentives for appropriate channelling of patients in the system. Great Britain and The Netherlands do apply this principle.
- Finally, the relevant information on the patient's problem should accompany the patient as he or she travels between the different levels in the system.
- Medical techniques should be allocated to different health system tiers according to their ever changing capacity.

Minimal Activities Package

This concept has had a meteoric rise in LMICs since the 1993 WB report 'Investing in Health' promoted it. It described the prioritized activities of public services concentrating on highly efficient disease-control activities. In this sense it would have been more appropriate to label it the 'maximal package of activities' gathering the only activities to be financed by (inter)national solidarity and the only ones tolerated in public services under the GATS (see Conclusions).

What would then be the basis for a genuine 'minimal (not maximal) package of activity'? If each level's functions must be specific and its structures identical, then it is possible to describe a set of minimum activities common to all structures of a given level – such as the Minimum Activities Package (MAP). The MAP of a level is the standard medical output common to all structures bearing the same name in a given country. The definition of the MAP is important for planning purposes; more specifically for a rational resource allocation minimizing opportunity costs. This implies that an efficient set of activities needs to be defined, matching the technologies and skills of each tier.

The WB has adopted the concept of 'essential clinical package': 'the most important factors in selecting the essential package should be the relative cost-effectiveness of interventions, the size and distribution of the health problems affecting the population and the resources available' (World Bank, 1993). This rationale – cost-effectiveness – partly conflicts with another approach which consists of planning of the health services' package starting from the bulk of the intersection between the community's demands, on the one hand, and the needs defined by professionals on the other.

In fact, the two methods end up proposing a different array of activities (narrow versus broad package of activity), the former ruling out the possibility of delivering polyvalent curative care in public services. From this point of view, the public services of northern European health systems contrast strikingly with the US medical services. In Great Britain, for instance, Morrell (1989) has proposed curative outpatient care; care and follow-up of chronic patients; preventive care; the organization of an information system; antenatal consultations; under-five clinics; care for the elderly and vaccination and screening activities (Morrell, 1989). Today in the vast majority of LICs, polyvalent curative medicine is delivered in 'upper' tiers as if the health centres were not able to do so.

A broader scope of activities, including general practice curative care, has been advocated for first-line health services on the grounds of arguments developed in Section 5, Chapter 12.

The definition of the MAP of the peripheral units is also shaped on practical experiences, thus in a dynamic perspective. The MAP is a sum of activities that, once implemented in a given health centre, enables new interventions to be integrated without deeply modifying the organization or the cost of the structure. For instance, if a health centre is capable to provide continuous care for tuberculosis patients, it can also carry out the follow-up of AIDS and leprosy without major changes.

MAPs are fairly homogeneous. In Africa for instance, in theory, the health centre MAP should include curative care; under-five clinics; antenatal care; care and follow-up of chronic patients; nutritional rehabilitation; disease-control interventions, and family planning services. In practice, however, DSPs often exclude polyvalent curative care from the array of health centre activities. The MAP of a district hospital should include inpatient facilities with nursing expertise; a referral consultation; appropriate care for common medical and surgical emergencies (such as caesarean section, strangulated hernia, extra-uterine pregnancy, appendectomy); maternity cases where complicated deliveries can be dealt with, and laboratory and X-ray facilities. It is a 'minimal' package of activities in the sense that it can be expanded. Two mechanisms should found such an expansion:

- the identification of local epidemiological priorities (trypanosomiasis and leprosy may not be distributed evenly in all health centres of a district and possibly be totally absent in some);
- the community will to expand some activities (for example, to purchase a larger array of pain killers and to finance emergency referrals to the hospital).

Territorial responsibility and a discriminative responsibility for populations

The population for which a given facility is responsible must be clearly and explicitly defined. In addition tools should be designed so as to allow health centre staff to identify patients as being a member (or not) of that population. The following arguments support this position:

- a more equitable distribution of care is possible;
- an optimal ratio of population size per facility can be ensured;
- an explicit responsibility for the health care of a population can only be effective when it is clear for whom the staff are responsible; and,
- in addition to the argument of effectiveness, efficiency is important: a scatter of scarce resources over too large a population should be avoided; users must be brought to prefer to use 'their' facilities over any other.

These facilities must have a territorial responsibility, or a population defined on the grounds of free affiliation or subscription up to a maximum figure (as in the UK or in

The Netherlands) (Ministry of Welfare, 1992). In the developing world, though, territorial responsibility is easier to implement due to transportation difficulties. The health centre will offer the entire gamut of minimal package activities to this well-defined population. This population will be the health services' interlocutor and partner in a continuous process of dialogue: the health committee's 'constituency' is thus defined. A clear identification of the population for which the health centre takes an explicit responsibility allows for an evaluation of the services delivered (knowledge of a denominator). Finally, a geographic responsibility will allow organized communities to co-manage publicly oriented health facilities.

It is clear that it is simply not possible for a health centre to commit itself to deliver continuous, comprehensive, and integrated care to people not belonging to that well-defined population.

A population base

Simulations may be used to calculate the increase in fixed costs when the number of facilities on a given level is increased. The population base per facility should be neither too small nor too large. If it is too small, it will be incompatible with the country's resources. It will also threaten the technical quality of the care delivered. Figures of one health centre per 10,000 inhabitants and one district hospital per 150,000 to 300,000 inhabitants are advisable for countries with very limited resources (manpower, equipment, financial resources). Assessments of the workload and the fixed costs of health centres and hospitals support that planning basis. For instance, each year an urban health centre covering 10,000 people should be able to deliver approximately 12,000 curative consultations (30/day); 900 antenatal consultations (18/week), and full immunizations and under-five clinics for 400 children.

Integrating NGOs into the system

An integration of NGO hospitals in national planning has considerable advantages: it allows governments to save on investment and operating costs, and it links highly committed and skilled people in a national endeavour. The integration of NGOs should, however, be conditioned by the NGOs' agreement to accept overall and explicit responsibility for a well-defined population and to operate within a system perspective; this may go against the ideal of a charitable approach to health care where a spontaneous reaction to human suffering overwhelms rational planning and action, and it may antagonize proselytic missions given to denominational health facilities. To integrate NGO hospitals in a national coverage map assumes appropriate financing and (management and production) contracts (see Criteria in Section 5, Chapter 14). Finally, as a reminder, the best staff (if available) of an NGO could possibly strengthen the functioning of district executive teams (Section 5, Chapter 13), alongside others belonging to other not-for-profit organizations. This would be best done under the direction of a (MoH) district medical officer, because the ultimate responsibility for the health system (its 'stewardship') should lie with the state.

Health care strategies

Reshuffling the PHC strategy

The Alma Ata Conference of 1978 defined the PHC strategy by generous principles such as reliance on community participation, decentralization of services, harmony between the health services' characteristics and the country's resources, importance of cultural aspects, search for equity, and integration of vertical programmes (World Health Organization, 1978). On the basis of the principles we have outlined, it is possible to specify the interpretation of this concept as a strategy involving the reorientation of the entire health pyramid. Its main elements are:

- PHC implies the development of first-line health services (e.g., dispensaries, health posts or health centres) so as to make them accessible and functional through an improvement of curative care and by adding preventive activities to build the MAP. Later, health promotion activities can be added according to local possibilities and needs. PHC should not be reduced to social marketing, nor reduced to merely the delivery of disease-control interventions as suggested by Walsh and Warren as early as 1979 (Walsh & Warren, 1979). Neither does PHC mean the deployment of village health workers, since they are unable to deliver care that would complement the existing skills and expertise of communities themselves.

- Village health workers, however, can contribute to improving the action of first-line health services in remote or very scattered populations. Village health workers are to be seen as a specific solution for a specific, situational problem, but not more than that. PHC therefore should neither be confused with the mere implementation of disease-specific programmes nor with an isolated health promotion initiative such as construction of latrines. The principle of specificity is usually overlooked and planners often do not plan for urban health centres claiming that their function could be taken over by the existing hospitals. In Africa this leads to very poor urban first-line coverage. Another common mistake is the development of vast first-line infrastructures (clinics) in urban settings, justified by the huge size of the population covered. There are two alternative options:

    - to increase the number of units while reducing dramatically their size and population; as argued above, this would definitely benefit the quality of care provided;
    - to nest mini-health centres in a large (urban) structure, each of them operating with their own staff and defined population (like in Costa Rica).

- The second element of this strategy lies in the reorientation of hospital functions. The operations of hospitals should be redirected to complement that which is being undertaken in the health centres (according to the principle of the specificity of each level). These structures should increase their technology progressively to solve more problems of referred patients, and at the same time reduce their first-line activities. Hence, the PHC strategy does not mean a denial of technology; rather, this technology should be provided to the appropriate structure within the health system. Nor should PHC be an exclusive choice between dispensaries and hospitals. On the contrary, the strategy implies a complementarity between hospitals and dispensaries. Furthermore, hospitals should support lower tiers with in-service training activities and short-term rotations (to optimize knowledge transfer within health systems), with evaluation, rationalization, and adaptation of clinical guidelines. They should make accessible (part of) their laboratory and imaging activities to patients sent by first-line care providers.

- The third element is participation. The health centre really is the most appropriate level for community participation to take place. Indeed the technical dimension of decisions made in a hospital inevitably transforms participation into community manipulation.

Participation is a means to allow the population's demands (and not only professionally defined needs) to be taken into account. Participation can only take place if a process of continuous dialogue between health services and the community exists, and if there is some co-management of health infrastructures. The existence of such a dialogue is obviously dependent on the extent to which the services provided are accepted by the people – the extent to which they respond to the people's demands. Only then may a participatory management of resources, a planning of activities fitting people's preferences, a development of self-sufficiency, and autonomy become possible.

District health systems

The provision of PHC has stumbled against the lack of good resource management and knowledge of the particularities of the terrain. This has led to the conclusion that decision making should be decentralized (Vaughan et al., 1984). For several years, the WHO has advocated a pivotal role for the district in service management and planning (Pan American Health Organization, 1988; World Health Organization, 1987).

In fact, the district concept derives from two rationales: on the one hand, the implementation of PHC strategy, requesting a decentralized management; and, on the other hand, the organization of integrated systems, which implies that one single team manages, simultaneously, the district hospital and the network of dispensaries. At the district level the operational pyramid should closely overlap the administrative one so as to enable professionals to identify deficiencies in health structures and to correct them through managerial changes.

In a broader sense, this managerial change requires one to centralize and decentralize techniques from health centres to hospital and vice-versa along the lines of continuous evaluation and resource fluctuation; and carry out activities on an integrated basis or a non-integrated basis, by health centres and mobile teams, respectively, according to evaluation and political pressures. There is thus a very strong case for considering the hospital as an element à part entière of the district: district management also means district hospital management. Figure 15.1 summarizes the activities of a district.

This scheme allows us to visualize:

- the responsibility of the district and its health centres for a geographically well-defined population;
- the delivery of a set of activities to be implemented in each dispensary (the MAP);
- the logistical and organizational functions that allow each unit to deliver these activities;
- the hierarchical relationships;
- the patient flow in the system (referral and counter-referral).

This scheme does not show, however, some of the functions the district hospital fulfils: indeed, very often the hospital is the place where medical assistants and students are trained, where first-line services are evaluated, where standardized clinical pathways are designed, and where epidemiological surveillance is centralized. In addition it is often the venue where district decision makers meet.

A district may also have a mobile team to deliver vertical disease-control activities (see Section 2, Chapter 4), for emergency interventions (such as outbreaks of disease), and for preventive activities targeting communities living too far from a health centre.

District executive team	District hospital
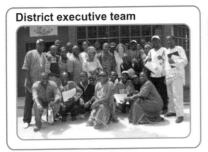	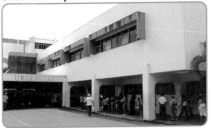

District mobile team	1. Admissions and outpatient consultations (internal medicine, paediatrics, obstetrics / gynaecology, surgery, ICU)
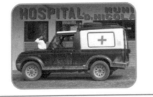	2. Capacity to handle emergencies in medicine and surgery
	3. Advanced diagnostics (laboratory, X-ray, ultrasound)
	4. Logistics

Solves ± 5% of health problems

Health centre 1	Health centre 2	Health centre 3
	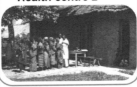	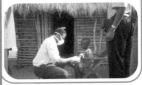
Health centre logistics	**Health centre logistics**	**Health centre logistics**
Drugs	Drugs	Drugs
Know how	Know how	Know how
Manpower	Manpower	Manpower
Finances	Finances	Finances
Operational activities	**Operational activities**	**Operational activities**
Health promotion	Health promotion	Health promotion
Participation	Participation	Participation
Family planning	Family planning	Family planning
Nutritional rehabilitation	Nutritional rehabilitation	Nutritional rehabilitation
Care for chronic patients	Care for chronic patients	Care for chronic patients
Under-5 medicine	Under-5 medicine	Under-5 medicine
Antenatal care	Antenatal care	Antenatal care
Curative care	Curative care	Curative care

Solves ± 90% of health problems

Target populations defined by a coverage map

Figure 15.1. The activities of a district. ICU, intensive care unit.

The size of most districts in sub-Saharan Africa could vary between approximately 150,000 and 300,000 inhabitants and count from 10 to 30 health centres. If the resources available increase, it may be justified to pool them at a smaller scale: districts could then progressively become smaller without going below a threshold where technical quality of care becomes endangered.

In conclusion, the 'reference system,' described as early as 1966 by Jolly and King, as a group of dispensaries and a reference hospital, corresponds to the district (Jolly & King, 1966). However, if the whole is to function in an integrated way, then it is crucial that this group of structures is managed as a system. A team of health professionals, gathering both 'hospital' and 'district' staff, has a key role to play in that process. A consistent district management team is not only a more effective and efficient management body than an isolated district medical officer, it is also a more appealing and challenging way of working for local health professionals. The supervision of health centres should be undertaken across organizations, horizontally rather than vertically, so that it increases learning and cooperation across health centres and permits a better understanding of public purpose.

References

Adekolu-John E. O. (1979). The role of dispensaries in community health care in the Kainji Lake area of Nigeria. *Journal of Epidemiology and Community Health*, **33**(2), pp. 145–9.

Armstrong D. (1979). The emancipation of biographical medicine. *Social Science & Medicine*, 13A(1), pp. 1–8.

Chiphangwi J. (1987). Antenatal care in a district hospital. *Tropical Doctor*, **17**(3), pp. 124–7.

Criel B. & Van Balen H. (1993). Paying for the Kasongo hospital in Zaire: A conceptual framework. *Health Policy and Planning*, **8**(1), pp. 61–71.

De Boer C. N. & McNiel M. (1989). Hospital outreach community-based health care: The case of Chogoria, Kenya. *Social Science & Medicine*, **28**(10), pp. 1007–17.

Groupe d'Etude pour une Réforme de la Médecine (G.E.R.M.). (1971). *Pour une politique de la santé*. Bruxelles: La Revue Nouvelle, Numéro spécial 1971 p. 10.

Gwatkin D. R., Berman P., & Burger S. E. (1986). Health posts: Are they contributing to better health? *PHN Technical Note*, **86**(4).

Jolly R. & King M. (1966). *The Organisation of Health Services*. In: King M., ed. *Medical Care in Developing Countries*. Nairobi: Oxford University Press.

Kasongo Project Team. (1981). Le Projet Kasongo; une expérience d'organisation d'un soins de santé primaires. *Annales de la Société Belge de Médecine Tropicale*, **60**(S1), pp. 1–54.

Macinko J., Montenegro H., & Nebot C. (2007). *Renewing Primary Health Care in the Americas: A Position Paper of the Pan American Health Organization/World Health Organization (PAHO/WHO). 2007*. Washington, DC: Pan American Health Organization/World Health Organization (PAHO/WHO).

Ministry of Welfare, Health and Cultural Affairs, The Netherlands. (1992). Choices in health care. A review of a report by the government committee in health care. *Journal of the Royal College of Physicians of London*, **26**(4), pp. 390–2.

Morrell D. (1989). The new general practitioner contract: Is there an alternative. *British Medical Journal*, **298**(6679), pp. 1005–7.

Pan American Health Organization. (1988). *Development and Fortification of Health Local System in National System Transformation*. Washington, DC: Pan American Health Organization. CD33/14.

Van Lerberghe W. & Lafort Y. (1990). *The Role of the Hospital in the District: Delivering or Supporting Primary Health Care?* Geneva: World Health Organization. WHO/SHS/CC/90.2.

Van Lerberghe W. & Pangu K. A. (1988). Comprehensive can be effective: The influence of coverage with a health centre network on the hospitalisation patterns in the rural area of Kasongo, Zaire. *Social Science & Medicine*, **26**(9), pp. 949–55.

Vaughan P., Mills A., & Smith D. (1984). The importance of decentralised management. *World Health Forum*, **5**(1), pp. 27–9.

Walsh J. A. & Warren K. S. (1979). Selective primary health care: An interim strategy for disease control in developing countries. *New England Journal of Medicine*, **301**(18), pp. 967–74.

World Bank. (1993). *World Development Report 1993: Investing in Health*. Oxford: Oxford University Press.

World Health Organization. (1978). Declaration of Alma-Ata. In: *Report of the International Conference on Primary Health Care, Alma Ata, USSR, 6–12 September 1978*. Geneva: World Health Organization, pp. 2–6.

World Health Organization. (1987). *Report of the Interregional Meeting on Strengthening District Health Systems Based on Primary Health Care, Harare, Zimbabwe, 3 to 7 August 1987*. Geneva: World Health Organization. WHO/SHS/DHS/87.13, Rev.1.

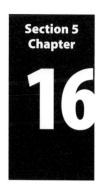

Section 5
Chapter

16

Principles for alternative, publicly oriented health care policies, planning, management and delivery

A code of good practice for the management of disease-control programmes

This chapter is extracted from:

Unger J.-P., De Paepe P., Green A. A code of best practice for disease control programmes to avoid damaging health care services in developing countries. Int J Health Planning and Management 2003; 18: S27-S39.

Continuing with some of the essential tenets in the management and delivery of health care, we suggest some principles, designed to avoid aspects of disease-control programmes. These have caused much consternation and challenge for both health practitioners and policy makers, facing different pressures, from donors and the public.

From our own research over the past three decades, we are able to tentatively propose four essential principles that might help avoid disease-specific programmes putting unnecessary pressure on quality health care systems. Through this we also suggest means to improve access to CHC in LMICs.

Disease-control activities should generally be integrated, with the exception of certain well-defined situations. They should be integrated in health centres, which offer patient-centred care

As discussed above, justification for this requirement is two-fold. The early detection of chronic diseases (such as tuberculosis and AIDS) and of acute conditions (such as severe malaria, childhood acute respiratory infections, diarrhoeal diseases) is hindered by low primary care utilization rates. In practice patient loyalty can only be created by good quality primary care. In addition improved doctor/patient communication should result in enhanced continuity of care and better cure rates. Still, there are exceptions for which a vertical organization is still appropriate (see above).

Disease-control programmes should be integrated in not-for-profit health facilities

The arguments for this are three-fold:

- Access to privately delivered health care financed by user charges in LICs is severely restricted (Ensor, 1997; McPake, 1997; Mouyokani et al., 1999).
- Attempts to modify behaviour in private practice to comply with national guidelines have faltered in developing countries (Hong et al., 1993). Private practitioners are frequently reluctant to implement national health policy guidelines (Lönnroth et al., 1999) or to refer their patients to public facilities when they encounter serious public health problems (Figueras & Saltman, 1998).

- The capacity of health authorities to regulate and control private health facilities is the cornerstone of disease-control integration in the private sector. It is doubtful whether health authorities in developing countries have the skills and resources to do this effectively; they already struggle to exert stewardship and control in the public sector. Figueras and Saltman acknowledge that the success of reform strategies in Europe required 'the availability of public health skills to assess health needs, evaluate interventions and monitor outcome' (Figueras & Saltman, 1998). The management skills and resources required for contracting out disease-control programmes seem well beyond the capacity of most developing countries, including those of middle income.

Disease-control programmes should plan to avoid conflict with health care delivery

Programme managers should prepare, in advance, a protocol for damage control, specifying how the programme will integrate 'on the ground,' how it will improve access to health care in host facilities, and how it will leave health facilities strengthened.

To protect the balance of health care functions (the 'minimum package of activities' that PHC centres in the developing world are expected to provide) from disruption or interference due to the integration of disease-control programmes, this protocol should:

- not only foresee the provision of adequate resources to health facilities in order to host programme activities, but compensate for the extra burden programmes place on them – which implies transparency in use of programme resources;
- plan a realistic timetable for results, compatible with PHC priorities. This may involve slower build-up of coverage to ensure disease-control sustainability. Bearing in mind the principle of diminishing returns, disease eradication programmes should be embarked upon with extreme caution;
- accept a degree of flexibility in the use of programme investments and permit the diversion of resources from a programme to, for instance, general functional improvements in PHC. One example may be that of microscopes, supplied as part of a tuberculosis control programme, which may be used to detect urinary tract infections. Similarly, for ethical reasons, drugs supplied as part of a particular programme should not be denied to any needy patient on the grounds that their condition is outside the programme's remit;
- develop the interface between health care professionals and the specific category of users targeted by the programme. For example, micro-nutrient delivery requires high coverage rates of under-five clinics; reduction in AIDS vertical transmission requires antenatal care and utilized maternity services; and the early detection of tuberculosis requires outpatient clinics with acceptable utilization rates.

Regarding human resources: 'Programmes often rely on the continued provision of incentives to attract and retain high-calibre staff to ensure that key activities are carried out.' We suggest that the best staff available locally should not be 'acquired' by the programme sponsors. Instead consideration should be given to recruiting experienced staff and offering them posts in district health management teams, with a joint responsibility to improve health care services, whilst implementing disease-control programmes.

The administration of disease-control programmes should be designed and operated to strengthen health systems

We have already suggested why indirect programmes with their lines of command going down to the health care units should be avoided, and why administrative integration should go together with operational integration (Figure 16.1).

Though naturally discussed with disease-control specialists at every stage, decisions on the integration of disease-control activities should be left to polyvalent health service managers, such as those of district management teams whose activities are not limited to the control of one or a few diseases.

The task of programme officers is to bring technical assistance to health professionals. This support should be delivered through health care middle management. Their duties also encompass operational research on the implementation of the disease-control programme. Programme officers who do not have the capacity to perform these tasks are not suited to the job. The lack of skilled personnel in developing countries is particularly acute at the peripheral level. This is why district bureaucracies should, in many instances, be able to re-deploy middle managers who are health professionals and return them to clinical responsibilities. They might be advantageously replaced with regional or national programme officers covering large territories and acting as advisors to district medical officers.

Vertical and indirect programmes do not mix well with plans to decentralize power to districts. When health centres consist mainly of a collection of vertical programmes, scope for local decision making is very limited and strategic decisions may remain with central government. Operational integration should always go together with administrative integration and

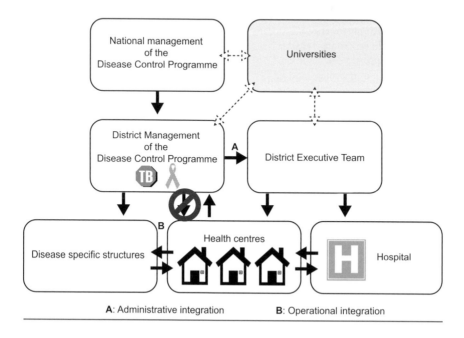

A: Administrative integration   B: Operational integration

Figure 16.1. Administrative and operational integrations. Desirable health systems relationships in case of operational and administrative integration. TB, tuberculosis.

thus complement the decentralization process. Greater autonomy should be granted to health service middle managers, because integrating disease-control programmes with health services requires continual mutual adjustments among highly skilled personnel. Administrative decentralization is also desirable because of geographical and socio-cultural heterogeneity within a country – for example, access to health care and user participation demands autonomy and decision making capacity at the periphery.

Local universities could be invited to participate in programme design, training and evaluation. By acting in partnerships like these, programme sponsors can facilitate the transfer of expertise and technology.

Finally, programme management control systems should be simplified, in order to avoid an unnecessary bureaucratic burden on health professionals.

Conclusion

As a conclusion for this section, there is a need to acknowledge the inevitable tensions in applying (health care delivery, managerial, planning and policy) principles belonging to a set. No such ensemble can per se determine the physiognomy of health systems. While some tensions between different principles were explored in this section, many will in the first instance require knowledge, experience, and the creativity of individual professionals. It will also need political decisions to be made about the principles and the value of health care by communities, regions and states. In our view there is no more important a stake in social existence, than health care policy that can have such a major impact on the individual and on households.

References

Ensor T. (1997). What role for state health care in Asian transition economies? *Health Economics*, 6(5), pp. 445–54.

Figueras J. & Saltman R. B. (1998). Building upon comparative experience in health system reform. *European Journal of Public Health*, 8, pp. 99–101.

Hong Y. P., Kim S. J., Lee E. G., Lew W. J., & Bai J. Y. (1993). Treatment of bacillary pulmonary tuberculosis at the chest clinics in the private sector in Korea. *International Journal of Tuberculosis and Lung Disease*, 3(8), pp. 695–702.

Lönnroth K., Thuong L. M., Linh P. D., & Diwan V. K. (1999). Delay and discontinuity – a survey of TB patients' search of a diagnosis in a diversified health care system. *International Journal of Tuberculosis and Lung Disease*, 3(11), pp. 992–1000.

McPake B. (1997). The role of the private sector in health service provision. In: Bennet S., et al., eds. *Private Health Providers in Developing Countries: Serving the Public Interest?* New York: St. Martin's Press

Mouyokani J., Tursz A., Crost M., Cook J., & Nzingoula S. (1999). An epidemiological study of consultations of children under 5 years of age in Brazzaville (Congo). *Revue d'Épidémiologie et de Santé Publique*, 47(Supplement 2:2), pp. 115–31.

A public health, strategic toolkit to implement these alternatives

Introduction to Section 6

Two policies conflict over the semantics of 'access.' For international aid agencies and Global Health Initiatives, access means 'people's use of disease-specific interventions' (Gwatkin et al., 2005), but for NGOs and government services acting as 'outlets' (Mills & Hanson, 2003) access refers to compliance in disease-control programme interventions (Hardon et al., 2009; Kumaresan et al., 2001; WHO Department of Reproductive Health and Research & United Nations Population Fund, 2003). As in the current chapter some academic institutions (Geneva University Hospitals, 2006; Olivier de Sardan & Jaffré, 2003) and NGOs (Marriott, 2009) have emphasized access to CHC (family and hospital medicine) as the core of the meaning of access.

In parallel with the principles highlighted in the previous section, strategies to improve access to good quality, comprehensive care in participatory, publicly oriented services are presented in this section. Although these strategies might appear somewhat prescriptive, they are in fact derived from professional experience that needs to be adapted in different contexts.

There is a combination of reflection and empirical evidence in this section. The first chapter advocates patient-centred care for general practitioners in LMICs where often there is no such tradition. The second chapter (Parts 1 and 2) reports field experiences in improving access to general practice in public services (in Ecuador, Chapter 18, Part 1), and access to drugs (in Senegal, Chapter 18, Part 2). We have also considered the thorny issue of the purchase of medicines by users of health services. This is a contested issue that has created polarization between donors and public health activists and between the public and their governments. But it needs to be addressed, since it is an important element of effective public provision.

We are fully aware that under-resourcing is a major issue (tax-based and/or social insurance) and would propose that in the absence of, or the limited availability of, national funds the possibility of supplementation by international sources will need to be considered. These would not go to disease-specific programmes, to date much favoured by donors, but to provide new forms of supply-side financing for MoHs and their facilities, alongside existing contracted not-for-profit facilities.

Additional national resources and the re-direction of current international funds would be a significant factor for securing universal access to CHC. These call for networking and lobbying in (inter)national arenas with support from civil society organizations (social and political) to support the case for CHC.

Chapter 19 examines if, and to what extent, managed care techniques used to improve efficiency in the commercial environment are specific to this setting or not. It then scrutinizes the alternative techniques available to improve the quality of health care in publicly oriented services. In its second part, it elaborates one such reflexive technique – The interface flow process audit. Finally, Chapter 20 discusses how public health courses can contribute to universal access to CHC and how public health academic entities can acquire the related expertise and knowledge.

References

Geneva University Hospitals. (2006). *Geneva Forum: Towards Global Access to Health. Programme and abstract book.* Geneva: Geneva University Hospitals.

Gwatkin D. R., Wagstaff A., & Yazbeck A. S. (2005). *Reaching the Poor With Health, Nutrition, and Population Services. What Works, What Doesn't, and Why.* Washington DC: The World Bank. RA418.5.P6R43.

Hardon A., Davey S., Gerrits T., & Hodgkin C. (2009). *From Access to Adherence: The Challenges of Antiretroviral Treatment.* Geneva: World Health Organization.

Kumaresan J., Bosman M., Bumgarner R., et al. (2001). *Global TB Drug Facility. A Global Mechanism to Ensure Uninterrupted Access to Quality TB Drugs for DOTS Implementation.* Geneva: World Health Organization. WHO/CDS/STB/2001.10a.

Marriott A. (2009). *Blind Optimism: Challenging the Myths About Private Health Care in Poor Countries.* Oxford, United Kingdom: Oxfam International.

Mills A. & Hanson K. (2003). Expanding access to health interventions in low and middle-income countries: Constraints and opportunities for scaling-up. *Journal of International Development*, **15**(1), pp. 1–131.

Olivier de Sardan J. P. & Jaffré Y. (2003). *Une Médecine Inhospitalière: Les Difficiles Relations Entre Soignants Et Soignés Dans Cinq Capitales D'Afrique De L'Ouest.* Paris: Karthala.

WHO Department of Reproductive Health and Research & United Nations Population Fund. (2003). *Measuring Access to Reproductive Health Services.* Geneva: World Health Organization. WHO_RHR_04.07.

17

A public health, strategic toolkit to implement these alternatives

Person-centred care: a key to strengthening health care and systems in low- and middle-income countries?

Adapted from the original article 'A plea for an initiative to strengthen family medicine in public health care services of developing countries,' by Jean-Pierre Unger, Monique Van Dormael, Bart Criel, Jean Van der Vennet and Paul De Munck, International Journal of Health Services, 32(4), 799–815, 2002.

Introduction

Thirty years after Alma Ata, PHC activists might have strong grounds for optimism. Both evidence (Starfield et al., 2005) and policy guidance (World Health Organization, 2008) now point in the same direction. Starfield and collaborators cleared all doubts about the superior contribution of primary care to health and equity, a conclusion reconfirmed by both the Commission on Social Determinants of Health's Knowledge Network on Health Systems (Gilson et al., 2007) and the Commission's final report (Commission on Social Determinants of Health, 2008). The 2008 World Health Report promoted PHC as 'coordinator of a comprehensive response (to people's expectations and needs) at all levels' and some major donor agencies followed suit.

People in need of health care in LMICs might have a different perception. A slum dweller in India consulting in an urban PHC centre might find a doctor once a week, without any other drugs than those for a handful of identified TB patients. A Quechua woman anywhere between Colombia and Chile might not be able to find a doctor speaking her language. In sub-Saharan Africa any patient able to convince a health worker that their illness is other than malaria belongs to the happy few. More than 30 years after Alma Ata, what is called primary care in LMICs often remains deficient, or there is no care at all.

In this chapter we argue that person-centredness[1] – as delivered through family medicine – is a core condition for strengthening health care in LMICs. Indeed PHC can contribute to equitable care through improving access on the one hand and by empowering people on the other. But this ideal situation can only be achieved when quality of care is optimized (De Maeseneer et al., 2007). Whilst this might appear to be the situation in some countries such as Thailand or even Brazil, person-centred care has been largely restricted to the articulate and the better off. We argue that participatory health care, including PHC, will need to broaden this through careful planning, better resourcing and a respect for the democratic right of all citizens. This is by and large not the case in LMICs, where poor quality of care – particularly the lack of a

---

[1] From around 2005, the expression 'person-centredness' is increasingly replacing the formerly common 'patient-centredness.' We welcome this shift from patient to person-centredness, as it avoids both bio-medical bias and the intrinsic contradiction between the term 'patient' and the essential person-centred care dimension of seeing the 'patient-as-person.'

person-centred perspective in primary care practice – is omnipresent and constitutes a major determinant of low demand for public health services (Audibert & de Roodenbeke, 2005; Haddad et al., 1998). The following analysis of standards of best practice of family medicine, delivered by general practitioners in HICs, provides a framework for identifying deficiencies and for developing strategies for improving PHC in LMICs. Even if primary care in LMICs is often delivered by medical assistants – nurses or auxiliaries (as in Africa), or non-generalists (including paediatricians and gynaecologists, as in Latin America) – analysis of best practice can fuel reflection about professional identities and roles of all primary care practitioners (Dugas & Van Dormael, 2003). Besides, family medicine is part of health care delivery reform in a growing number of LMICs, including Vietnam, Egypt, Morocco, Tunisia, Thailand (Williams et al., 2002) and most Latin American nations. Family medicine networks have been launched in East and Southern Africa (De Maeseneer et al., 2006). Our 'public' emphasis is not on government-owned facilities per se, but on all publicly oriented, primary care institutions – that is to say with policies characterized by a quest for social profit, equity, solidarity, well-being, and patient autonomy (Giusti et al., 1997).

Standard of best practice in family medicine

Quality of care in general practice remains an ill-defined concept (Winefield et al., 1995). In England characteristics that have been used to define good general practice are: 'excellence in diagnosing and treating established illness; in preventing the onset of illness; in enabling patients to understand and make sense of their illness in meeting patients' wants, and in business efficiency' (Toon, 1994). While this definition applies to all care-givers, Starfield (Starfield, 1994) offers specific operational criteria to define primary care: the elements of first contact, continuity, comprehensiveness, and a coordination of synthesis function. Another dimension often attributed to good general practice is the improvement of patient autonomy. Clients' demands and satisfaction criteria provide useful insights into the definition of quality. A study undertaken in England, Greece, Yugoslavia and the former Soviet Union showed that key dimensions of satisfaction with primary care include the nature and quality of the doctor–patient relationship as well as the practitioner's professional skills (Calnan et al., 1994). A systematic literature review on patients' priorities with regard to primary care revealed that, of a total of 57 options, the most frequently mentioned characteristics were provision of information, a humane attitude and the competence of the doctor (Wensing et al., 1998). While patients in different HICs might have differing views on some aspects of care, they most of all share a claim for good doctor–patient communication and accessibility of care (Grol et al., 1999). In a LIC, Haddad and colleagues reached similar conclusions and proposed the following taxonomy of perceived quality: technical competence, good interpersonal relations, availability of resources and services, and accessibility and effectiveness of care. A recent Canadian study (Wong et al., 2008) found that, although patients discuss accessibility most frequently, domains most associated with satisfaction are interpersonal communication and continuity of care.

In the second half of the twentieth century, family medicine became the gold standard of general practice – at least in Europe, North America and Australia. Family medicine had emerged as a professional response to the need for comprehensive personal care in the context of increasing specialization of care following World War II. In 1991 the World Organization of Family Doctors (WONCA) described the family physician as 'a generalist who accepts everyone seeking care, whereas other health providers limit access to their services on the basis of age, sex and/or diagnosis,' who 'cares for the individual in the context of the family, and the family in the context of the community, irrespective of race, culture or social class' (Bentzen et al., 1991). Similarly, the American Academy of Family Physicians states that 'the family medicine process is unique. At the centre of this process is the patient–physician relationship, with the patient viewed in the context of the family' (American Academy of Family Medicine, 1992). Indeed, family medicine in most HICs had steadily espoused a specific model of doctor–patient interaction. Family medicine borrowed this concept from the eminent psychotherapist Carl Rogers,[2] who had stated that 'it is the quality of the interpersonal encounter … which is the most significant element in determining effectiveness' (Rogers, 1962). In 1969 Enid Balint outlined 'patient-centred medicine' as 'another way of medical thinking' (complementary to what she termed 'illness-orientated medicine'), whereby the patient 'has to be understood as a unique human-being' (Balint, 1969). In McWhinney's terms 'the physician tries to enter the patient's world, to see the illness through the patient's eyes' (McWhinney, 1989). Stewart and colleagues (Stewart et al., 2003) delivered a detailed description of patient-centred methodology in six interconnecting components:

- exploring the person's experience of the health problem;
- understanding the person as a whole;
- finding common ground for management of the health problem;
- integrating health prevention and promotion;
- enhancing the doctor-patient relationship; and
- being realistic about personal limitations, time and resources.

Mead and Bower (Mead & Bower, 2000) summarized patient-centredness in five key dimensions:

- a bio-psychosocial perspective (understanding a person's illness beyond conventional disease taxonomies);
- the 'patient-as-person' (understanding the patient as a unique experiencing individual within a unique context);
- sharing power and responsibility;
- a therapeutic alliance; and
- the 'doctor-as-person' (in self-awareness of a doctor's subjectivity).

By the end of the twentieth century, person-centredness was well established as a standard of best practice in family medicine, primarily in HICs. Accordingly, we now witness a boom of activity in studying, promoting and teaching person-centred care. Discussion on how to measure person-centredness is ongoing (Heritage & Maynard, 2006; Mead & Bower, 2002). Yet, the body of evidence indicating positive impact of person-centredness on patient satisfaction, adherence to treatment, and health outcomes is steadily growing (Brown et al., 2003). Beyond its impact on outcomes, person-centredness is arguably a dimension of health care quality in its own right (Berwick, 2009). To promote person-centred care through family medicine WONCA – constituted in 1972 – now has 97 member organizations in 79 countries (WONCA, 2007). Person-centred practice is increasingly taught in undergraduate and postgraduate medical education in HICs.

---

[2] Rogers' approach to psychotherapy is best known as 'client-centred therapy' since 1951, although he earlier called it 'non-directive therapy.' In the 1980s, he replaced 'client-centred' with 'person-centred,' preceding the shift from 'patient-centred care' to 'person-centred care' by two decades.

Primary care practice in low- and middle-income countries

Primary care staff in LMICs generally concentrate on specific programmes: antenatal care, under-five child clinics and immunizations, family planning, nutritional rehabilitation, and disease control. Patient management gets less attention. The energy devoted to preventive programmes, together with poor resource management, resulted in the diminished importance of curative care in public facilities during the 1980s and 1990s. This was in line with the 1993 World Development Report, which stated that, in poor countries, public facilities should deliver only 'essential clinical services' (World Bank, 1993), which meant a curative solution for a few well-defined diseases. The purpose of such concession to the public service in its competition with the private sector may have been to integrate disease-control programmes (such as prevention of diarrhoeal diseases and acute respiratory infections) into health care delivery. Obviously, patients must be present at health centres if candidates for these programmes are to be recruited, but this approach effectively limits the ability of staff to meet patient demand within the public sector.

Ministries of health tend to define primary care staff as 'good' when they create links between programmes, enabling patients to access the right programme for their health status at the right time. However, if only five or six preventive programmes and 'elementary' curative care services are available, then the person-centred principle is of limited relevance. All that is required is a small number of parameters to enable staff to channel the patient to the appropriate programme (Is she pregnant? Does she want to postpone the next pregnancy? Is the child vaccinated?). In practice primary care staff in LMICs rarely build generic preventive activities into curative care (with the exceptions of immunization and DOTs). Only in exceptional cases do they set up prevention programmes that are not part of a national programme.

The implementation of prevention programmes tends to be dominated by quantitative objectives. Together with the frequent, and often inappropriate, use of standardized guidelines, this helps to explain why communication between patients and primary care providers is, on the whole, so poor in clinical practice in developing countries. A clear example of this is the so-called 'post-consultation' we witnessed in Ecuador – auxiliaries explaining their condition and treatment to the patients, in compensation for the doctors who did not. Overall primary care providers in LMICs do not sufficiently take into consideration the individual dimension of care. We need to understand the factors underlying this situation before any solutions can be identified.

Reasons for the neglect of person-centred care

In Africa – and also to a large extent in Latin America and Asia – health care for the poor has usually been the object of central planning, since few doctors voluntarily choose to live and work in poor and deprived environments (except in some church-related health care institutions). A century ago, family practice still lacked the legitimacy to be exported by the colonial powers to the colonies, or to be imported by the already independent Latin countries (Van Dormael, 1997). In Africa and Asia colonial medicine was mainly featured with hospitals and disease-control programmes (sometimes managed in military style, as in French Western and Equatorial Africa). Medical specialists controlled undergraduate medical education, because general practice was considered unscientific (Flexner, 2002).

The 1978 Alma Ata conference boosted PHC, but fell short of stressing the importance of responding to individually expressed needs. Soon after, MoHs in LMICs concentrated their funding on disease-control programmes along the lines of SPHC (Walsh & Warren,

1979), criticized for its inefficiency and lack of acceptability in recipient communities (Unger & Killingsworth, 1986). Their bureaucratic justification continued to emphasize guidelines and instructions, in marked contrast to the professional rationale prevailing in HICs, which promoted individual decision making (Van Dormael, 1995). The emphasis on only a few programmes in LMICs was further reinforced by the argument that – with the medical assistants and nurses in charge of PHC services having such low levels of education – this was all that could realistically be delivered. However, positive experiences with African medical assistants, given appropriate training and supervision, suggest that the educational level per se is not a valid reason for basing primary care on just a few programmes (Darras et al., 1981).

This is not to deny the impact of some disease-control programmes, notably those for children under five – where a significant impact on life expectancy can be achieved – and to a lesser extent those for expectant mothers. However, the limited scope of such programmes is a serious handicap. Most significantly, the concentration on specific disease-control programmes meant that, for a vast majority of MoHs, other childhood complaints and adult pathologies, including psychosocial problems, were not considered part of primary care responsibilities.

Vertical programmes integrated into primary care services could have been compatible with a bio-psychosocial approach. In Europe family doctors benefited from standards improving their handling of specific complaints and diseases. In LMICs, however, a lack of vision undermined programme integration. In practice the integration process has contributed to unsustainable outputs and a deterioration of quality of care. Furthermore, downgrading the duties of primary care staff to merely meeting technical standards in narrow domains has restricted professional identity and motivation (Unger, 1991). While some level of rationalization is needed to support sound decision making, excessive rationalization works against person-centred care. Rationalization affected clinical practice, requiring health staff to be disease-oriented rather than responsive to individual complaints.

Clinical education in LMICs followed the old hospital-based patterns of HICs. Undergraduate studies rarely exposed students to criteria such as efficiency, problem-solving, and use of appropriate primary care means and technology. Excessive dependence on radiology and laboratory tests undermined the use of medical history and clinical examination. Health workers were not taught to use experience to address health problems caused or made worse by psychological and social factors and, therefore, were often unaware of possible psychosomatic conditions. The biomedical model – applied to a restricted range of conditions – remained predominant in medical education of LMICs.

From the 1980s, concurrent with an increasingly global promotion of the principles of person-centred care, family medicine finally made its entry into the curricula of medical schools in LMICs. At first this happened mainly in countries where national policy adhered clearly to social goals. Consequently, the uptake of family medicine was no easygoing process in the era of structural adjustment. In Nicaragua, for example, a postgraduate course in family medicine was introduced in the last years of the first Sandinista government, but discontinued soon after a neoliberal government came to power (Zamora & Zuniga, 1992). By and large in LMICs the introduction of family medicine led to a new speciality and not to the reinforcement of general practitioners, as had been the case in Europe. Often trained in hospital settings only, many of those specialist family doctors never started working in health centres but rather stayed in the outpatient department of hospitals. This is, however, not the case everywhere. In Mali, for example, community-owned health centres are increasingly staffed with family doctors (Coulibaly et al., 2007).

Strategies to improve primary care

This chapter concludes by advocating a range of strategies for improving the quality of care in publicly oriented services. Public services still represent an important part of health care delivery in many LMICs. Even in countries with predominant private service provision, such as India and Bangladesh, many NGOs operate along the lines of public services. Public, and other publicly oriented services, need to develop appropriate strategies for improving the quality of care they provide, and improving primary care is key to doing so. Focusing on publicly oriented services is both a value-based and a logical choice, as addressing private for-profit services is unlikely to yield the desired results (Brugha & Zwi, 1998). A range of strategies is required, in addition to changes in the undergraduate curriculum, which can take more than 15 years to have an effect (Boelen, 1991).

A number of strategies for improving PHC and introducing person-centredness are outlined below.[3] Not all are applicable in every situation, but they can be drawn upon once a diagnosis has been made of the local or national situation. They should be treated as hypotheses to be tested in the context of action research, under the aegis of MoHs, research institutions, community representatives, international agencies, and professional organizations.

In-service development of person-centred care

In-service demonstration of person-centred care should be offered to primary care staff in pilot facilities. Attempts to improve the provider-patient interaction have been effective in HICs (Liaw et al., 1996) as well as in LMICs (Henbest & Fehrsen, 1992). Several techniques are available (see Section 6, Chapter 19, Part 1).

Improvement of health staff motivation

Although material benefits and a decent income certainly contribute to staff motivation, these by themselves are not sufficient to improve quality of care (Nitayarumphong et al., 2000). Less materialistic issues should also be addressed. These can include an open discussion of a political approach to development and the grounds on which the health professional is attempting to get social recognition. The nature of relations with patients and recognition by the local community are all the more essential in rural practice where opportunities to develop alternative social networks are limited (Dieleman et al., 2003). Job satisfaction – another important constituent of motivation – can be enhanced by working on the living environment, individual factors, and self-confidence as a professional (Franco et al., 2002). One way of improving the latter is by narrowing the gap between the clinical techniques mastered by the staff and the available equipment. Another way of enhancing professional identity is by organizing exchanges between primary care staff from different places (Van Dormael et al., 2007).

Improvement of the organization of primary care delivery

In HICs, improved management of primary care practice has a limited impact on actual performance (Ram et al., 1998), but the relationship is likely to be more important in LMICs where organizational deficiencies are more prominent. Techniques such as managed care and interface flow process audits will be discussed in the next chapters.

---

[3] Specific techniques relating to these strategies will be dealt with in the following chapters.

Changes in health policy

Primary care does not take place in a vacuum; a supportive policy is needed. MoHs in LMICs can create national directorates for primary care practice, to steer in-service training and sector planning amongst other goals. Promotion of person-centredness in public primary care requires a strong political will. In the absence of this interim strategies can be based on mid-level managers through international projects. International agencies have a big responsibility here, just as they had a major role in driving primary care into a corner. At a local level there are also possibilities for building a community counter-power to curb health professionals and civil servants. This would help tackle the larger issue of the limited control by lower social classes over service delivery and help launch health professionals into a dialogue with communities for setting up publicly oriented health services.

Conclusion

What can we expect from these changes? A better relationship between practitioners and patients could pave the way for renewed community interest in public PHC services. It could also halt the deterioration of public services, increase accountability and bridge the divide between publicly owned and other publicly oriented services.

It took half a century of continuous effort to recognize the value of person-centredness in family medicine in HICs – a process involving conceptualization, information and advocacy, professional organization, and staff and curriculum changes in universities. LMICs can build upon these achievements and take advantage of the fact that person-centred family practice has now been conceptualized in such a way that it can be taught, adapted to the local context, and implemented.

References

American Academy of Family Medicine. (1992). *Family Medicine, Scope and Philosophical Statement*. Costa Mesa, CA: American Academy of Family Medicine.

Audibert M. & de Roodenbeke E. (2005). *Utilisation des services de santé de premier niveau au Mali: analyse de la situation et perspectives*. World Bank, African Region: Human Development Department.

Balint E. (1969). The possibilities of patient-centered medicine. *The Journal of the Royal College of General Practitioners*, 17(82), pp. 269–76.

Bentzen B. G., Bridges-Webb C., Carmichael L., et al. (1991). *The Role of the General Practitioner/Family Physician in Health Care Systems: A Statement From WONCA*. Singapore: WONCA.

Berwick D. M. (2009). What 'patient-centered' should mean: Confessions of an extremist. *Health Affairs (Millwood)*, 28(4), p. W555–65.

Boelen C. (1991). *Changer l'éducation médicale*. Genève: OMS. WHO/EDU/91.200.

Brown J. B., Stewart M., & Ryan B. L. (2003). Outcomes of patient-provider interaction. In: Thompon T. L., et al., eds. *Handbook of Health Communication*. Mahwah, NJ: Lawrence Erlbaum Associates, pp. 141–62.

Brugha R. & Zwi A. (1998). Improving the quality of private sector delivery of public health services: Challenges and strategies. *Health Policy and Planning*, 13(2), pp. 107–20.

Calnan M., Katsouyiannopoulos V., Ovcharov V. K., Prokhorskas R., Ramic H., & Williams S. (1994). Major determinants of consumer satisfaction with primary care in different health systems. *Family Practice*, 11(4), pp. 468–78.

Commission on Social Determinants of Health. (2008). *Closing the Gap in a Generation: Health Equity Through Action on the Social Determinants of Health. Final report of the Commission on Social Determinants of Health*. Geneva: World Health Organization.

Coulibaly S., Desplats D., Kone Y., et al. (2007). Une médicine rurale de proximité: l'expérience des médecins de campagne au Mali [Neighbourhood rural medicine: An experience of rural doctors in Mali]. *Education for Health (Abingdon, England)*, **20**(2), p. 47.

Darras C., Van Lerberghe W., & Mercenier P. (1981). The Kasongo project; lessons from an experiment in the organisation of a system of primary health care. *Annales de la Société Belge de Médecine Tropicale*, **60**(Supplement).

De Maeseneer J., Hugo J., Hunt V. R., & True R. (2006). Flemish council funds family medicine network in East and South Africa. *WONCANews*, **32**(1), pp. 5–7.

De Maeseneer J., Willems S., De Sutter A., Van de Geuchte I., & Billings M. (2007). *Primary Health Care as a Strategy for Achieving Equitable Care*. Ghent: University of Ghent.

Dieleman M., Cuong P. V., Anh L. V., & Martineau T. (2003). Identifying factors for job motivation of rural health workers in North Viet Nam. *Human Resources for Health*, **1**(1), p. 10.

Dugas S. & Van Dormael M. (2003). *La construction de la médecine de famille dans les pays en développement*. Studies in Health Services Organisation & Policy (SHSOP) 22. Antwerp: Institute of Tropical Medicine. pp. 1–352.

Flexner A. (2002). Medical education in the United States and Canada. From the Carnegie Foundation for the Advancement of Teaching, Bulletin Number Four, 1910. *Bulletin of the World Health Organization*, **80**(7), pp. 594–602.

Franco L. M., Bennett S., & Kanfer R. (2002). Health sector reform and public sector health worker motivation: A conceptual framework. *Social Science & Medicine*, **54**(8), pp. 1255–66.

Gilson L., Doherty J., Loewenson R., & Francis V. (2007). *Challenging inequity through health systems. Final report Knowledge Network on Health Systems*. Geneva: WHO Commission on the Social Determinants of Health.

Giusti D., Criel B., & de Béthune X. (1997). Viewpoint: Public versus private health care delivery: Beyond the slogans. *Health Policy and Planning*, **12**(3), pp. 192–8.

Grol R., Wensing M., Mainz J., et al. (1999). Patients' priorities with respect to general practice care: An international comparison. European Task Force on Patient Evaluations of General Practice (EUROPEP). *Family Practice*, **16**(1), pp. 4–11.

Haddad S., Fournier P., Machouf N., & Yatara F. (1998). What does quality mean to lay people? Community perceptions of primary health care services in Guinea. *Social Science & Medicine*, **47**(3), pp. 381–94.

Henbest R. J. & Fehrsen G. S. (1992). Patient-centredness: Is it applicable outside the West? Its measurement and effect on outcomes. *Family Practice*, **9**(3), pp. 311–7.

Heritage J. & Maynard D. W. (2006). Problems and prospects in the study of physician-patient interaction: 30 years of research. *Annual Review of Sociology*, **32**, pp. 351–74.

Liaw S. T., Young D., & Farish S. (1996). Improving patient-doctor concordance: An intervention study in general practice. *Family Practice*, **13**(5), pp. 427–31.

McWhinney I. (1989). The need for a transformed clinical method. In: Stewart M. & Roter D., eds. *Communicating With Medical Patients*. London: Sage Publications, pp. 51–64.

Mead N. & Bower P. (2000). Patient-centredness: A conceptual framework and review of the empirical literature. *Social Science & Medicine*, **51**, pp. 1087–110.

Mead N. & Bower P. (2002). Patient-centred consultations and outcomes in primary care: A review of the literature. *Patient Education and Counseling*, **48**(1), pp. 51–61.

Nitayarumphong S., Srivanichakorn S., & Pongsupap Y. (2000). Strategies to respond to health manpower needs in rural Thailand. In: Ferrinho P. & Van Lerberghe W., eds. *Providing Health Care Under Adverse Conditions*. Antwerpen: ITG Press, pp. 55–72.

Ram P., Grol R., van den Hombergh P., Rethans J. J., van der Vleuten, V, & Aretz K. (1998). Structure and process: The relationship between practice management and actual clinical performance in general practice. *Family Practice*, **15**(4), pp. 354–62.

Rogers C. R. (1962). The interpersonal relationship: The core of guidance. *Harvard Educational Review*, **32**(4), pp. 416–29.

Starfield B. (1994). Is primary care essential? *Lancet*, **344**(8930), pp. 1129–33.

Starfield B., Shi L. Y., & Macinko J. (2005). Contribution of primary care to health systems and health. *Milbank Quarterly*, **83**(3), pp. 457–502.

Stewart M., Brown J. B., Weston W., McWhinney I. R., McWilliam C. L., & Freeman T. R. (2003). *Patient-Centered Medicine: Transforming the Clinical Method*. Abingdon, UK: Radcliffe Publishing.

Toon P. D. (1994). What is good general practice? A philosophical study of the concept of high quality medical care. *Occasional Paper Royal College of General Practitioners*, (65), p. i-55.

Unger J. P. (1991). Can intensive campaigns dynamise front line health services? The evaluation of an immunisation campaign in Thies health district, Senegal. *Social Science & Medicine*, **32**(3), pp. 249–59.

Unger J. P. & Killingsworth J. R. (1986). Selective primary health care: A critical review of methods and results. *Social Science & Medicine*, **22**(10), pp. 1001–13.

Van Dormael M. (1995). *Médecine générale et modernité. Regards croisés sur l'occident et le tiers monde*. Thèse de doctorat en sciences sociales, Université Libre de Bruxelles.

Van Dormael M. (1997). *La médecine coloniale, ou la tradition exogène de la médecine moderne dans le tiers monde*. In: Van Lerberghe W., Kegels G., & De Brouwere V., eds. Studies in Health Service Organisation & Policy. Antwerp: ITG Press, pp. 1–39.

Van Dormael M., Dugas S., & Diarra S. (2007). North-South exchange and professional development: Experience from Mali and France. *Family Practice*, **24**(2), pp. 102–7.

Walsh J. A. & Warren K. S. (1979). Selective primary health care: An interim strategy for disease control in developing countries. *New England Journal of Medicine*, **301**(18), pp. 967–74.

Wensing M., Jung H. P., Mainz J., Olesen F., & Grol R. (1998). A systematic review of the literature on patient priorities for general practice care. Part 1: Description of the research domain. *Social Science & Medicine*, **47**(10), pp. 1573–88.

Williams R. L., Henley E., Prueksaritanond S., & Aramrattana A. (2002). Family practice in Thailand: Will it work? *The Journal of the American Board of Family Practice*, **15**(1), pp. 73–6.

Winefield H. R., Murrell T. G., & Clifford J. (1995). Process and outcomes in general practice consultations: Problems in defining high quality care. *Social Science & Medicine*, **41**(7), pp. 969–75.

WONCA. (2007). WONCA: World Organization of National Colleges, Academies and academic associations of general practitioners/family physicians. http://www.globalfamilydoctor.com/aboutWonca/aboutwonca.asp?refurl=aw.

Wong S. T., Watson D. E., Young E., & Regan S. (2008). What do people think is important about primary health care? *Health Care Policy*, **3**(3), pp. 89–104.

World Bank (1993). *World Development Report 1993: Investing in Health*. Oxford: Oxford University Press.

World Health Organization (2008). *The World Health Report 2008 Primary Health Care – Now More Than Ever*. Geneva: World Health Organization.

Zamora N. & Zuniga L. (1992). *Medicina Integral En Nicaragua Revision Hospital Carlos Marx 1987–1992*. Managua: Silais Oriental.

A public health, strategic toolkit to implement these alternatives

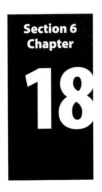

18 Improving access

Pierre De Paepe, Edgar Rojas, Luís Abad, Patrick Van Dessel and Jean Pierre Unger

Part 1: Access to curative care in first-line health services: an experience in Ecuador

Introduction

In LMICs it is generally acknowledged that access to curative care could be improved if primary care health services were strengthened and new health centres opened when required,[1] if in addition skilled teams are organized in these services and if resource allocation does not discriminate against primary care as has historically been the case in many LMICs. Some publications also focus on the importance of good doctor–patient communication, as highlighted in Chapter 17 of this section, to improve access and to ensure effective integration of health services (Haddad & Fournier, 1995; Litvack & Bodart, 1993). There are also important technical dimensions of supporting primary care health services, including sustainable drug supplies in public services (Hanson & Gilson, 1993) (see Part 2 of this chapter).

However, while many publications analyze the determinants of service utilization and the impact of services on health status, little has been published on how to actually improve access to health care because the discussion to date has been part of a larger neoliberal policy framework, that views comprehensive care as rhetoric as well as in isolation from publicly oriented health services.

The following Part 1 describes a study based on empirical research and interventions in several sites which was implemented by an international team to improve access to curative health care in a network of MoH health centres (primary care health services) in Ecuador between 1993 and 1998. Its objective was to explore alternative ways of providing quality CHC in public health facilities which suffered from severe budgetary constraints.

During the 1990s the policy environment in Ecuador was hostile to any enterprise related to public provision, as a result of the implementation of neoliberal health policies. The latter was however to prove fatal to the country's economy and health care system. In 1990 the country's public expenditure on health was 3.7% of its GNP[2] but by 1997 it was even lower having been cut to a mere 2.7% of its total government budget. As a

---

[1] At relatively low cost as has been argued in Section 5, Chapter 12, by contrast to the high cost disease-specific programmes that have been the trend over the past 3 decades. This approach has been successfully applied in a number of countries such as Nicaragua and Zimbabwe in the 1980s, Costa Rica, Cuba, among others.

[2] INCAE/Progresec. Cuadernos de economía N° 6. Data provided by Cepar in 1997.

result access to health services fell sharply, and was made even worse by a concentration of health professionals in urban centres (Merino, 2007), a lack of drugs, poor steward-ship, political nominations for health posts reinforcing job instability, low salaries, and dual employment of physicians in public and private clinics. By 2002 some 30% of the Ecuadorian population were not able to make use of health services in case of illness, and social security funded health services (IESS) admissions and outpatient consultations also dropped by 35% between 1996 and 2003 (Pan American Health Organization & Consejo Nacional de Salud – CONASA, 2007). The demise of health services was reflected in an increase in maternal mortality by 10% between 1990 and 2002 (Hermida, 2007), even though maternal care was meant to be free. The already severely impoverished population suffered increasing out-of-pocket health expenditures, rising from 34.2% to 38.1% of total household expenditure, over the period when the research was implemented (1993 to 2003) (World Health Organization, 2006).

The experience in Ecuador is an illustration of the possibilities for (and limitations of) an intervention to be successfully undertaken in countries where even governments have little or no commitment to improving access to health care. The intervention illustrates some of the challenges that local action in the health sector may face in a hostile setting dominated by neoliberal policies in the health sector for some time.

Methodology

The methodology for the basis of intervention undertaken was action research (Lewin, 1946), which departs from traditional, descriptive studies of health-seeking behaviour as it relies on a set of hypotheses and considers research as a cyclical process of planning, learning and action, which seeks concurrently to solve an immediate problem as well as strengthening the capacity of an organization. The researcher here is implicitly involved in decisions and opera-tions as opposed to playing the role of bystander, as is often the case with more traditional research methodology.

The objective of action research is a dynamic one: to bring about change, to generate new knowledge (and, accessorily, to explain a phenomenon). The steps of action research as uti-lized are summarized in Figure 18.1.

Background

The intervention for access to comprehensive care is based on the experiences to improve access in Ecuador by the Primary Health Care (PHC) Project from 1993 until 2003 (those

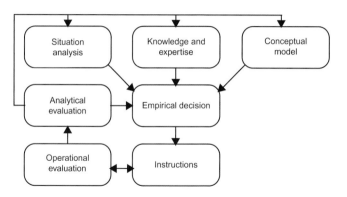

Figure 18.1. Stages of action research. *Source:* Nitayarum-phong, S., Mercenier, P. (1992). Ayutthaya research project: Thailand experiences on health systems research. Life sciences and technologies for develop-ing countries; methodology and relevance of health systems research; research reports. Paper presented at contract holders meeting, 8, 9 and 12 April. pp. 55–78. Centre International de l'Enfance (CIE), Paris.

Table 18.1. Demographic and socio-economic context of the research intervention in Ecuador, 1995

Province	Health District	1995 population	Ecosystem	Population living at poverty level (%)
Quevedo	Quevedo	228,751	Coast	43
Cañar	Cañar	67,325	Central Andean Mountains	29
Cañar	Azogues	97,386	Central Andean Mountains	29
Morona santiago	Macas	58,292	Central Andean Mountains	64
Napo	Tena	80,954	Central Andean Mountains	33
Pastaza	Puyo	28,443	Eastern Amazonia	45
Research area	N/A	561,151	N/A	N/A
Ecuador	N/A	11,223,020	N/A	48

Note: N/A means 'not applicable.'

Source: Encuesta de Condiciones de Vida, Ecuador 1995/1996.

presented here were led between 1993 and 1998). The PHC Project was carried out under a long-term bilateral development cooperation agreement between Ecuador and Belgium. It was led in six health districts with a total population of 561,151 in 1995 – which was about 5% of the country's population.

The location for research and the selection of the health districts was chosen to reflect the diversity of the ecosystems of Ecuador. They are represented in Table 18.1 and Figure 18.2.

In the period between 1999 and 2000, Ecuador suffered a severe economic crisis, with GDP contracting by more than 6% (Central Intelligence Agency, 2009). Poverty increased significantly over this period. Ecuador's infant mortality rate, for example, fell by 35% between 1970 and 1981, but in 1988 it was still at the high level of 40/1,000 live births excluding the possibility of under-registration (UNICEF, 2009).

Under-utilization of curative care – local factors

In the selected districts (Table 18.1) medical officers were asked to diagnose the under-utilization of curative care specific to each health centre. They did this with an ad hoc analytical frame incorporating the indicators for utilization. They analyzed possible ways to improve access through a set of strategies for improvement. This analytic process was carried out through a cycle of evaluation and learning over a 10-year period and by different stages, as illustrated by Table 18.2 (p. 214).

The proposed model for access to health care considers different criteria to be put in place simultaneously: geographical, medical, intra-institutional, psycho-socio-cultural, chronological and financial. The intervention undertaken was based on the following hypotheses:

1. Firstly, improving access to quality comprehensive care in primary care public health services is possible – under budgetary constraints and in an otherwise hostile

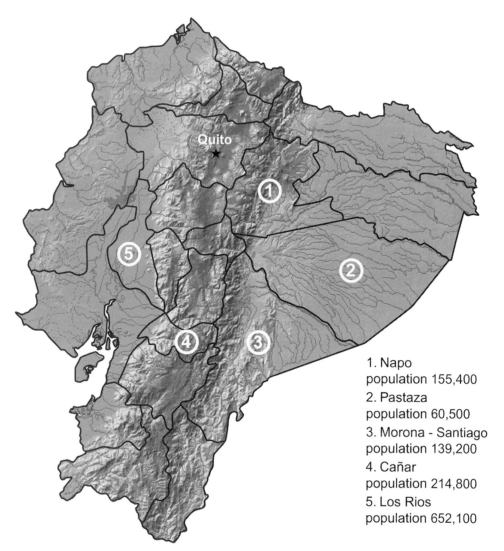

1. Napo
population 155,400
2. Pastaza
population 60,500
3. Morona - Santiago
population 139,200
4. Cañar
population 214,800
5. Los Rios
population 652,100

Figure 18.2. Location of the PHC project initial interventions in Ecuador (1993–1997). Population statistics date from 1999. *Source:* http://www.populstat.info/Americas/ecuadorp.htm.

environment – if health staff become motivated to engage in a participatory dialogue with patients individually and with the community as a whole.

2. Secondly, in order for a community to support its primary care public health service it needs to have a positive relationship with the health care providers.

3. Thirdly, we wondered if it was possible to motivate health staff in public health services to engage in delivering quality health care and open up for dialogue without economic incentives, on the basis of a better recognition of their work.

4. Fourthly, that it is not necessary to have access to external funds in order to obtain better access to quality CHC but only external guidance.

5. Fifthly, that it is feasible for the public sector to fund and monitor such a strategy.

Table 18.2. Model of analysis and strategic orientation

Type of accessibility	Indicators	Strategies for improvement
Total	New curative consultations per year per inhabitant. Proportion of population with at least one curative consultation yearly. For hospitals inpatient wards: admission rates.	Community participation in decision making process. Promotion of publicly oriented services. Improvement in quality of care and services. Permanent and stable presence of staff. Where needed appropriate task shifting between GPs, nurses, and not GPs.
Geographical	% of total population living at less than 5 km from health centre. Natural obstacles (mountains, rivers, etc.) on the way to a health centre	Redistribution of health teams in smaller health centres. Association of NGOs to the public services network. Changes in preventive consultations. Training of community-based promoters in isolated zones.
Pharmaceutical	% of prescriptions bought outside the health centre. Range of pharmacy stocks interruptions.	Variants of the Bamako Initiative.[1] Ongoing provision of drugs financed with cost recovery.
Intra-institutional	Average duration of consultation. Average time of stay in health centre and obstacles encountered within.	Reorganization of patient flow, task delegation, introduction of health appointments, limiting writing time during consultation, rationalization of information system, priority access to patients from within the centre's responsibility zone.
Psycho-social and cultural (obstacles perceived by the users)	Results from observation of consultation, post-consultation findings from patients through interviews	SOAP method[2], in-service training, intervision[3], supervision[4], promotion of person-centred care, evidence-based medicine, intercultural abilities of hired personnel, human resources stability
Chronological	Degree of compatibility of opening hours with users' activities. Patients refused during consultation hours	Standardizing opening hour schemes, providing also non-financial incentives for personnel
Financial	Price of sickness episode according to family income[5]	Improvement of health centres' problem solving-capacity. Cost control (e.g., rationalization of prescription). Modalities of payment that favour solidarity (prepayment and fee per sickness episode). Exoneration for indigents. Cross-subsidization at district level.

Notes:
1 Bamako Initiative, see Part 2 of this chapter;
2 SOAP, method to structure consultations and medical records in first-line services, conceived to take into account the patient's viewpoint in order to enable negotiations between professionals and users on clinical decision making and follow up (Weed, 1969). This method includes the restructuring of curative consultations so as to clearly identify the patient's concerns (Subjective), the collection of physical signs and symptoms (Objective), a joint patient–doctor assessment of the condition (Assessment) and finally the agreement upon treatment and follow up planning (Plan); Is there a problem here in that you exclude all other factors in context as in the patient's background? Does it work to have such an exclusive clinical focus?;
3 Inter-vision: case review performed by peers to improve quality of care;
4 Supervision: in-service training method based on direct observation of clinical practice by an experienced peer;
5 Should be equivalent to 1 and 3 days of monetary income respectively for urban and rural dwellers.

Obstacles specifically linked to commercial insurance and care delivery

There are also other obstacles specifically linked to commercial insurance and care delivery (some have become widespread in Ecuador).

These include obstacles to care that are linked to commercial health insurance, for example, skyrocketing transaction and administrative costs (to the user and as opportunity cost for MoHs); obstacles to insurance affiliation and risk selection; obstacles to efficient market (local monopolies; lack of consumer information); insufficient package of insured/delivered benefits; inappropriate tier-specific classification of health activities; expensive co-payments; patients' ignorance of administrative procedures; information asymmetry; audits of authorization of payments delaying access to care; low insurance coverage rate; under-the-counter payments and bribes (such as votes against social insurance rights).

Finally, there are obstacles typical of commercial practices in public sector such as gifts and unofficial payments (Smith et al., 2005); ineffective follow-up of contracts with autonomously managed hospitals; sale of hospital drugs; biased distribution of social classification as a basis for tariffs and absenteeism. In the present experience only absenteeism has been tackled. Unofficial payments were an important problem in one of the intervention hospitals but did not prove to be vulnerable.

Improving strategies

At the inception of the research, criteria relating to the quality of care and health services organization were shared with health professionals. The quality criteria were presented in Section 5, Chapter 14.

In practice, part or all of the following strategies were used in the six health districts:

- Improved pharmaceutical access establishing a management system for medical drugs (see Part 2 of this chapter), based on user fees and with an exemption for the poor and characterized by co-management between community health committees and health teams.
- Improved financial access introducing flat user fees per sickness episode, including most costs related to first, subsequent, and referral consultations for the same health problem. Costs covered included consultation fee, drugs, clinical tests, health imaging, and possibly hospital expenditure in case of referral during a maximum of 15 days.
- Improved psycho-social access by testing techniques to introduce person-centred, bio-psychosocial care in the largest possible number of health centres, at the lowest possible cost (see Section 6, Chapter 19, Part 1). Techniques used were patient-physician communication, bio-psychological checklists, SOAP (subjective, objective, assessment, and plan) structure, and family files (see notes of Table 18.2 and Chapter 19, Part 1).
- Improved overall accessibility strengthening community participation and establishing a link between health professionals and the community through the creation of health committees. Their members were elected in community assemblies.

Evaluation of impact

From 1993 to 1996 utilization rates (as the proportion of users in the total population) significantly increased, although not evenly in every province (Table 18.3). The increase was related, in our view, to improved organization of the health centres, better dialogue with the local

Table 18.3. Trends in utilization of curative care (1993–2005)

	Quevedo	Cañar	Azogues	Macas	Tena	Puyo
Changes in proportion of users of primary care services in the whole population (1993–1996)	+17%	+ 93%	+25%	–9%	+272%	+13%
Utilization rate (new curative cases per inhabitant per year) (1996)	0.27	0.31	0.22	0.3	0.3	0.5
Changes in proportion of outpatient consultations in a hospital on total district consultations (1994–1996)	–3%	–17%	–6%	–4%	–0%	– 18%
Proportion of users of primary care services in the whole population (2001 and 2005)	Utilization indicators are on average 20% above the pre-intervention levels.					

Source: De Paepe, 1998.

community, and an adequate supply of drugs. On the other hand, the reasons for these uneven results were found in variable responses to the research protocols due to many health centres being closed because of lack of staff and in the fact that not every district reached a plateau in their performance at the same time. At subsequent controls in 2001 and 2005 the utilization rates continued to be sustained in two of the six districts. Excessive referrals and the undue utilization of hospital care (as a proportion of outpatient consultations in a hospital by district) shrank in five of the six hospitals over the same period, reflecting better access to, and quality of care in, primary care health centres. The results suggest at the least a good indication of sustained, although limited, effectiveness of implemented strategies to improve access to health care.

Lessons learned

We would venture the opinion that the research framework presented in this chapter can deliver a potentially useful tool for district executive teams. District teams needed to assess levels of accessibility to each particular health centre (and hospital) in their constituency, identify each specific mix of obstacles, set appropriate indicators, and address obstacles progressively. Lessons gleaned from this experience are outlined below.

Community participation and ownership

The development of community participation is a priority in public services aiming at the delivery of comprehensive care. Virtually all strategies for improvement put forward here – financial and drugs co-management, support to building infrastructures, organization of preventive consultations, and reorganization of activities and opening hour schedules – were made possible through a participatory dialogue. To better engage in this kind of participation a sound individual patient-physician dialogue is required, for the community to manifest its interest in its health centre, and for the physician to be able to enter into a dialogue with that community.

Co-payments

An apparent paradox in this case is that co-payments served to improve access to medical care, compared to those which were described as free consultations. This meant that the flat user fee per sickness episode (see above) was kept lower compared to the total price of diagnosis and treatment components incurred separately, minus the price of the consultation. To achieve such sharp flat fees the total cost per disease episode needed reducing. This was achieved through the rationalization of clinical decisions, and the introduction of between-patients, cross-subsidies for direct costs (feasible through the use of generic drugs). The co-payment was introduced in all the districts surveyed with an exoneration clause for the poor which involved also payment methods that favoured solidarity between (moderately and severely ill) patients (payment per episode) and between the healthy and the sick (community health insurance).

Co-financing

Partial community co-financing of primary care health services is a sustainable way of contributing to public services co-management and community empowerment. It requires, however, continuous core funding by governments. In the health centres of Puyo and Azogues districts these mechanisms prospered after the withdrawal of cooperation by Belgium, in spite of unfavourable national health policies and unstable governments.

Professional motivation and ownership

Full-time, exclusive dedication of doctors to publicly oriented services, decent salaries, job stability and career perspectives are known to be crucial to not-for-profit services. Unfortunately, these factors could not be influenced for research purposes. Physicians in Ecuadorian primary care services generally worked under unfavourable administrative rules which included short-term contracts, long working hours and a scheme of 1-year mandatory civil service for recent medical graduates, factors known to affect to some extent the commitment of physicians. Results would have been much more important had this constraint been lifted.

Professionalization of managerial functions in public services

Ten years have followed the end of the research intervention. Two of the six districts, Puyo and Azogues, have managed to sustain the intervention and improve their results. The role of a motivated and stable district management team appears to have been a key feature of the intervention. We learned from this intervention that the function of district medical officer should be professionalized, to include qualifying exams during professional careers.

Conclusion

Although marked in relative terms, the improvement in access to health care achieved by the strategies presented here were insufficient in absolute terms, because of an external constraint: the scarce allocation of doctors to health centres, many being closed because of lack of staff. This suggests that local initiatives need badly to be supported by a consistent national health policy and resources aiming to secure universal access to CHC (Groupe d'Etude pour une Réforme de la Médecine [G.E.R.M.], 1971; Mercenier, 1971; Unger et al., 2003).

Conversely, the design of national health policies can take advantage of local, pilot experiments. Firstly, with action research, they permit to elaborate health care models, managerial tools, and health development strategies that can be generalized by national authorities. Secondly, pilot experiments can be used to yield demonstration structures useful to convince policy makers. When successful, their health facilities can host teaching practices.

Finally, the strategies presented in this chapter have a domain of validity limited to publicly oriented health services; commercial facilities have little commitment to improving health care accessibility for the general population.

References

Central Intelligence Agency. (2009). *CIA Factbook Ecuador*. https://www.cia.gov/library/publications/the-world-factbook/geos/ec.html.

De Paepe P. (1998). *5 Años proyecto APS, análisis de conceptos, metodología y resultados 1993–1998*. Convenio Ecuatoriano Belga.

Groupe d'Etude pour une Réforme de la Médecine (G.E.R.M.). (1971). *Les lignes de force d'une politique de santé. In: Pour Une Politique De La Santé*. Bruxelles: La Revue Nouvelle, pp. 9–17.

Haddad S. & Fournier P. (1995). Quality, cost and utilisation of health services in developing countries. A longitudinal study in Zaire. *Social Science & Medicine*, **40**(6), pp. 743–53.

Hanson K. & Gilson L. (1993). *Cost, Resource Use and Financing Methodology for Basic Health Services. A Practical Manual*. New York: United Nations Children's Fund. N°16.

Hermida C. (2007). Mortalidad materna. In: *La Equidad En La Mira: La Salud Pública En Ecuador Durante Las Últimas Décadas [Eyes on Equity: Public Health in Ecuador During the Last Decades]*. Organización Panamericana de la Salud en Ecuador. [in Spanish]. Quito: World Health Organization, pp. 57–60.

Lewin K. (1946). Action research and minority problems. *Journal of Social Issues*, **2**(4), pp. 34–6.

Litvack J. I. & Bodart C. (1993). User fees plus quality equals improved access to health care: Results of a field experiment in Cameroon. *Social Science & Medicine*, **37**(3), pp. 369–83.

Mercenier P. (1971). *Les objectifs de l'organisation médico-sanitaire. In: Pour Une Politique De La Santé*. Bruxelles: La Revue Nouvelle, pp. 67–72.

Merino C. (2007). Los recursos humanos en el campo de la salud. In: *La Equidad En La Mira: La Salud Pública En Ecuador Durante Las Últimas Décadas [Eyes on Equity: Public Health in Ecuador During the Last Decades]*. Organización Panamericana de la Salud en Ecuador. [in Spanish]. Quito: World Health Organization, pp. 222–37.

Pan American Health Organization & Consejo Nacional de Salud – CONASA. (2007). *La Equidad En La Mira: La Salud Pública En Ecuador Durante Las Últimas Décadas [Eyes on Equity: Public Health in Ecuador During the Last Decades]*. [in Spanish]. Quito: Ecuador.

Smith P. C., Preker A. S., Light D. W., & Richard S. (2005). Role of markets and competition. In: Figueras J., et al., eds. *Purchasing to Improve Health Systems Performance*. Geneva: World Health Organization, pp. 102–21.

Unger J. P., Marchal B., & Green A. (2003). Quality standards for health care delivery and management in publicly oriented health services. *International Journal of Health Planning and Management*, **18**, pp. S79–S88.

UNICEF. (2009). *Info by Country: Ecuador*. http://www.unicef.org/infobycountry/ecuador.html.

Weed L. L. (1969). *Medical Records, Medical Education and Patient Care*. Chicago: Year Book Medical Publishers.

World Health Organization. (2006). *The World Health Report 2006: Working Together for Health*. Geneva: World Health Organization.

Part 2: Improving access to drugs in publicly oriented services: an experience in Senegal

Adapted from: Unger J.-P., Mbaye A. M., Diao M. Finances and Drugs at the Core of District Health Service Rehabilitation. A Case-Study in Senegal: the Kolda District. Health Policy and Planning 1990; 5(4): pp. 367–377.

Introduction

Access to drugs is essential for accessibility to care in any setting. This article examines one experience from Senegal from the angle of health services management. It was conducted to explore how health professionals in charge of publicly oriented hospitals and health centre networks can contribute towards improving access to essential drugs within health services – drugs which were not being subsidized by the government or any other agency. The experience echoes the Bamako Initiative (1986–1996), a WHO- UNICEF programme to sustainably improve access to drugs and curative care in LMIC public services. It has since generated scores of publications – many in favour of continuing with patient payments, as part of the dominant policy paradigm covered in this book so far, while others who support universal health care provision have been vehemently against such a model. This paper thus departs from the hundreds of publications addressing the issue of the supply of medicines in LMICs by a managerial approach and a political concern for public services.

Nowadays, multilateral donor agencies do fund access to drugs in LICs and fragile states, although this access continues to remain quite poor. Twenty years previously, however, the situation was very different. In 1987 WHO and UNICEF launched the Bamako Initiative (BI), a joint programme in some 35 countries which aimed at securing a sustainable supply of drugs in MoH services. NGO health facilities were thus not targeted by the initiative. A second and equally important objective was to contribute towards making public services more democratic, while also promoting the community co-management of these services – which then as now continues to be resisted by professionals and civil servants (Morgan, 2001). The BI explicitly aimed at counter-balancing the power of civil servants and health professionals over users of services and communities where services were located (Diallo et al., 1996; Hanson & Gilson, 1993; Knippenberg et al., 1990). While this objective was certainly a laudable one, if the BI had addressed publicly oriented services as a whole instead of an exclusive focus on MoH facilities, and also hospitals instead of health centres only, it might have contributed to democratizing all of them.

The experience in Kolda, described here, did not depart totally from the essential features of the BI. In the latter, for example, an initial investment enabled the provision of essential and generic drugs to health centres. However, these were to be renewed through user fees. This investment was subject to the acceptance among health professionals of the need to rationalize prescriptions and to introduce co-management with community participation in their facilities. Consequently, the BI managerial tools addressed local financial and pharmaceutical management, organization of community participation, and rationalization of prescription (Newbrander et al., 2001). These relatively complex tasks were supposed to be routinely known amongst health service managers. However, the parameters of a district strategy that was to be conducted by district management teams were neither as well established nor as well known.

Over a period of 9 years, the BI markedly improved (Knippenberg et al., 1997) health services utilization in three countries. In Benin, where it was most successful, service utilization rates increased by a factor of 7 (Levy-Bruhl et al., 1997).[1] This result appeared paradoxical, especially to its opponents, since the BI was based on user fees. This paradox may be explained by the use of cheap, essential generic drugs and low prices on the international market obtained by purchasing large quantities of drugs. The total cost of sickness episodes to patients was therefore significantly lower than it would otherwise have been.

Pharmaceutical management in Kolda – public services in the 1980s

Kolda is the name both of a town (with a population of then 35,000) and a district (population 184,000). The district, which was predominantly agricultural, had a small 40-bed hospital, 15 government dispensaries, and a few catholic dispensaries. Financing of public services in Senegal largely depended on government funds and revenue from user fees. The former was grossly inadequate. Between 1982 and 1986 government contributions to Kolda health district remained at USD 0.05 per inhabitant per year. User fees were managed by local community committees and were also insufficient. Drug shortage was common, but this was also due to structural problems – an ineffective National Pharmacy organization, the difficulty of health districts to purchase drugs on international markets and poor local management. The key managerial weaknesses were as follows:

- The drug stock recovery rate, in theory permitted by user fees, was quite poor because only a small proportion (less than one-third) of these funds was spent on buying medicines.
- The list of medicines to be purchased was inefficient and included many injectable products and linctuses as well as substances of dubious benefit.
- Health centres bought many products from local retailers, at prices 5 or 10 times higher than charged by wholesalers in Dakar.
- In the health centres in which medicines were ordered on a monthly basis, the health committees tended to hoard their resources.

Management strategy

The strategic priority in Kolda district was to abolish the use of prescriptions issued by the hospital and dispensaries for the purchase of drugs at private pharmacies.

The key elements of the pharmaceutical strategy (described in Figure 18.3) included:

- establishing a limited stock of medicines;
- setting up (financial and pharmaceutical) management control systems;
- organizing a district pharmacy for the hospital and health centres. Stock record cards, with 'warning' levels for reordering based on rates of consumption and delivery times, were introduced in the district pharmacy. Ordering was based on monthly consumption rates;
- granting access to the pharmacy to the hospital services; and

---

[1] The BI failed in several other countries, due to nepotism and incompetence at district level – sometimes medicines intended for use by communities being sold privately. Such factors are likely to hamper any health policy and are not specific to the BI. Rather the community participation enabled by the BI permitted improved control on civil servants in many instances. In some the community representatives were themselves corrupt.

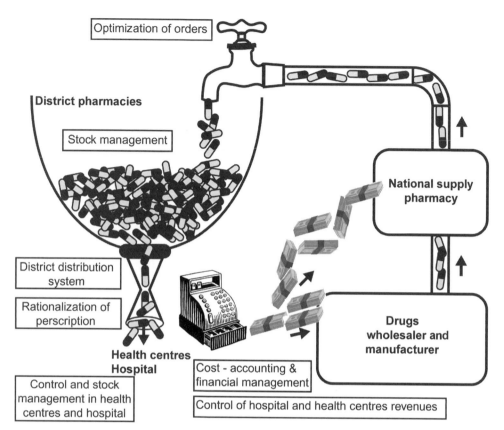

Figure 18.3. Visualizing the relations between components of the managerial strategy.

- extending this opportunity to the health centres as stock in the pharmacy increased, and upon acceptance of reforms by health centre staff.

The 'parameters' for rationalizing the prescription of drugs by health professionals were as follows:

- An accepted list of medicines was drawn up and negotiated with the district doctors.
- The hospital pharmacy was reorganized to a district pharmacy.
- Standardized therapeutic schemes for the commonest syndromes and symptoms were drawn up.
- Prescribers were trained to be empathic to their patients, and medicine stores were established in the various departments of the hospital.
- When all this had been done, hospitals stopped issuing prescriptions for use in private pharmacies, except where patients insisted on vitamins or injections and could not be persuaded otherwise.

Finances were also reorganized:

- Community activities (such as village dances, fairs and lotteries) and local government support made it possible to supplement the quite limited funds provided by the government for the purchase of medicines. Repayment of debts by the health district enabled some health centres to purchase considerable quantities of medicines.

- The district team also set limits for cash advances, introduced a system of auditing, and neutralized health centre committees who had been reluctant to spend their funds on drugs (community participation sometimes gives rise to misappropriation or 'freezing' of funds).
- Notice was given that during 12 months neither health centres' methods of management nor financing were changed (as were those of the hospital). During this period, they were not granted access to the district pharmacy in the hospital.

Results[2]

Progress varied in the different types of institutions – with the highest gain accruing to the district hospital. Expectedly, the increase in access to, and use of, the hospital was much greater than the rate for the health centres. In January 1988 the dispensary for major endemic diseases became the first recipient of a capital advance (literally a pump) for the purchase of medicines. Thanks to this, and also to good technical supervision, its volume of consultations showed a particularly sharp increase. Receipts from user fees in Kolda hospital between 1985 and 1987 showed that, in 2 years, revenue from this source nearly trebled. However, in spite of this substantial progress, the district's total revenue, expressed in francs per inhabitant per year, remained low. Finally, the increase in recurrent expenditure on medicines followed the total increase in revenues and, in the case of the hospital, the increase in the share of income devoted to medicines.

Discussion

Several lessons may be learned from the Kolda experience.

Lessons for local health systems management

The experience allowed the parameters of a district strategy for securing access to drugs in publicly oriented services to be more systematically organized.

The scheme stopped prescriptions being issued by publicly oriented facilities, for use in private pharmacies – a crucial factor in securing use of health services by the population as well as acceptance from health services staff to reform and improve the public services.

The experience showed that, in some instances, the reorganization of a second-line hospital can be the first stage in a strategy designed to improve access to drugs in the facilities network – while it is acknowledged that health centres are crucial to health development. The value of this approach lies in the amount of money released by reforms confined to one big institution. Its disadvantage is the risk of diverting patients resident in a town away from the health centres to the hospital. Counter-reference of patients should thus be planned at a later stage.

The rationalization of financing and of pharmaceutical management must take place simultaneously with the investment. This will mean that staff will see the need for financial control, a *sine qua non* condition to the sustainable supply of medicines. Also, an increase in tariffs without a simultaneous improvement in services proved unacceptable to the population.

The health service may be under-used for reasons other than shortage of medicines (see Section 6, Chapter 18, Part 1). Financial and pharmaceutical reorganization must therefore form part of a more complex district strategy. This complexity, as well as the quality of

---

[2] For detailed information on cash flows, utilization rates and other quantitative data, see the original article.

management required, makes it essential that district medical officers should have in-service public health training and receive technical supervision directed towards problem-solving.

The merging of pharmaceutical stocks in dispensaries and hospitals, as opposed to the separate sale of medicines, makes it possible to adopt a system of fees for sickness episodes, a method much more amenable to continuity of care than fee-for-service, and which reduces the risk of over-prescribing that is intended to increase the income of health professionals (Association pour la promotion de la santé de Pikine et al., 1988).

Lessons for national policies

The specific features of Senegalese health policy, which determined the successes and failures recorded in Kolda, may have lessons for other countries.

The district management team can transfer the benefits of the hospital to the health centres or, conversely, use incomes from the dispensaries to provide additional finance for the hospital. This possibility underlines the importance of having the district teams responsible for two tiers of the health system and of adopting a systemic management style.

The MoH must ensure that the district management team receives the technical supervision they require. This must be conceived as a tool for continuous education – not control. While control is needed, its mechanisms should be clearly separated.

The Ministry of Health or of Finance must give public service units freedom to manage the funds earned (together with user representatives). This local independence must not, however, be used as a pretext for cutting government contributions to district finances.

During the experience period, the increase in price was greater than the inflation rate in the case of many essential medicines (tetracycline, aspirin). The prices of non-essential medicines however had been reduced. Pricing was designed to maintain the drug companies' profits, i.e., to maintain the use of non-essential drugs. The supply of cheap medicines to districts depends on a consistent pharmaceutical policy: in particular a national supply pharmacy must be established; essential medicines must be free of tax; international invitations to tender must be even-handed, and the price of essential medicines must be negotiated with producers and importers.

The district also moderately increased its independence from government funding. However, in rural health centres, the improvement in supplies made possible by the release of hoarded resources and the repayment of the hospital's debts was of uncertain sustainability. Again, this shows the need for an effective, national supply system of essential generic drugs to hospitals and health centres belonging to the publicly oriented sector.

Rebuilding drug stocks and improving pharmaceutical management takes time. International cooperation should be adjusted to the pace of a district's development and should not seek to speed it up in order to comply with their external budgetary constraints.

The population had little confidence in community health workers (Walt et al., 1989) because their knowledge is often much the same as the empirical knowledge of lay community members. Priority in pharmaceutical investment should therefore go to professionally staffed health institutions. This is especially important in the context of revamped PHC, at a time where many academics re-interpret it as merely an additional, unprofessional layer in the health care pyramid. PHC is much more than that: it is meant to radically amend the structure and functioning of the entire health care system – starting from health centres and peripheral hospitals.

In Senegal, the temporary effect of intensive immunization campaigns and the inability of health centres to maintain proper levels of cover beyond the initial intensive phase have shown the inappropriateness of integrating specialized programmes in inappropriate circumstances (Unger, 1991). Recruitment of the target population should be achieved by continual contacts between the health service and individuals during curative consultation – designed to offer discretionary, individual health care – and with the community. In other words a sustainable access to general, essential drugs in publicly oriented services is needed to improve access to care and thus to disease-specific detection and prevention. It constitutes an alternative to the distribution of food (Loevinsohn & Loevinsohn, 1987) or propaganda designed to arouse enthusiasm for preventive activities (Manoff, 1985).

While improvements in pharmaceutical and financial management are a priority for all districts, this shouldn't be conceived as a vertical vision of the strengthening of health systems (Marchal et al., 2009; Smith & Bryant, 1988). Priorities must be decided at district level and may be different for each particular institution, e.g., to take account of local resources.

References

Association pour la promotion de la santé de Pikine, Coopération technique belge, & Ministère de la Santé du Sénégal. (1988). *Projet Pikine: soins de santé primaires en milieu urbain 1986–7*. Dakar, Senegal.

Diallo I., McKeown S., & Wone I. (1996). Bamako boost for primary care. *World Health Forum*, 17(4), pp. 382–5.

Hanson K. & Gilson L. (1993). *Cost, Resource Use and Financing Methodology for Basic Health Services*. A Practical Manual. New York: United Nations Children's Fund. N° 16.

Knippenberg R., Levy-Bruhl D., Osseni R., Drame K., Soucat A., & Debeugny C. (1990). The Bamako initiative: Primary health care experience. Children in the tropics: Review of the International Children's Centre. *Children in the Tropics*, 1990(No. 184–185), pp. 94.

Knippenberg R., Soucat A., Oyegbite K., et al. (1997). Sustainability of primary health care including expanded program of immunizations in Bamako initiative programs in West Africa: An assessment of 5 years' field experience in Benin and Guinea. *International Journal of Health Planning and Management*, 12, pp. S9–S28.

Levy-Bruhl D., Soucat A., Osseni R., et al. (1997). The Bamako initiative in Benin and Guinea: Improving the effectiveness of primary health care. *International Journal of Health Planning and Management*, 12(Supplement 1), pp. S49–S79.

Loevinsohn B. P. & Loevinsohn M. E. (1987). Well child clinics and mass vaccination campaigns: An evaluation of strategies for improving the coverage of primary health care in a developing country. *American Journal of Public Health*, 77(11), pp. 1407–11.

Manoff R. K. (1985). *Social Marketing: New Imperatives for Public Health*. Praeger: Abbey Publishing.

Marchal B., Cavalli A., & Kegels G. (2009). Global health actors claim to support health system strengthening: Is this reality or rhetoric? *PLoS Medicine*, 6(4), e1000059.

Morgan L. (2001). Community participation in health: Perpetual allure, persistent challenge. *Health Policy and Planning*, 16(3), pp. 221–30.

Newbrander W., Collins D., & Gilson L. (2001). *User Fees for Health Services: Guidelines for Protecting the Poor*. Boston: Management Sciences for Health.

Smith D. L. & Bryant J. H. (1988). Building the infrastructure for primary health care: An overview of vertical and integrated approaches. *Social Science & Medicine*, 26(9), pp. 909–17.

Unger J. P. (1991). Can intensive campaigns dynamise front line health services? The evaluation of an immunisation campaign in Thies health district, Senegal. *Social Science & Medicine*, 32(3), pp. 249–59.

Walt G., Perera M., & Heggenhougen K. (1989). Are large-scale volunteer community health worker programmes feasible? The case of Sri Lanka. *Social Science & Medicine*, 29(5), pp. 599–608.

Section 6
Chapter

19

A public health, strategic toolkit to implement these alternatives

Improving clinical decision making

Jean-Pierre Unger, I. Vargas and M. L. Vázquez

Part 1: Non-managed care techniques to improve clinical practice

Introduction

In recent years managed care became a promise of cost control and reduction of unnecessary services utilization, especially in countries with very limited resources. Most LMICs included it early in their reform packages (Tollman et al., 1990). In spite of scarce empirical evidence on the implementation of managed care techniques in this setting (Luck & Peabody, 2002) and intense debates surrounding their introduction in countries such as the USA (Christianson et al., 2005; Simonet, 2005), these techniques were increasingly exported to LMICs.

In this chapter we briefly analyze the results of the introduction of managed care techniques in different environments, explore issues related to the resulting loss of autonomy in clinical practice and offer alternative techniques to improve quality of health care.

What is managed care and what are its results?

The literature offers different approaches and definitions of managed care, probably because it does not convey one single, common concept, but a set of principles and interwoven practices (born in the 1980s in the USA to control costs).

Managed care techniques aim at providing incentives for productivity and efficiency while improving quality of services. They should be distinguished from the organizations which implement them. In this chapter we will attempt to focus on the former and address, in the first instance, clinical mechanisms designed to improve clinical decision making.

Clinical managed care techniques include (http://pohly.com): adjusted drug benefit lists; benchmarks (goals chosen by comparisons with other providers, by consulting statistical reports available, or drawn from the best practices within the organization or industry and used in quality improvement programmes to encourage improvement of care efficiency); standard case management and standard of care (diagnostic and treatment process that a clinician should follow for a certain type of patient, illness, or clinical circumstance); clinical or critical pathways (a 'map' of preferred treatment/intervention activities, which outlines the types of information needed to make decisions, the timelines for applying that information, and what action needs to be taken by whom, developed by clinicians for specific diseases or events); clinical practice guidelines (utilization and quality management mechanism designed to aid providers in making decisions about the most appropriate course of treatment for a specific clinical case); disease management (a coordinated system of preventive, diagnostic, and therapeutic measures intended to provide cost-effective, quality health care for a patient population who have or are at risk for a specific chronic illness or medical condition); formulary (an approved list of selected pharmaceuticals and their appropriate dosages felt to be the most useful and cost-effective for patient care); step therapy (drug plans may require an enrollee to try one drug before the plan will pay for another drug. Step therapy aims to control costs by requiring that enrollees use more common drugs which are usually less expensive).

Besides clinical tools, managed care techniques also include economic incentives for physicians and patients (e.g., to select less costly forms of care); audits of medical necessity of specific services; controls on inpatient admissions and lengths of stay; and selective contracting with health care providers.

As far as typology is concerned, some managed care techniques directly act upon demand (such as authorization to pay), while others modify the supply (utilization review; limits to prescription, tests, examinations and references; risk sharing; clinical guidelines; per capita payments; and gate keeping) (Vargas Lorenzo, 2009). A study (Remler et al., 1997) suggests that the key determinant in selecting one or another type of mechanism is the degree of integration between insurance and provision of health care. Where purchaser and provider functions are vertically integrated, the dominant mechanism is control of health care utilization with restrictions on medical practice. Where there is a split between purchaser and provider, demand modifiers which are to prevent excessive usage and capitation are favoured.

The advantages and disadvantages of managed care techniques may be summarized as follows (Vargas Lorenzo, 2009). Some authors (Landon et al., 2004) argue that these techniques contribute to organizations' efficiency in lowering premiums and co-payments, solving problems of information asymmetry, and improving care quality, e.g., with:

- control over resources use (Peiró, 2003);
- reduction of inappropriate demand (audits and authorization of examination requests);
- risk transfer from insurer to provider;
- rationalization of expenditure and prevention (Vargas, 2002).

Other authors emphasize the downside of managed care with limited access being the main problem (Gold, 1998). A literature review of studies comparing US managed care organizations with traditional insurance models (Miller & Luft, 2002) has shown that the former has a poorer record than the latter in securing access, on indicators such as:

- the proportion of enrollees with a regular source of care;
- difficulties to contact the usual care provider;
- difficulties to get an appointment;
- unmet needs; and
- necessity to travel more extensively to access health care.

On the other hand, compared to traditional health insurances, HMOs offered a wider coverage as both premiums and co-payments were lower (Miller & Luft, 2002). Numerous reviews have also shown negative opinions amongst US health professionals and insurance contributors (Christianson et al., 2005; Simonet, 2005). Mentioned difficulties included halting or prevention of the reimbursement of prescribed drugs, tests, admissions, references and longer waiting lists to consult specialists (Christianson et al., 2005; Simonet, 2005).

Yet another, but little studied, problem with managed care techniques is the loss of professionals' control and autonomy of clinical decision making, which is linked to the standardization of clinical practice – creating a motive for dissatisfaction amongst professionals, who have been compelled to use them (Mechanic, 2001). It has been argued that this form of standardization may harm the quality of care, because it limits the professional's capacity to adjust to unexpected patients' needs, which is not uncommon in health services (Shortell et al., 2009). The organization's theory maintains that normalization of work processes, skills and outputs are not appropriate to those uncertain situations – mobilizing interwoven or reciprocal sequences of professionals' interventions and requiring to process a large amount of information (Galbraith, 1973; Mintzberg, 1988). In health care environments such scenarios are numerous – unexpected changes in a patient's condition, variable response to medical intervention, co-pathology (Young et al., 1998) – when health care cannot be planned and is more effectively delivered where and when the information is issued.

As a conclusion, one could say that the technique is not the problem in itself, but the goals that are set and the context in which it is used. GPs operating as gate-keepers, for instance, can be used to improve access to the health care system and continuity of relationship (Starfield, 1998), as well as network efficiency (Ortún & Gervás, 1996). However, private insurers and managed care organizations such as HMOs do not use them to improve access, but rather to control references to specialists, admissions, and medical procedures and thereby control costs (Ellsbury et al., 1990). With regard to the context, mechanisms such as capitation fees could incentivize efficiency and integration of prevention and curative care in environments where providers' payment was based on fees for services, and as such, inducing demand. But in developing countries with low services productivity, these mechanisms may reduce the provision of necessary services, and at the end of the day, provoke health status deterioration and increase disease-related costs – more than in industrialized countries where, acknowledgedly, these undesirable outputs may also occur even with social security systems.

Managed care techniques are not only met in private organizations but also in public systems, where they may constrain access as well – probably when their objectives are unbalanced. For instance gate keeping can result in waiting lists even in (MoH) public services, when its objective is to control references to specialists and not to secure utilization of the most appropriate health care facility. Authorizations to pay do not only prevail in (privately managed) HMOs but also in social insurance and national health systems. Commercial private and social insurance organizations would then differ by the degree of access to care permitted rather than by the techniques used to rationalize it.

Therefore, at first glance, managed care techniques appear not specific to one particular organizational context. Furthermore, they may convey positive or negative effects according to the purpose of their utilization – whether it is mainly cost control in health care delivery or not, which is probably *more often* the case in commercial than in MoH environments.

We contend that this conclusion holds for economic incentives and organization techniques meant to control costs – they are 'neutral' so to speak – but that clinical techniques designed to improve care effectiveness and efficiency can be placed on a continuum between antipodes which will make them more or less prone to commercial versus social use – even if they cannot be clearly dichotomized.

Is there a criterion to analyze the techniques designed to improve clinical decision making, a criterion which helps distinguish those merely prone to be used in publicly oriented medical practice and organizations?

We consider one example of such a criterion – therapeutic freedom versus standardization – and the gradient between these two poles. We then analyze how the choice for each of them depends on the rationale of health care organizations and their context – amongst an otherwise effective regulatory environment.

Standardization of clinical decision making (under the form of clinical guidelines for instance) has been advocated for improving the problem-solving capacity of health care providers and control costs. In first-line services this is specially needed in contexts where GPs' tasks are shifted to nurses and medical assistants, as is generally the case in sub-Saharan Africa. However, this *may* run against the flexibility required to tackle unexpected patient needs, in particular bio-psychosocial needs met in family medicine practice, and demands as detected when delivering patient-centred care (Section 6, Chapter 17).

Besides, rationalization of clinical decision making may impact negatively on providers' motivation. The more clinical decisions are standardized, the less the care provider's freedom. Such freedom is of special importance to professionals because their identity has been forged throughout lengthy and difficult studies. When decision making becomes over-standardized, they often feel that their skills and judgement are under-used and that a computer could do the job as well.

However, at the side of financial incentives, the health professional's existential commitment is pivotal to guarantee the delivery of CHC. This is so true that forging this commitment is the *raison d'être* of medical ethics (be it Hippocratic or Ayurvedic) (Sharma & Dash, 2006) – while deontology looses relevance when clinical decisions are fully predictable.

While mainstream managed care techniques stress standardization as a tool of cost control, of contracting out, and ultimately of commodification, alternative techniques balancing rationalization of clinical decision making and therapeutic freedom are needed to secure a non-profit health care delivery and management (Section 5, Chapter 14). These are now examined.

Non-managed care techniques to improve clinical decision making: a practical guide

Clinical decision making

Problems with clinical decisions and their implementation in LMICs can be classified into two categories.

Firstly, manual skills of doctors and nurses are unevenly distributed in LMICs. For instance, some GPs can perform a caesarean section, while others do not even know how to insert an intra-uterine device, perform a nasal tamponage or incise a whitlow. In these regions few development projects have set out to improve the surgical skills of district hospital health professionals (Lett, 2000; Loutfi et al., 1995; Sohier et al., 1999) or to develop family practice (Atherton et al., 1999). In fact the vast majority of in-service training was restricted to disease-control interventions, usually building on agreed-upon standards. As in Europe (Grol et al., 1994) their common denominator has often been mechanistic, simple clinical criteria – as is often used in quality assurance (Björk et al., 1992; Forsberg et al., 2000; Omaswa et al., 1997).

Secondly, the signs, symptoms and tests that GPs and nurses use are more tailored to hospital settings than to first-line practice. However, the predictive values of the tests are a function of disease prevalence, which, for serious conditions, tends to be much lower in the GP's case mix than in the hospital.

To correct these weaknesses, some strategies are well established:

- In-service training supervision of junior doctors by experienced doctors via direct observation of consultations is pivotal to correcting individual weaknesses in clinical practice.
- Hospital rotations are useful to local know-how/do-how transfer. To maximize learning opportunities self-managed, 1-week spells in hospital wards can be structured as a list of manual techniques to be acquired versus learning progresses ('seen, done, known').
- Staff expected to use standards should be involved in the design of local adaptation of guidelines, algorithms and decision trees if they are to use them effectively.

There are also ad hoc techniques readily available such as:

- Intervision, which is a review of difficult cases management performed by peers to improve quality of care.
- The Internet now enables many district medical officers and hospital doctors to access evidence-based medical sites.
- An interactive training programme in tropical medicine exists on CD-ROM, which can be distributed to all doctors.[1]

Development of patient-centred care in first-line services

Strategies to improve patient–doctor interactions have proved effective in Europe (Liaw et al., 1996) as well as in developing countries (Henbest & Fehrsen, 1992). Here follows a summary of available techniques.

- GPs' biomedical approach to disease can be modified by sound theories on disease aetiology (to enlarge the scope of determinants beyond the biomedical) and by audit-oriented observations (to identify deficiencies in care) (Public Health Research and Training Unit of the ITM, 1989).
- One can teach GPs criteria for the quality of care, such as continuity,[2] the quest for patient autonomy, and the need to medicalize a problem (or not).
- In-service demonstration of patient-centred care should be offered to doctors in pilot facilities.
- Dialogue can become an intellectual challenge if relevant techniques are taught. Training in communication can rely on a psychiatrist with expertise in the doctor-patient relationship, and aide-mémoires of special patients' problems can be designed to systematically explore psychosocial and psychosomatic disorders (such as sexual problems, drug addiction, alcohol dependence). Personal experience of one of the authors in Ecuador (Section 6, Chapter 18), based on these strategies, showed changes in the care provider's willingness to deliver holistic care.

---

[1] This CD-Rom is distributed freely by the ITM to not-for-profit entities which demand it. Contact: Prof J. Van den Ende, Institute of Tropical Medicine, Department of Medicine, Nationalestraat 155, 2000 Antwerpen, Belgium.

[2] Tools to improve continuity of care for chronic patients include defaulters tracing systems (device for schedule of due dates, ad hoc home visits, improved doctor–patient communication, standardization of criteria to actively trace defaulters, communication lines with patients wherever they live), appropriate evaluation (e.g., with the Piot model); care free at the point of delivery or at least fee per sickness episode; ad hoc information system.

- Balint groups[3] permit the exchange of experiences and an analysis of how the doctor's feelings can interfere with case management. It remains to be seen whether these techniques are applicable to doctors in cultures that are not inclined to introspection, or whether other approaches, building upon traditional knowledge of social relationships, would be more relevant to the context of developing countries.
- Quantifiable methods of evaluating psychological care are achievable in general practice (Crossley et al., 1992).
- Problem-oriented medical records, such as the SOAP method,[4] can be used to structure the consultation (Weed, 1969).

Promotion of patient-centred care in hospital settings

Holistic nursing is the equivalent of patient-centred care in a hospital. Its promotion requires Taylorian organization – one specific task for each staff member – to be transformed in many hand-crafted workshops, similar to the work practices adopted by the Volvo Company in the 1980s. In each ward the most qualified residents (a nurse or an MD) can be responsible for a certain number of patients directly rather than for tasks. Their job involves making decisions in symptomatic (as opposed to aetiologic) treatments, psychological follow-up, coordinating with other professionals, planning hospital stays, monitoring clinical parameters and maintaining contact with families and first-line practitioners (Figure 19.1). Specialist doctors are then used as consultants to make diagnosis and treatment decisions. This model requires team-work, ad hoc training, supervision and evaluation to enable task delegation. It also requires enough nursing or resident staff and may therefore not be applicable

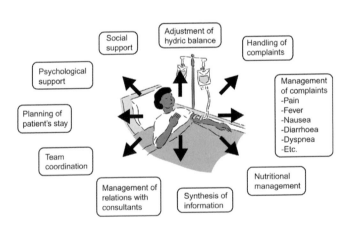

Figure 19.1. Tasks to be shifted to experimented nurses (and thus to be standardized, supervised and evaluated) in LMIC hospitals – to whom patients rather than tasks are delegated.

---

[3] A Balint group is a small group of caregivers who meet regularly for case discussion under the guidance of a qualified group leader, in order to better understand and make use of the caregiver–patient relationship in a therapeutic and professional way. The Balint method is called so in honour to the pioneering work of Michael and Enid Balint in the 1950s.
[4] SOAP is a problem-oriented method for making notes, whereby S stands for subjective data obtained from the care-seeker; O refers to objective data acquired by observation, inspection, or testing; A relates to the assessment of the patient's current situation and progress made throughout the course of treatment; and P represents the actual patient care plan.

in some rural hospitals. Holistic nursing schemes have succeeded in community nursing (Leedam, 1972; Simmons, 1975). AIDS programme managers and specialists were the first in the disease-control community to rediscover holistic, integrated nursing because of their staff needs (Bennett et al., 1995) and the specific bio-psychosocial care requirements of their patients (Pratt, 2003).

Coaching health professionals to secure continuing medical education and psychological support

Coaching health professionals adds to traditional continuing medical education (Sekerka & Chao, 2005):

- a possibility to assess individual and group learning needs, based on in-service observation and discussion of medical practice and health care;
- psychological support to professionals and teams; and
- organizational changes coordinated with in-service training.

Coaching relies on methodologies such as education-oriented supervision (which should not be understood as a control), intervision and action research (see Section 6, Chapter 18). Coaches are health professionals with lengthy experience of services organization who regularly visit a limited number of health centres and hospital wards and subtly attend clinical activities (with patient consent). Once they identify key problems, an agreement on a corrective approach is quested between supervisor and supervisee.

Conclusion

We suggested that the WHO concept of strengthening health systems with six building blocks lacks a commitment towards the delivery of CHC. The present chapter adds an array of techniques to improve related clinical skills as part and parcel of CHC.

These techniques depart from managed care practices (and indeed are, to our best knowledge, exceptionally used in commercial settings) by their preoccupation for a balance between rationalization of clinical decision making and doctors' therapeutic freedom. Such balance is needed because in many instances, standardization of clinical decision making will enhance the problem-solving capacity of doctors and nurses, while therapeutic freedom facilitates their professional identity and motivation to deliver care of good quality.

The existence of a gradient along this line between managed care and non-managed care techniques suggests that, in publicly oriented services, circumstances may justify the use of techniques which could be classed in the managed care category. For instance, dichotomous algorithms may be used to shift doctors' clinical responsibilities to nurses in African public services. They should be applied with flexibility, leaving room for bio-psychosocial care and negotiations with patients. Possibly, they could even be amended with the participation of their end users, namely doctors and nurses.

Although decent income, and possibly a mixture of incentives (fee for services, salary and capitation, as in the UK), are important to build professionals' motivation, the organization mission, the environment (in particular the national health policy and regulatory capacity), and non-managed care clinical techniques are central to secure access to CHC.

References

Atherton F., Mbekem G., & Nyalusi I. (1999). Improving service quality: Experience from the Tanzania family health project. *International Journal for Quality in Health Care*, 11(4), pp. 353–6.

Bennett L., Miller D., & Ross M. (1995). *Health Workers and AIDS: Research, Intervention and Current Issues in Burnout and Response*. Chur, Switzerland: Harwood Academic Publishers GmbH.

Björk M., Johansson R., & Kanji N. (1992). Improving the quality of primary care services in Angola. *Health Policy and Planning*, 7, pp. 290–5.

Christianson J. B., Warrick L. H., & Wholey D. R. (2005). Physicians' perceptions of managed care: A review of the literature. *Medical Care Research and Review*, 62(6), pp. 635–75.

Crossley D., Myres M. P., & Wilkinson G. (1992). Assessment of psychological care in general practice. *British Medical Journal*, 305(6865), pp. 1333–6.

Ellsbury K., Montano D., & Krafft K. (1990). A survey of the attitudes of physician specialists toward capitation-based health plans with primary care gatekeepers. *QRB Quality Review Bulletin*, 16(8), pp. 294–300.

Forsberg B., Barros F. C., & Victora C. G. (2000). Developing countries needs more quality assurance: How health facility surveys can contribute. *Revue de littérature*, pp. 193–6.

Galbraith J. R. (1973). *Designing Complex Organizations*. Boston: Addison-Wesley Longman Publishing Co.

Gold M. (1998). Beyond coverage and supply: Measuring access to health care in today's market. *Health Services Research*, 33(3), pp. 625–52.

Grol R., Baker R., Wensing M., & Jacobs A. (1994). Quality assurance in general practice: The state of the art in Europe. *Family Practice*, 11(4), pp. 460–7.

Henbest R. J. & Fehrsen G. S. (1992). Patient-centredness: Is it applicable outside the West? Its measurement and effect on outcomes. *Family Practice*, 9(3), pp. 311–7.

Landon B. E., Zaslavsky A. M., Bernard S. L., Cioffi M. J., & Cleary P. D. (2004). Comparison of performance of traditional Medicare vs. Medicare managed care. *Journal of the American Medical Association*, 291(14), pp. 1744–52.

Leedam E. J. (1972). *Community Nursing Manual: A Guide for Auxiliary Public Health Nurses*. Singapore: McGraw-Hill.

Lett R. (2000). Canadian network for international surgery: Development activities and strategies. *Canadian Journal of Surgery*, 43(5), pp. 385–7.

Liaw S. T., Young D., & Farish S. (1996). Improving patient-doctor concordance: An intervention study in general practice. *Family Practice*, 13(5), pp. 427–31.

Loutfi A., McLean A. P., & Pickering J. (1995). Training general practitioners in surgical and obstetrical emergencies in Ethiopia. *Tropical Doctor*, 25(Supplement 1), pp. 22–6.

Luck J. & Peabody J. W. (2002). When do developing countries adopt managed care policies and technologies? Part II: Infrastructure, techniques, and reform strategies. *American Journal of Managed Care*, 8(12), pp. 1093–103.

Mechanic D. (2001). The managed care backlash: Perceptions and rhetoric in health care policy and the potential for health care reform. *Milbank Quarterly*, 79(1), p. 35.

Miller R. H. & Luft H. S. (2002). HMO plan performance update: An analysis of the literature, 1997–2001. *Health Affairs (Millwood)*, 21(4), pp. 63–86.

Mintzberg H. (1988). *La Estructura De Las Organizaciones*. Barcelona: Ariel Economía.

Omaswa F., Burnham G., Baingana G., Mwebesa H., & Morrow R. (1997). Introducing quality management into primary health care services in Uganda. *Bulletin of the World Health Organization*, 75(2), pp. 155–61.

Ortún V. & Gervás J. (1996). Fundamentos y eficiencia de la atención médica primaria. *Médicina Clínica (Barcelona)*, 106(3), pp. 97–102.

Peiró S. (2003). De la gestión de lo complementario a la gestión integral de la atención de salud: gestión de enfemedades e indicadores de actividad. In: Ortún V., ed. *Gestión Clínica y Sanitaria*. Barcelona: Masson, pp. 17–89.

Pratt R. (2003). *HIV and AIDS: A Foundation for Nursing and Healthcare Practice*. London: Hodder Arnold.

Public Health Research and Training Unit of the ITM. (1989). The training of district medical officers in the organisation of health services: A methodology tested in Senegal. *Health Policy and Planning*, **4**, pp. 148–56.

Remler D. K., Donelan K., Blendon R. J., et al. (1997). What do managed care plans do to affect care? Results from a survey of physicians. *Inquiry-the Journal of Health Care Organization Provision and Financing*, **34**(3), pp. 196–204.

Sekerka L. E. & Chao J. (2005). Peer coaching as a technique to foster professional development in clinical ambulatory settings. *Journal of Continuing Education in the Health Professions*, **23**(1), pp. 30–7.

Sharma R. K. & Dash V. B. (2006). *Caraka Samhita*. Varanasi, Chowkamba Press.

Shortell S. M., Gillies R. R., Anderson D. A., Erickson K. M., & Mitchell J. B. (2009). *Remaking Health Care in America*. 2nd edn. San Fransisco: Jossey-Bass.

Simmons J. A. (1975). *Nursing Psychiatrique: Guide De Relation Infirmière-Client*. Montréal: Éditions HRW.

Simonet D. (2005). Patient satisfaction under managed care. *International Journal of Health Care Quality Assurance Incorporating Leadership in Health Services*, **18**(6–7), pp. 424–40.

Sohier N., Frejacques L., & Gagnayre R. (1999). Design and implementation of a training programme for general practitioners in emergency surgery and obstetrics in precarious situations in Ethiopia. *Annals of the Royal College of Surgeons of England*, **81**(6), pp. 367–75.

Starfield B. (1998). Primary Care. *Balance Between Healthcare Needs, Services and Technology*. New York: Oxford University Press.

Tollman S., Schopper D., & Torres A. (1990). Health maintenance organisations in developing countries: What can we expect? *Health Policy and Planning*, **5**(2), pp. 149–60.

Vargas Lorenzo I.(2009). *Barreras en el acceso a la atención en salud en modelos de competencia gestionada: un estudio de caso en Colombia, Bellaterra*, España: Universidad Autónoma de Barçalona.

Vargas L. I. (2002). La utilización del mecanismo de asignación per cápita: la experiencia de Cataluña. *Cuadernos de Gestión*, **8**(4), pp. 167–78.

Weed L. L. (1969). *Medical Records, Medical Education and Patient Care*. Chicago: Year Book Medical Publishers.

Young G. J., Charns M. P., Desai K., et al. (1998). Patterns of coordination and clinical outcomes: A study of surgical services. *Health Services Research*, **33**(5), pp. 1211–36.

Part 2: Interface flow process audit. The patient's career as tracer of quality of care and system: an experience from Belgium

Adapted from: Unger J.-P., Marchal B., Dugas S., Wuidar M. J., Burdet D., Leemans P., Unger J. Interface flow process audit: using the patient's career as a tracer of quality of care and of system organisation. International Journal of Integrated Care May 2004; Vol. 4. ISSN 1568–4156 – http://www.ijic.org/.

Introduction

The technique presented here is a reflexive, versatile method which produces several advantages from a public health perspective. It helps to improve the quality of care and rationalize the organization of local health services, especially the cooperation between primary and secondary care professionals. It enables clinicians to realize that they are working within a system and that many patients require a continuum of care. It helps them to be self-critical and reflective about their own decisions and to enter into a continuous process of improvement. Also it identifies local weaknesses in knowledge dissemination and in the general organization of health services.

Several drawbacks attached to tracer condition and selected procedure audits oblige clinicians to rely on external evaluators. Interface flow process audit is an alternative method enhancing integration of health care across institutions and is useful for regular in-service self-evaluation. Bridging the primary-secondary care gap, the interface flow process audit's focus on the patient's career combined with the broad scope of problems that can be analyzed are particularly powerful features.

The following paper presents this methodology, created to permanently improve health service organization through the identification of clinical deficiencies. In such audits the patient career serves as tracer of the weaknesses of the system.

In recent years, quality of care has become a top priority on the policy agenda in many countries. In the UK this concern resulted in the introduction of the clinical governance concept (Shekelle, 2002). Although audit has been firmly established as a key element of clinical governance in the National Health Service (NHS) and in various quality assurance initiatives in other countries, audits in which the audit loop is effectively closed remain rather rare (Gnanalingham et al., 2001). Indeed, despite the enthusiasm of policy makers for quality assurance and improvement, health professionals in all countries and across all types of health systems found it hard to support these efforts (Shekelle, 2002).

Background

The barriers to implementing effective audits have been well described: lack of resources, lack of expertise or support in audit design, problematic relationships between audit team members, and organization-related impediments (lack of cooperation between management and clinicians, lack of clarity about lines of authority and accountability, lack of time and organizational culture). Other factors include divergent views of the participants on the objectives of audit and their general attitude towards audit (Baker et al., 1995; Berger, 1998; Johnston et al., 2000;

Szecsenyi, 1996). Shekelle summarizes it well: resistance to quality improvement programmes is rooted in the professionals' distrust of the criteria by which quality is measured; the perception that audit and other quality improvement initiatives primarily aim at blaming health professionals and the fact that resources almost never follow responsibility to take on additional time-consuming duties (Shekelle, 2002). But as important, the author points to the fact that there are no role models on how to implement effective quality improvement programmes.

The manner and degree to which professionals of different levels are involved in audit may have an influence on the degree of ownership and usefulness of the results. Medical audit was conceived in the USA as an instrument to assist health professionals to analyze and evaluate clinical care. Initially, in one-way audit – an external form of audit – specialists of one group investigated the quality of care offered by another group (Baker, 1994). The literature offers numerous examples of one-way audits of general practice, led by specialists (for example in obstetrics [Bryce et al., 1990], diabetes [Singh et al., 1984], and hypertension [Bulpitt et al., 1982] and vice-versa). Clinical audit, where multidisciplinary teams of health professionals aim to improve the quality of care, may be more effective in bringing about change within organizations by surpassing the narrow borders of specific specialities.

Also, the focus and range of the audit design may have consequences for its relevance from a systems perspective. Clinical microsystems can be defined as small groups of health professionals and providers responsible for the care for a well-defined population. The structure and strategies of microsystems have an influence on health system performance and on patient outcomes. Despite this, management of health care human resources mostly focus on the individual level, or on the level of work units defined by professional occupation, when dealing with design of units or analysis of performance (Mohr & Batalden, 2002).

Specific features

The interface flow process audit (IFPA) integrates two models of audit. Creating links across the primary and secondary care interface is getting increasingly more attention in industrial countries, as it is recognized that improved streamlining of the patients' careers may have a positive impact both on quality of care and on cost containment (Kvamme et al., 2001; Szecsenyi, 1996). This concern is taken into account by the interface audit component, that has been defined as 'complete audit cycles conducted by professionals from both primary and secondary care working together as a team to improve quality' (Wright & Wilkinson, 1996). Any aspect of the interface between first line and second line can be the subject of audit: referral systems, coordinating chains of care and communication between hospitals and general practitioners (Eccles et al., 1996).

This type of audit may potentially strengthen the clinical microsystems, in that its health professionals analyze the journey of the patient through the system in order to improve quality of care.

The second component of interface flow process audit is based on the flow-process model, which is used to identify the hurdles a patient meets during his journey through the health system. As such it should add the patient's perspective to the auditing process. 'The stages in the patient's use of the service are broken down into steps. The problems a patient may encounter at each step are identified, studied and solutions looked for. This emphasis on the patient's perspective makes flow process audit particularly valuable' (WHO Working Group of Quality Assurance, 1994). We would, however, say it offers the patient's perspective rather indirectly, as the patient is usually not participating in person.

The IFPA uses critical incidents as an entry point for auditing local health systems. Critical incidents, sometimes referred to as significant events, are unforeseen, rare and not necessarily negative events occurring in the course of a case management (Kasongo Project Team, 1981; Westcott et al., 2000). Their detection and analysis may allow systematic failures of a process or an organization to be identified, similar to the principles underlying root cause analysis, a technique widely used in the US health care industry and non-health care industries to find and eliminate the cause of a quality problem in an effort to prevent its recurrence. The interface flow process audit has already been used to improve the quality of patient care in different settings (Kasongo Project Team, 1981), but to our knowledge not yet as a method to improve (local) health system organization.

The Belgian experience

In practice, the IFPA required the establishment of a team of hospital physicians of a general hospital in Brussels and general practitioners regularly referring patients to this hospital (Unger et al., 2003). This team greatly coincided with an existing clinical microsystem. The number of participants varied between 3 and 20 attendants per session. Initially, a public health specialist experienced in general health service organization would be the best person to lead the audits. Their role was to facilitate and introduce the audit methodology, to encourage critical questioning of the actual process and the integration of public health criteria in decision making, and finally to advise the team on organizational changes to improve quality of care and service organization.

A technical support and coordination team was established to follow up the proposed changes, to check their implementation, and to prepare the audit meetings. This team met monthly and included local general practitioners, some (referral hospital) specialists, and a public health coach. The patient's case analysis required from one to three 1-hour sessions. The following are the questions examined during the flow process audit.

First-line health and non-health services

Was there any delay in the patient getting a consultation? Was the care offered comprehensive, in particular bio-psychosocial? Was the care continuous? How has the independence of the patient been enhanced by the process? How was the suffering of the patient dealt with? Was the patient appropriately derived to the hospital? Was a proper differential diagnosis defined? Was the care effective and efficient? Was an appropriate team of professionals managing the case? Were non-medical (social and psychological) services adequately used? What services were used following discharge? How was prevention and promotion personalized for this patient?

Clinical decision making and diagnosis

Which tests were of doubtful usefulness? Which tests were forgotten? Are there reasons to believe that some tests were carried out badly (paradoxical results, for example). Were there any cheaper alternatives that should have been considered? Were the signs and symptoms strong enough to make a diagnosis? Were certain laboratory tests or medical imaging unnecessary? Was the use of tests during the course of the illness justified by the illness? Are there reasons to suspect false positives (for example, ineffective treatment) or false negatives (diagnosis delayed, unexplained death, repeated tests with conflicting results)? Considering the symptoms, were the important diseases eliminated (those dangerous, not spontaneously self-limiting diseases, causing considerable suffering or leading to death)? Were evidence-based medicine sites and the literature in general used?

Choice of treatment

What was the hypothetical diagnosis? What result was one hoping to achieve? Was there consistency between the treatment and the diagnosis? Was treatment up to the norms described in the literature? Did one forget to deal with the suffering and problems experienced by the patient by concentrating solely on the aetiology of suffering? How effective was the treatment (side effects – iatrogenic – avoidable?)? Did an avoidable complication, a sequel, or a death occur? Could the same result have been achieved more rapidly? What were the signs and symptoms used to evaluate this? Was there any scope for reducing medication (duplication and doubtful efficacy of certain drugs)? Were there cheaper alternatives to the drugs used?

Nursing

Were there any critical incidents that might suggest poor quality of nursing (treatment badly or incompletely administered, delay in the execution of orders, sterilization errors, and nosocomial infections)? Were there any known psychological problems that could have been avoided with better nursing care?

Type of hospital admission

Was admission delayed? Was the length of stay too short or too long? What could have been done to reduce the length of stay (better collaboration from the family, improving equipment at the primary care level, better work organization and earlier access to a specialist)? Was the choice of department (emergency ward, outpatient clinic, medical ward, surgical ward) appropriate? What measures were taken on discharge of the patient? How can the hospital contribute to strengthening primary care in order to improve the quality of the implementation of these measures?

Global evaluation of the results

How to assess the treatment results (outpatient follow-up, at primary care, or hospital level) in terms of the general state of the patient (deceased, cured, appropriate continuing care) and of the evolution of the dominant symptom (disappeared, improved, identical, increased)? With hindsight, was the treatment useful? (in other words does the hospital offer techniques also available to general practitioners or health centres?) With hindsight, what were the justifications for admission? Could a better result have been obtained had there been better collaboration from the family? Better equipment? Training for the doctor? Easier access to a specialist? Better work organization? Preliminary operational research? Technical supervision? Was the psychological distress properly addressed?

Examples of shortcomings identified by IFPA with one patient audit

These are some of the shortcomings identified at different levels during a particular audit led in Brussels in 2003. Considering quality of clinical care, it showed that in the clinical decision making process not enough attention was paid to the patient's complaints and symptoms. Non-relevant tests, with a long waiting list, contributed to an unacceptable length of stay. As to service organization, identified weaknesses include delays in delivering urgent results to general practitioners, inefficient use of diagnostic tests (automatic request of D-dimer test, inappropriately used Leg Ultrasound Scan, uninformative ventilation/perfusion scan results), the use of an inappropriate laboratory technique (latex D-dimer test), and inadequate training of staff in the emergency unit. This analysis was followed by measures to improve quality of care: differentiating urgent from non-urgent tests regarding the results feedback sent by the hospital laboratory to the general practitioners, the introduction of enzyme-linked immunosorbent D-dimer tests, and the standardization of reporting of ventilation/perfusion scan results. The interface flow process audit enabled some gaps between actual medical practice and best practice to be filled by continuing medical education in areas such as clinical epidemiology, rationalization of disease control, and utilization of evaluation criteria (cost-efficiency, patient's viewpoint, and uncertainty).

Synthesis: How to assess the measures undertaken to correct or improve the system?

Conclusion

IFPA thus offers a number of theoretical advantages over traditional designs of audit. It enables a comprehensive evaluation of quality of care, allowing identification of a wide range of problems across organizational borders, as opposed to the tight focus of tracer condition audit. The interface flow process audit proved to be an initiative that 'usefully explores the possibilities of supporting development of guideline-retrieval systems customized for individual general practitioners or practices' (Langley et al., 1998). This too contrasts with tracer condition audit, which often results in an unmanageable amount (Hibble et al., 1998) of insufficiently used (Christakis & Rivara, 1998; Grol et al., 1998) guidelines, designed without the involvement of their users.

Participants generally confirm that the IFPA helps them to analyze the quality of case management both at primary and secondary care level. This suggests that the method avoids one category of professionals (for instance general practitioners) being judged by another (specialists) on the basis of standards that are not shared by both parties. Furthermore, improved contacts between general practitioners and hospital specialists help to strengthen local care structures. Bridging the primary-secondary care gap, its focus on the patient's career combined with the broad scope of problems that can be analyzed are powerful features.

References

Baker R. (1994). What is interface audit? *Journal of the Royal Society of Medicine*, **87**(4), pp. 228–31.

Baker R., Robertson N., & Farooqi A. (1995). Audit in general practice: Factors influencing participation. *British Medical Journal*, **311**(6996), pp. 31–4.

Berger A. (1998). Why doesn't audit work? [editorial]. *British Medical Journal*, **316**(7135), pp. 875–6.

Bryce F. C., Clayton J. K., Rand R. J., Beck I., Farquharson D. I., & Jones S. E. (1990). General practitioner obstetrics in Bradford [published erratum appears in BMJ 1990 May 26; 300(6736): 1394]. *British Medical Journal*, **300**(6726), pp. 725–7.

Bulpitt C. J., Daymond M. J., & Dollery C. T. (1982). Community care compared with hospital outpatient care for hypertensive patients. *British Medical Journal (Clinical Research Ed)*, **284**(6315), pp. 554–6.

Christakis D. A. & Rivara F. P. (1998). Pediatricians' awareness of and attitudes about four clinical practice guidelines. *Pediatrics*, **101**(5), pp. 825–30.

Eccles M. P., Deverill M., McColl E., & Richardson H. (1996). A national survey of audit activity across the primary-secondary care interface. *Quality in Health Care*, **5**(4), pp. 193–200.

Gnanalingham J., Gnanalingham M. G., & Gnanalingham K. K. (2001). An audit of audits: Are we completing the cycle? *Journal of the Royal Society of Medicine*, **94**(6), pp. 288–9.

Grol R., Dalhuijsen J., Thomas S., Veld C., Rutten G., & Mokkink H. (1998). Attributes of clinical guidelines that influence use of guidelines in general practice: Observational study. *British Medical Journal*, **317**(7162), pp. 858–61.

Hibble A., Kanka D., Pencheon D., & Pooles F. (1998). Guidelines in general practice: The new Tower of Babel? *British Medical Journal*, **317**(7162), pp. 862–3.

Johnston G., Crombie I. K., Davies H. T., Alder E. M., & Millard A. (2000). Reviewing audit: Barriers and facilitating factors for effective clinical audit. *Quality in Health Care*, **9**(1), pp. 23–36.

Kasongo Project Team(1981). Le Projet Kasongo; une expérience d'organisation d'un soins de santé primaires. *Annales de la Société Belge de Médecine Tropicale*, **60**(S1), pp. 1–54.

Kvamme O. J., Olesen F., & Samuelson M. (2001). Improving the interface between primary and secondary care: A statement from the European Working Party on Quality in Family Practice (EQuiP). *Quality in Health Care*, **10**(1), pp. 33–9.

Langley C., Faulkner A., Watkins C., Gray S., & Harvey I. (1998). Use of guidelines in primary care – practitioners' perspectives. *Family Practice*, **15**(2), pp. 105–11.

Mohr J. J. & Batalden P. B. (2002). Improving safety on the front lines: The role of clinical microsystems. *Quality & Safety in Health Care*, **11**(1), pp. 45–50.

Shekelle P. G. (2002). Why don't physicians enthusiastically support quality improvement programmes? *Quality & Safety in Health Care*, **11**(1), pp. 6.

Singh B. M., Holland M. R., & Thorn P. A. (1984). Metabolic control of diabetes in general practice clinics: Comparison with a hospital clinic. *British Medical Journal (Clinical Research Ed)*, **289**(6447), pp. 726–8.

Szecsenyi J. (1996). Improving care at the primary-secondary care interface: A difficult but essential task. *Quality in Health Care*, **5**(4), pp. 191–2.

Unger J. P., Criel B., Dugas S., Van der Vennet J., & Roland M. (2003). Workshop 13: EUPHA section on health services research: In search of best innovations: Comparative methods in health services research. The Local Health Systems (LHS) project in Belgium [Abstract]. *European Journal of Public Health*, **13**(4), p. 26.

Westcott R., Sweeney G., & Stead J. (2000). Significant event audit in practice: A preliminary study. *Family Practice*, **17**(2), pp. 173–9.

WHO Working Group of Quality Assurance. (1994). *Report of the WHO working group on quality assurance*. Geneva: WHO. WHO/SHS/DHS/94.5.

Wright J. & Wilkinson J. (1996). General practitioners' attitudes to variations in referral rates and how these could be managed. *Family Practice*, **13**(3), pp. 259–63.

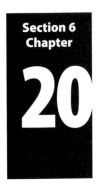

**Section 6
Chapter**

20

A public health, strategic toolkit to implement these alternatives

Reorienting academic missions: how can public health departments and public health teaching in particular best support access to good quality comprehensive health care?

Adapted from: Jean-Pierre Unger, Patrick Van Dessel. Teaching and training of health professionals. Health and Development. July 2009, special issue. 'Equal opportunities for health: Action for development.' Conference. CUAMM, Padova, June 2009–06–16A: 50–55.

Introduction

Improving the autonomy of LMIC health sectors from donor dependence and influence requires not only sufficient government financing, but also the broadening and transfer of knowledge within these countries. The managerial skills to run publicly oriented services and the conceptual framework needed by them to assess health policies were the subject of Sections 5 and 6. In Chapter 19 we explored some techniques of knowledge transfer from hospitals to health centres and vice-versa. In this final chapter of this section we examine how academic and public health departments can best contribute to the break from commercially motivated health policies, in preparing health professionals in publicly oriented services to improve access to comprehensive care.

Schools of public health, especially those concerned with LMIC, rarely treat health care delivery and medicine as a priority domain of study. Rather, they tend to concentrate on disease control and focus on policies related to this, and therefore teach in the main epidemiology, demography, statistics, and management of disease-specific programmes and their resources.

This is no mean paradox, since recent studies show that access to comprehensive care is probably the most important determinant of health. For instance, among women in Poland, up to 80% of premature deaths were related to conditions amenable to medical care (Nolte et al., 2002).

Nowadays, some authors put at up to 30 years life expectancy gains attributable to preventive and curative health services in the USA during the twentieth century (Shapiro, 2005). In industrialized countries, with improvements in public health (both environmental interventions and prevention) largely completed, medical care became undisputedly the major determinant of life expectancy (Bunker, 2001).

In practice, these arguments amount to a plea for schools of public health to bridge the gap that has traditionally split public health and medicine. In the present chapter we will provide an overview of the content of such public health courses which address medicine and CHC in the main, elaborate on their pedagogic methods, and describe the type of practice and research needed to consolidate links between teaching and practice. Finally, we will identify obstacles to relevant public health knowledge management and its production in an academic environment.

Public health management

In this chapter we call 'public health management' (PHM) a body of knowledge that could be used in order to contribute to universal access to quality comprehensive care and to develop those health services expected to deliver them.

Since universal access to CHC is mainly a stated LMIC government objective, health professionals who endorse this objective feel a moral obligation as citizens to try and influence national health policies. They cannot be satisfied with being only the executers of policies and plans to such professionals, and the desire to influence national policy is a managerial issue, just as is the optimization of the use of resources. While the audience of public health courses are often health system managers and policy makers, PHM courses in our view should be open to any health professional who wants to amend health services and systems from wherever they are posted, since ultimately they are likely to be able to influence how health care is delivered on the basis of evidence and experience.

For their part, good policy makers should strive to design policy as part of a cycle which includes regulation, control, and health care delivery (a 'top-down' approach, in combination with an assessment of the policy implementation, a 'bottom-up' phase).

Since this view allocates policy responsibilities to field practitioners and managerial ones to policy makers, it blurs the borders between health care management and policy – which is why health management and policy should be taught together.

Content overview of courses in public health management

The objectives of most such courses may be described as aiming at preparing health professionals to understand, apply, and promote the principles of PHM in improving access to and quality of comprehensive care delivery, developing publicly oriented services and in influencing national policies. The courses also encourage professionals to learn how to control and regulate health services with commercial activities. In practice graduates of such courses should thus be capable of analyzing real life health services and to design and implement strategies to develop local health systems in different environments.

The competencies required by health professionals to promote not-for-profit health services and systems – ex-students of public health management courses (Buron et al., 1995) – may be classified into four different levels as described by Malglaive, an authority in adult pedagogy (Malglaive, 1990).

Theoretical knowledge

The PHM theoretical knowledge is made of a distinct set of quality criteria (Section 5) which reflects publicly oriented values and system thinking. Because these criteria are inter-related, their sum can be viewed as a reference analytical framework for health system analysis rooted in history. For instance, the balance between Bismarckian and Beveridgean financing in European health systems has to be understood in the light of social and political factors. The consequences of these mechanisms on the quality of care can be analyzed using the standards described in Section 5, Chapter 14, as well as with criteria specific to neoclassic economics, for instance. Alongside the determinants of health systems, theoretical knowledge also describes research methods (e.g., action- and operational research).

Practical knowledge

Professionals require concepts and a theoretical framework to reduce uncertainty and enhance their creativity and efficiency in decision making. The teaching strategies are adapted to local situations and aim to complement their experience and sense of responsibility. The practical knowledge is made of a meta-theory of such strategies or meta-strategies (Mintzberg et al., 1998). They can be described and assessed, and are specific to principles (Section 5, Chapter 12). These meta-strategies adjust objectives to available resources by a sequence of analysis, decision, action, and evaluation. For instance, it is possible to classify the expected output of district (general) hospitals at the level of public expenditure on health. Meta-strategies consider relevant elements in an environment where the configuration of the health system is the most important element. For instance, those strategies designed to strengthen health services will not be identical in professional bureaucracies and divisionalized health systems (Section 5, Chapter 13). Consider the following example.

> The link between health services and the population.
> In France, Belgium, and Germany, there is no attempt to stabilize the relationship between a patient and his/her doctor (except on occasions where financial incentives are provided to GPs to hold patient files). In The Netherlands and the UK people are obliged to select a doctor for a defined period of time. In Costa Rica the same is defined by a map of geographical coverage. In the USA clients of HMOs, on the other hand, have to use a limited number of health centres and hospitals.

Finally, meta-strategies also address the management of several resources together – as in the Bamako Initiative (Section 6, Chapter 18, Part 2) or in hospital management.

Empirical knowledge

The PHM empirical knowledge helps to implement health interventions and specific managerial procedures. This knowledge is needed to design detailed strategies (e.g., antenatal care in Chad or in Chile; care to chronic patients and defaulters tracing systems in France or in Vietnam; introduction of family files in GP practice in Cuba or in Ecuador). Ideally, the design of such strategies should rely on the use of action research and be preceded by field tests.

Know-how

The know-how enables the gathering of attitudinal and manual skills – which cannot be described purely through written instruction. They are needed in the delivery of care (e.g., to perform a caesarean section or to deliver a patient-centred care consultation) and management (e.g., in supervising family doctors).

These four levels of competencies are not sequential but rather inter-linked, which is why PHM courses need to offer a mix of them (Figure 20.1).

Professional and academic competencies

We now examine why public health students require a mix of professional training and academic teaching and why, subsequently, teachers of public health should be continuously, and

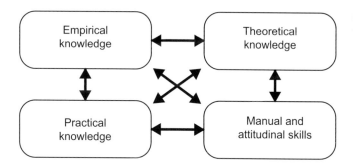

Figure 20.1. Relationships of Malglaive's categories of knowledge.

actively, involved also in the delivery of health care and have knowledge of the management of organizations.

The term 'academic' refers to knowledge produced by scientific methods. Traditional clinical epidemiology is an example of academic knowledge. It helps, for instance, to know the sensitivity, specificity, and predictive values of a sign (e.g., Lassègue sign in the diagnosis of meningitis) or a symptom (e.g., chronic cough in the diagnosis of pulmonary tuberculosis).

The term 'professional' applies to knowledge used in professional practice. It is produced by repeated experience. When semi-quantitative methods in clinical epidemiology are used to define thresholds justifying the use of a medical test or an image (X-ray, scan), they fall in the professional domain. Other examples are provided by the management of a district (made up of a network of health centres and a referral hospital) or psychiatric care.

In PHM, four essential features characterize professional knowledge:

- Concepts that are being taught need to be meaningful for action. In other words they should help health managers to practice what they preach: to implement their own decisions, as well as those made by communities and/or by 'decision makers.'
- Theory and practice – from the teacher's viewpoint, explaining knowledge merely drawn from books and papers may be insufficient. He/she should have real life experience if they are to identify relevant problems, be credible and be able to illustrate concepts in relation to practice. Thus, teachers of PHM in ideal circumstances should continue to be involved in health services and policy circles throughout their professional career. In general relevant concepts and examples can thus be derived from personal attempts to change an organization or a policy, from praxis.
- Defining strategy – illustrations from a wide variety of situations allows the domain of relevance of a particular strategy to be more clearly defined. In order to assess strategies inputs, processes and outputs, reflexive methods (such as audits and evaluation indicators) are needed but not necessarily in the realms of scientific demonstration.
- Professional knowledge will often require field demonstrations and visits to pilot health care services.

In conclusion, three out of the four public health competencies are professional in essence, belonging to the realms of the empirical, practical knowledge and know-how – a context that is often unrecognized.

The fourth competency, 'theoretical knowledge,' is the only purely academic knowledge. It has also specific relevance in PHM:

- It builds on inter-disciplinary, rather than multi- or mono-disciplinary teaching (Morin, 1979). For instance, economics alone will not provide satisfactory tools to study and enhance the motivation of health professionals: the professional culture also needs to be addressed – by sociological methods, for example.
- It builds on human sciences methods.
- When directed to adults, even the teaching of academic knowledge (say, epidemiology) cannot be merely ex-cathedra. The professional background and experience of students should be used as the raw material for a course enhanced by group work, participatory teaching, and problem-based learning. These pedagogic methods will increase the likelihood that concepts that are taught will be translated into practice.

In conclusion, it may be said that the transmission of health management and policy know-how loses its relevancy when academic teaching is not linked to professional training. As stated by Mintzberg, 'Were management a science or a profession, we should teach it to people without experience. It is neither' (Mintzberg, 2004).

Acquiring relevant knowledge

Figure 20.2 provides a meta-model which summarizes the strategic choices to be made by public health academic units to produce knowledge, while at the same time attempting to influence health care delivery, its management and, as the theme of this book, its policy.

What then is the best way of defining research priorities in PHM? The most important criterion is that the research projects should contribute to the development of the health services and/or policies where they are undertaken within a public health department. Research projects should also be geographically and functionally complementary to each other and progressively cover all clinical, managerial and social action aspects of health service organization and policy.

Health-systems research has very particular features that serve as the basis for its workability. We have argued that this is often not fully appreciated within the biomedical research community. Health-systems management differs from mere disease control in that it addresses a much wider array of decisions and resources as well as political and social influences. This difference leads us to three epistemological considerations.

Firstly, health-systems research needs to address strategic management – an academic discipline already established in business and public administration (Mintzberg et al., 1998).

Secondly, strategic models contributing to system analysis and managerial decision making are usefully derived from scientific management (Meyer, 2000). To study and rationalize managerial and clinical decisions (Barker, 1995) action research (Section 6, Chapter 18)

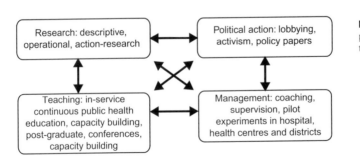

Figure 20.2. Activities of a public health academic unit and their relationships.

can be used to establish best courses of action. Generalization of action research conclusions requires teamwork, lengthy follow-up of field projects, intellectual exchanges, and coordination with ex-alumni networks.

Thirdly, relevant models for health-services management generally build on methods belonging to social, political and managerial sciences, and, to a lesser extent, on epidemiology and medicine. As said above health-systems management requires reciprocal changes in several methods and disciplines, being interdisciplinary rather than multidisciplinary in essence.

Obstacles in an academic environment

Some publications highlight the contribution of research in reinforcing vertical strategies and programmes in the health sector and pinpoint the deficiencies of evidence-based policy making for strengthening health systems (Behague & Storeng, 2008). The reason is easy to understand. Academic staff involved in health services have to pay the price, measurable in terms of their effort and academic opportunity cost. This field experience is rarely valued by the research and teaching bureaucracies. In particular these public health research workers need to overcome two main obstacles to the development of professional knowledge in an academic milieu.

Firstly, most international research funding agencies have relentlessly aimed at privatizing health education and research, and at increasing joint ventures in health education programmes. This has had two consequences:

- While government subsidies to universities have shrunk, private grants have been provided to departments which accept the agenda of private interests (e.g., of Foundations). International competitive research grants are also allocated to the best academic units, as judged by their publications even though some 'objective' criteria were required for this task. However, only the impact factor of publications – a criterion which favours privately owned journals, to the detriment of open-access ones – became the universally accepted yardstick, while research content and perspective was often or largely overlooked by evaluation committees. Except in some North European countries, we learn that reading a scientific paper is not always considered a relevant exercise for its evaluation.

- Research grants were conditioned on careful project description, with plans laid out for a period of 3 to 4 years – often at the expense of the flexibility needed to determine research objectives and methods. This type of rigid planning does have drawbacks for action research, which requires a more dynamic hypothesis. Furthermore, it prevents the utilization of often valuable unexpected research results.

Secondly, interdisciplinary research in health policy and management runs against individual academic career prospects. In general public health academics tend to focus their research and teaching on one resource (e.g., human resources, financing) or one system deliverable (e.g., AIDS, maternal health), because this is more compatible with academic research and publications. This factor has been denounced by E. Morin, among others, as a key obstacle to inter-sectoral research (Morin, 1990).

In conclusion, in the absence of political will and appropriate research and teaching policies, the development and teaching of knowledge in PHM will continue to require from researchers a strong commitment rooted in some kind of existential social motivation. This will allow us to link public health to philosophy, politics and ideology in as much as health care and health policy are political entities rather than technical ones. Such a social configuration in this view would enable the professional's life to become immensely rewarding – making him/her an actor rather than a spectator of his/her study object.

References

Barker C. (1995). Research and the health services manager in the developing world. *Social Science & Medicine*, **41**(12), pp. 1655–65.

Behague D. P. & Storeng K.T. (2008). Collapsing the vertical-horizontal divide: An ethnographic study of evidence-based policymaking in maternal health. *American Journal of Public Health*, **98**(4), pp. 644–9.

Bunker J. P. (2001). Symposium – The role of medical care in contributing to health improvements within societies. *International Journal of Epidemiology*, **30**(6), pp. 1260–3.

Buron A., Unger J. P., & Van Damme W. (1995). L'apprentissage dans la formation d' adultes. Le cas de la formation des médecins généralistes. *Annales de la Société Belge de Médecine Tropicale*, **75**(Supplement 1), pp. 13–25.

Malglaive G. (1990). *Enseigner à Des Adultes*. Paris: PUF.

Meyer J. (2000). Qualitative research in health care. Using qualitative methods in health related action research. *British Medical Journal*, **320**(7228), pp. 178–81.

Mintzberg H. (2004). *Managers Not MBAs: A Hard Look at the Soft Practice of Managing and Management Development*, 1 edn. San Francisco: Berrett-Koehler Publishers.

Mintzberg H., Lampel J., & Ahlstrand B. (1998). *Strategy Safari: A Guided Tour Through the Wilds of Strategic Management*, 1 edn. New York: Free Press.

Morin E. (1979). La Paradigme Perdu. *La Nature Humaine*. Paris: Sevil.

Morin E. (1990). *Introduction à La Pensée Complexe*: EME Editions Sociales Françaises.

Nolte E., Scholz R., Shkolnikov V., & McKee M. (2002). The contribution of medical care to changing life expectancy in Germany and Poland. *Social Science & Medicine*, **55**(11), pp. 1905–21.

Shapiro J. (2005). Stunning update: U.S. life expectancy gains continuing to erode. http://www.clickpress.com/releases/Detailed/1413005cp.shtml.

Conclusions

A failure at large

International health and aid policies share a large responsibility for the breakdown of the health systems of many LMICs. The fact that two decades of neoliberal policy systematically undermined access to quality health care services for a majority of the world population receives insufficient attention. The consequences in terms of avoidable suffering, ill health, debt, poverty, and death are largely overlooked.

Consider avoidable death attributable to MDG-related conditions, representing only a fraction of premature mortality:

- More than 530,000 women die of conditions linked to pregnancy every year (World Health Organization, 2007b);
- Pneumonia and diarrhoea still kill 3.8 million children under five each year;
- 2 million people died of AIDS in 2007 (UNAIDS, 2008);
- 1.6 million people died of tuberculosis in 2005 (World Health Organization, 2007a);
- Between 700,000 and 900,000 children die of malaria in Africa every year.

Overall, avoidable suffering is responsible for 9.3 million deaths every year, an amount close to the yearly death toll of World War II. Arguably, we face a need for a policy shift that re-establishes the right to access quality health care. Such a policy shift would have a positive impact on a broad array of suffering, including and beyond ill health and death (Yamin, 2008).

Consider migration as an example. While HICs oppose human trafficking (U.S. Department of State, 2008) (for human rights reasons) and illegal migration (of unqualified workers and their families), they fail to support policies to improve living conditions in LMICs. At the onset of the twenty-first century about 50% of LICs could not secure access to health care for their populations (Department of Economic and Social Affairs, 2000). In the region of Kayes (Mali) and neighbouring zones in Senegal, people rely on remittances from their migrated townsmen to cope with health care costs. At the same time the death toll related to migration from West Africa to Europe is countless (United Nations High Commissioner for Refugees, 2005). Even in an MIC, such as Colombia, up to one-third of the population still lacks access to health care services (Vargas Lorenzo, 2009). Migration might not be a solution for them: in the USA – the favoured recipient country for Latin American migrants – one in four individuals lacks timely access to optimal care (University of Pennsylvania School of Medicine, 2009).

Consider poverty. While the mutual linkage between ill health and poverty is now firmly established (Commission on Social Determinants of Health, 2008) and international agencies strive to reduce poverty in LMICs for already a decade, catastrophic health expenditure remains the single most important source of poverty in many parts of the world (Kawabata et al., 2002; Van Doorslaer et al., 2007).

Consider the efficiency of international aid on health and take the HIV/AIDS pandemic as an example. While the international donor community managed to dramatically increase HIV/AIDS-specific funds – up to half of total official development assistance (ODA) in 2008 – AIDS-specific mortality remains stable (UNAIDS, 2008). Global HIV incidence remains equally unaffected: while the rate of new infections falls in some countries, this trend is offset by increases in new infections in others.

Consider bureaucratization and regulation. While HICs and international agencies started promoting neoliberal policies on the premise that government services were plagued by bureaucracy, disease-specific administrations destabilized LMICs' health systems and government services, compounded by a wealth of administration related to the management of disease-specific programmes and projects. In MICs – where private health care delivery was intensively promoted – regulation of the private sector proved insufficient. Government administrators were incapable of controlling prices, introducing generic prescriptions, registering staff, accrediting health facilities, and correctly supervising management contracts. In many ways the capacity required by governments to develop effective regulation proved even more difficult than to provide services on their own (Mills et al., 2001).

A large part of the public health community – and health economists in particular – actively supported the current international health and aid policies. The plethora of publications advocating privatization and commodification of health care is overwhelming, certainly if compared with the paucity of critical papers in scientific journals. This is not to say that critical scholars and activists in LMICs did not gather evidence against neoliberal health policies: their findings were unfortunately either neglected or ignored.

Learning from the impact of health policies

International health and aid policies surfed the successive neoliberal waves of the Reagan/Thatcher era in the 1980s, the Bush/Major era in the 1990s, and the Bush/Blair era in the last decade. They achieved the backing of the medico-pharmaceutical complex, of corporations involved in marketing private health insurance, and of the Bretton Woods institutions. In its highly influential 1993 WDR the WB dismissed 'the provision of CHC in public services' as irrelevant (World Bank, 1993). This report placed the Bank in a powerful position as the global policy maker in health, outmanoeuvring the WHO. It also paved the way for a generation of publications depicting public health care as inefficient, bureaucratic and unresponsive. The commodification of health care unfolded in such innovations as the purchaser–provider split, in the autonomous management of public hospitals, the contracting-out of health services, and different forms of managed care. While nominally supporting the strengthening of health systems, academics and policy makers increasingly supported the fragmentation and commodification of health services as an evidence-based way forward (Behague & Storeng, 2008).

Despite mounting criticism and evidence of failure, the Bretton Woods institutions and bilateral aid agencies continue to condition their loans to LMICs on the acceptance of limiting public health service delivery to disease control (Smith & MacKellar, 2007). International bureaucracies dependent on disease control – the Global Health Initiatives amongst others – continue to resist genuine attempts to redirect policies. The proportion of their resources allocated to LMIC health systems strengthening contrasts with their declarations of intent.

Obstacles to policy changes are also related to the economic entities created during the last 15 years. Harvard professors Bossert and Hsiao for example helped to push through the neoliberal health reform in Colombia a decade ago, a country which reserved a central place for private insurance in health financing. Yet they now argue that private health insurers, whatever their drawbacks, are too dominant in the financial sector to envisage a return to a social insurance and care delivery system (Ronderos, 2009). This statement probably also holds true for HICs such as the US and The Netherlands.

Because of their very *raison d'être*, multilateral economic organizations are unlikely to learn from failure in health care access and end the deadlock in MDGs in health. In addition the GATS negotiations threaten to enforce privatization of health care and open LMIC markets to HIC-based corporations. The GATS Article 1.3c says that 'a service supplied in the exercise of governmental authority means any service which is supplied neither on a commercial basis, nor in competition with one or more service suppliers.' It prevents governments and non-commercial agents from providing subsidized goods in the health sector for which there is market demand (Unger et al., 2004), and eventually makes the privatization of curative care compulsory, with only some disease control left for public sectors. Subsidies to publicly oriented services owned by ministries of health, city councils, and NGOs could thus be barred on the grounds of GATS article 1.3c. As a consequence access to general care could further decline for the poorest of this world. Obviously, politicians who endorse such agreements carry a heavy moral responsibility.

Reasons for optimism

Even in an economically non-supportive environment, various stakeholders could actively promote socially motivated health care delivery: health workers (provided they receive a decent salary) and professional organizations, public health teachers and researchers, non-profit NGOs, trade unions, and other civil society movements. A wider scope than the health sector only is needed to identify potential allies and to lobby for a social cause.

The 2008 financial and economic collapse and its ongoing consequences provide a momentum to do so. The collapse of pension funds highlighted one inconvenience of worldwide privatization of insurance, and led to the re-nationalization of private social security funds in an MIC such as Argentina. In the USA business firms finally realized that their employees' private health insurance weighed heavily on the price structure of their goods. Some of them joined health and political activists to lobby against the medical and insurance industry. In the UK medical associations renewed their defence of public services, when they discovered how managed care undermined their therapeutic freedom and their income. In continental Europe trade unions and mutual sickness funds, together with health activists, have mobilized to preserve and expand public services.

Linking personal, professional, social, and political identities

Accessible, continuous, integrated, and patient-centred care are essential features of medical deontology. As such health-service organizations and professional bodies should aim to ensure that health care delivery meets these criteria. This will only happen if teachers and activists bridge the existing gap between individual medicine and public health. Overcoming the segmentation of health care provision is a prerequisite for the fulfilment of a social rationale in health services, to which health care professionals can effectively contribute. Both motivation and skills are essential for the latter.

As we have argued before, skills can be expanded in many ways. One additional and useful way forward would be the inclusion of public health in the medical curriculum and in the development of schools of public health in medical faculties wherever possible. This would open up avenues for practice in health-service organization for undergraduates.

Increasing the motivation of heath professionals is a less straightforward task. Decent remuneration is important but not the only factor, as the unfavourable outcomes of managed care and performance-based payment illustrate. Managed care and pay-for-performance have received worldwide promotion on the premise that human behaviour is driven by personal gain (Stocker et al., 1999). In other words that every Homo sapiens is entirely Homo economicus. Right or wrong, this assumption overlooks a core characteristic of the economic man: he or she will avoid work whenever possible. Consequently – and more overtly so in LMICs – managed care arrangements and performance-based financing have hardly been able to control fraud or to motivate health professionals to deliver patient-centred care, not to mention their dubious impact on quality of, and access to, care (Eldridge & Palmer, 2009). Extrinsic motivation (as provided by decent remuneration) is an essential building block of motivation. But when applied blindly (as in performance-based financing) it might even crowd out intrinsic motivation, and eventually reduce motivation (Frey, 1998). This also happens when remuneration of subgroups of health workers (as in public health administration and disease-control programmes) is excessively higher than in other subgroups, leading to internal brain-drain. Examples in the real world are plentiful. In Zambia, for instance, young health workers often opt for a career in a financially more rewarding donor-dependent programme, rather than for public service (Schatz, 2008), though knowing that their medical skills will be underused by an employer interested in mere disease control.

Intrinsic motivation can be seen as the outcome of personal, professional, social and political identities of a human being. As such it can include elements of self-interest. It is complementary, not opposed to extrinsic motivation. Getting the balance of elements is essential to achieve decent health care. Motivation is indeed both an internal and a transactional process, in a broader societal and political context (Franco et al., 2002). Supportive leadership is a key factor supporting the motivation of health workers (Mbindyo et al., 2009). Professional bodies endorsing social values can also be key in improving motivation; even where organizational goals or government policies are at odds with a social rationale. Worldwide examples of success are the Thai Association of Rural Doctors, the Brazilian Association of Postgraduates in Collective Health (ABRASCO, Associação Brasileira de Pós-Graduação em Saúde Coletiva), and the UK Royal College of General Practitioners. Linking politics and care, they have all been able to defend universal access to patient-centred care and to provide a motivating environment for their members.

From policy to politics

LMICs and states as different as Botswana, Brazil, Costa Rica, Cuba, Kerala (India), Sri Lanka, Swaziland, Tamil Nadu (India), Thailand, and Zimbabwe have all been able to deliver quality care with a social goal. Reflecting on these experiences offers material to re-think international health and aid policies, and to reconsider development per se. What political lessons can be derived from successful attempts to deliver publicly oriented health services?

Key lessons from the health sector to enable development[1] in the twenty-first century:

1. Health services with a social rationale can be viable, effective, and efficient. This also applies to education, social protection, and basic services such as water supply – all related to people's essential needs. Even in a market economy not all goods need to be commoditized.
2. There is a need to balance efficiency, effectiveness, responsiveness, and equity while organizing public oriented services.
3. Genuine community participation through co-management of health services offers an avenue to democratize both (local) governments and NGOs.
4. A dialogue between the actors involved – professionals, users, communities, and political and social organizations – is key to public sector development. Publicly oriented health care services are most viable when planned and developed from both the centre at MoH level (top-down) and peripheral professionals together with communities (bottom-up). Experiences such as that of Porto Alegre in Brazil show that top-down and bottom-up planning are complementary: direct democratic organization can enhance representative democracy.
5. Publicly oriented services – in health and other social sectors – should respond to people's needs, but also to their demand, for recognition of the public as the ultimate stakeholder.
6. The tight relationship between community participation and progress in health suggests that culture (in particular of minorities) should receive special attention in development, for the sake of democracy but also because diversity of cultures is an asset for each society – not because it is a constraint to implement health programmes.

Our proposed health policy is based on a political philosophy. It entails a 'poiesis' – the production of a work of lasting significance, the technical knowledge necessary for the craftsman to produce his work – and 'praxis', defined by Aristotle as implicit action meant to enhance the capabilities of people (the health professionals).

Let us examine the 'poiesis' first. The WHO constitution states that 'the enjoyment of the highest attainable standard of health is one of the fundamental rights of every human being ...' This standard is guilty of the sin of vagueness and impracticability as it requires health policies to act upon all environmental, political, social, and economical determinants of health. Instead the right to CHC of good quality is a short-term objective which can be adopted by health professionals and activists and contribute to practically adjust their activities (Institute of Tropical Medicine Antwerp, 2001). In the vast majority of the countries (which, unlike Costa Rica, do not have a strong unified publicly oriented health system) improving access to such care requires (enhanced) not-for-profit systems to be constructed on existing (often low-quality) not-for-profit health services while strategically planning alliances with social and political organizations. Such a stand treats states not only as a functional body (and implicitly as a Platonician/Hegelian moral ideal) but also, and above all, as a product of social dynamics.

What about the, praxis,? Our proposed health policy assumes a practical and theoretical attempt to reconcile professional, cultural, and political ethics. Indeed, as opposed to 'Realpolitik,' the design and implementation of publicly oriented health policies require applying ethical standards. There is a continuum between the responsibility and conviction ethics defined by Max Weber (Weber, 2002). More than others, doctors, nurses, and health managers need to rely on conviction ethics, which aims at making decisions based on an ideal. They cannot be satisfied with allocative ethics consisting of mechanical application of process rules.

---

[1] Some would say 'to enable Democratic Socialism'.

Our proposed publicly oriented health policy is political in the sense that it refers to actions (deeds) meant to challenge the structures of power and social organization from an ethical perspective. Its theory attempts to minimize the unforeseeable results of deeds through the development of an appropriate know-how and the subsequent engagement in action: poiesis and praxis.

References

Behague D. P. & Storeng K. T. (2008). Collapsing the vertical-horizontal divide: An ethnographic study of evidence-based policymaking in maternal health. *American Journal of Public Health*, **98**(4), pp. 644–9.

Commission on Social Determinants of Health. (2008). *Closing the Gap in a Generation: Health Equity Through Action on the Social Determinants of Health. Final Report of the Commission on Social Determinants of Health*. Geneva: World Health Organization.

Department of Economic and Social Affairs – Public Division. (2000). *Charting the Progress of Populations*. New York: United Nations. ST/ESA/SER.R/151.

Eldridge C. & Palmer N. (2009). Performance-based payment: Some reflections on the discourse, evidence and unanswered questions. *Health Policy and Planning*, **24**(3), pp. 160–6.

Franco L. M., Bennett S., & Kanfer R. (2002). Health sector reform and public sector health worker motivation: A conceptual framework. *Social Science & Medicine*, **54**(8), pp. 1255–66.

Frey B. S. (1998). *Not Just for the Money: An Economic Theory of Personal Motivation*. Ypsilanti, MI: Beacon Press.

Institute of Tropical Medicine Antwerp. (2001). *Declaration on 'Health Care for All.'* Antwerp: Institute of Tropical Medicine.

Kawabata K., Xu K., & Carrin G. (2002). Preventing impoverishment through protection against catastrophic health expenditure. *Bulletin of the World Health Organization*, **80**(8), p. 612.

Mbindyo P., Gilson L., Blaauw D., & English M. (2009). Contextual influences on health worker motivation in district hospitals in Kenya. *Implementation Science*, **4**, p. 43.

Mills A., Bennett S., & Russell S. (2001). *The Challenge of Health Sector Reform: What Must Governments Do?* Oxford: Palgrave Macmillan.

Ronderos M. T. (2009). Lo mejor y lo más débil del sistema de salud colombiano. http://www.semana.com/noticias-salud-seguridad-social/mejor-debil-del-sistema-salud-colombiano/125943.aspx.

Schatz J. J. (2008). Zambia's health-worker crisis. *Lancet*, **371**(9613), pp. 638–9.

Smith R. & MacKellar L. (2007). Global public goods and the global health agenda: Problems, priorities and potential. *Globalization and Health*, **3**(1), p. 9.

Stocker K., Waitzkin H., & Iriart C. (1999). The exportation of managed care to Latin America. *New England Journal of Medicine*, **340**(14), pp. 1131–6.

U.S. Department of State. (2008). *Trafficking in Persons Report*. Washington, DC: U.S. Department of State.

UNAIDS. (2008). *2008 Report on the global AIDS epidemic*. Geneva: UNAIDS. UNAIDS/08.25E / JC1510E.

Unger J. P., De Paepe P., Ghilbert P., & De Groote T. (2004). Public health implications of world trade negotiations. *Lancet*, **363**(9402), p. 83.

United Nations High Commissioner for Refugees. (2005). *UNHCR project to shed light on Africa-Europe transit migration*. http://www.unhcr.org/41ffa0f54.html.

University of Pennsylvania School of Medicine. (2009). *1 in 4 Americans Lack Access to Care During Medical Emergencies*. http://www.disabled-world.com/medical/medical-care.php.

Van Doorslaer E., O'Donnell O., Rannan-Eliya R. P., et al. (2007). Catastrophic payments for health care in Asia. *Health Economics*, **16**(11), pp. 1159–84.

Vargas Lorenzo I. (2009). *Barreras en el acceso a la atención en salud en modelos de competencia gestionada: un estudio de caso en Colombia, Bellaterra*. España: Universidad Autónoma de Barçalona.

Weber M. (2002). *Le savant et le politique*. Paris: Éditions La Découverte.

World Bank. (1993). *World Development Report 1993: Investing in Health*. Oxford: Oxford University Press.

World Health Organization. (2007a). *Fact sheet N°104: Tuberculosis*. http://www.who.int/mediacentre/factsheets/fs104/en/.

World Health Organization. (2007b). Maternal Mortality Ratio Falling Too Slowly to Meet Goal. http://www.who.int/mediacentre/news /releases/2007/pr56/en/print.html.

Yamin A. E. (2008). Will we take suffering seriously? Reflections on what applying a human rights framework to health means and why we should care. *Health and Human Rights*, **10**(1), pp. 45–63.

Glossary

Bio-psychosocial care. Health care which is delivered while taking into account three dimensions of the patient's life and experience: his/her biological condition (directly related or not to the disease – object of consultation), social circumstances (e.g., his/her family, labour, and income), and psychological features (e.g., his/her emotional status and impact of/on the treated pathology).

Commodification. To turn into or treat as a commodity, to make commercial.

Curative care. Curative care is conceived to quell symptoms, reduce probability of subsequent disability and death, and eliminate their aetiological cause. In the natural history of the progression of disease curative care falls between secondary prevention (which aims at an early detection of an established disease) and tertiary prevention (rehabilitation).

Discretionary care. This term is used for curative care delivered in answer to the demand of an individual patient, as opposed to care provided on the basis of collective needs defined by disease-control organizations and programmes (e.g., 'all patients with AIDS').

Health systems/services mission. Such mission is the *raison d'être* of health systems/services – a *consistent* set of values and objectives which ground the quality standards used by an organization to design or select its inputs, processes, and outputs.

Integrated health care. Health care which enables the mobilization of clinical techniques and prevention belonging to another activity package (for instance when a malnourished child is sent to a TB programme and vice-versa, according to his/her needs).

Integrated health systems. Health care systems are made up of two layers of health facilities which respond to specific criteria such as complementarity of functions and free access for the patient to care, as needed by them. Fragmented health systems, on the other hand, do not secure hospital access for patients referred to by first-line health services.

Integrated services. Operational integration of services refers to the delivery of disease-control interventions by the general staff of first-line services. Administrative integration refers to the transfer of authority over operationally integrated disease-specific interventions from disease-specific programme officers to polyvalent members of a district executive team.

Interface flow process audit. This is an audit process conceived to improve health care quality and the integration of services whereby evaluation of the patient's treatment ('flow process') in first- and second-line services is used to reveal weaknesses in organization and deficiencies in knowledge. This audit is called 'interface' because both GPs and specialists participate in the process.

Managed care techniques. These are techniques conceived to make clinical decision making more efficient (and effective). They are based on the strict use of diagnosis and treatment standards, financial incentives aimed at increasing productivity and efficiency of health care providers, and at modifying patterns of health services utilization.

Non-managed care techniques. Non-managed care techniques are polyvalent techniques which are meant to improve the effectiveness and efficiency of health care delivery that are not intervention specific. In general they are different from managed care techniques since they aim at a balance between freedom of clinical decision making and efficiency.

Piot Model. A mathematical model (a product of fractions) designed to assess the cure rate – and consequently the access to a continuum of care spanning from utilization of health care services to sensitivity to treatment (e.g., a particular regimen of tuberculostatics) – of patients suffering from a given condition (e.g., tuberculosis).

Polyvalent health care. This term is used throughout the book to describe health care not related to one particular disease-control programme (e.g., AIDS programme) or risk-specific programme (e.g., antenatal care). Polyvalent (or versatile or multifunction) health care encompasses family, community, and hospital medicine, including thereby health care belonging to specialties. Accordingly, polyvalent health care outlets are health centres and general hospitals.

Professional Bureaucracies (Mintzberg, 1993). These are health systems characterized by standardization of professional skills rather than output, a high degree of autonomy for working units, and weak vertical and horizontal integration (Mintzberg H. 1993. *Structure in Fives. Designing Effective Organisations.* New Jersey: Prentice-Hall Inc, Figure 1–2, p. 10).

Publicly oriented. In this book, we use this qualifier of health care delivery, management, and services as a substitute to 'with a social mission,' 'with a social benefit' or 'not-for-profit' – as opposed to commercially based care and health care services.

Target population. The target population of a health centre or a hospital is the population which is supposed to be served by these services. The need to define this arises from the necessity to specify the target population of preventive activities as well as to integrate curative and preventive activities.

Index

patient satisfaction, 202
specificity, principle of, 186
  planners overlook, 190
stability, political
  health care and, 159
  poverty threatens, 173
staff. *See also* health
      professionals
  competition for, 22
    disease control
        programmes and, 196
    DSPs, 8
    private sector and, 22
  DCPs demotivate, 53,
      205
  efficient use of, 52
  human resource policy, 44
  income, 44
  loss of skills, 29
  motivation, 23, 206
    improvement of access
        and, 213, 217
    increasing, 250
    managed care and, 227,
        228, 250
  PPM-DOTS, 60
  role in holistic care, 230
  status, 29
    Costa Rica, 75
stakeholders
  ethics code, 176
  socially motivated care
      promotion, 249
standardization
  clinical practice, managed
      care and, 227, 228
standards
  best practice in family
      medicine, 202–207
  clinical, machine
      bureaucracies, 165
  quality, publicly oriented
      services, 165, 176–182
status
  health professionals, 29, 182,
      206
  utilization of health care and,
      125, 126
stewardship as government
      role, 57, 178, 189, 196
  WHO defines, 6, 62,
      83
stigma
  access influenced by,
      tuberculosis, 60
  public provision carries in
      Lebanon, 140

Structural Adjustment
      Programmes. *See* SAP
subsidy
  disease control, health care
      delivery and, 44
  private sector, 117
  public
    Chile, 100
    GATS and, 30, 35, 83, 249
    India, 114
    Lebanon, 140, 141, 145,
        146–147, 148, 149, 150
    WHO report and, 6
supplier-induced demand, 7,
      134
    Lebanon, 141
support
  community, of public
      services, quality of care
      and, 168, 173
  of health professionals, 172
sustainability
  disease control, 196
  drug supply, 210, 219
  DSPs, 159
  funding, 167
  PPM-DOTS programme, 60
  problems with
    effects on health
        systems, 20
Sweden
  divisionalized system, 172
  health expenditure, 73
  social insurance, 74
Swedish International Devel-
      opment Cooperation
      Agency (SIDA)
  demand-based projects, 112

Tanzania, malaria programmes,
      39, 42
Tavistock Group, 176
taxation, health care funding,
      30
territorial responsibility,
      facilities, 188
Thailand
  family medicine, 202
  for-profit approach
      influences care in, 24
tracer
  pathologies, 25, 88
    audit, 238
  patient's career as, for audit,
      234, 235–238
trade
  agreements. *See also* GATS,

  Free Trade
    effect on health services, 6,
        74, 114, 115, 117, 119
    politicians responsibility
        for, 249
  GHIs and, 8
training
  clinical
    LMICs, 205–206
    informal providers, 43
    in public health, 240–245
    in-service, 44
      hospital role in, 190
      patient-centred care, 48
      person-centred care, 206
      supports clinical decision-
          making, 228–230
  medical
    Costa Rica, 75
    deterioration, 29
    India, 112
    person-centredness in,
        203, 205, 206
    professional bureaucracy
        and, 170
    to meet Hippocratic ideal,
        166
  PPM-DOTS programme, 58
  standards influence care, 205
treatment
  audit, 236–238
  discrepancies, effects on
      health systems, 20
  outcome rates, tuberculosis,
      59, 63
  rates
    Colombia, 87, 91
    Piot model and, 40, 44
    Piot model estimates, 38
  related to need, 128
  saving life vs. reducing
      morbidity, 161
  tuberculosis, 60
tuberculosis
  Chile, 102
  control, 19, 155
    assessment of
        programmes, 38
    barriers to care and, 134
    contracting out, 35, 88
    India, 113
  early detection, 156, 196
  incidence
    Colombia, 88
  mortality, 247
    Costa Rica, 26, 78
    MDG, 17